Lymphoedema

D0794890

Edited by

Robert Twycross
Karen Jenns and
Jacquelyne Todd

Foreword by

Terence Ryan

WITHDRAWN FROM STOCK

MEDICAL LIBRARY, CITY HOSPITAL

AUTHOR ..... TWYCROSS

BOOK No. 003527

CLASSMARK ..... WH 700 LYM

RADCLIFFE MEDICAL PRESS

© 2000 Robert Twycross, Karen Jenns and Jacquelyne Todd

Radcliffe Medical Press Ltd
18 Marcham Road, Abingdon, Oxon, OX14 1AA

All rights reserved. No part of this publication may be reproduced, stored in a retrieval system, or transmitted, in any form or by any means, electronic, mechanical, photocopying, recording or otherwise without the prior permission of the copyright owner.

British Library Cataloguing in Publication Data

A catalogue record for this book is available from the British Library.

ISBN 1 85775 377 1

Typeset by Advance Typesetting Ltd, Oxon
Printed and bound by TJ International Ltd, Padstow, Cornwall

Contents

Foreword   vii

Preface   ix

List of contributors   x

Medical abbreviations   xii

Useful addresses   xiii

1   The patient's perspective   1
      Madeleine Robertson Squire

2   How does tissue swelling occur?   11
      The physiology and pathophysiology
      of interstitial fluid formation
      Anthony Stanton

3   Classification of lymphoedema   22
      Vaughan Keeley

4   Clinical features of lymphoedema   44
      Vaughan Keeley

5   Pain in lymphoedema   68
      Robert Twycross

6 Psychosocial aspects of lymphoedema 89

Mary Woods

7 Management strategies 97

Karen Jenns

8 Skin management in lymphoedema 118

Nina Linnitt

9 Acute inflammatory episodes 130

Peter Mortimer

10 Exercise and lymphoedema 140

Karen Hughes

**11 Containment in the management
of lymphoedema** 165

Jacquelyne Todd

12 Manual lymphatic drainage 203

Albert Leduc and Olivier Leduc

13 Simple lymphatic drainage 217

Sarah Bellhouse

14   Pneumatic compression therapy   236
Tracey Bray and Justine Barrett

15   Drug treatment for lymphoedema   244
Robert Twycross

16   Novel treatments:

Transcutaneous electrical nerve stimulation   271
Alexander Waller and Michaela Bercovitch

Low-level LASER therapy   282
Robert Twycross

17   Surgery and lymphoedema   285
Tom Carrell and Kevin Burnand

18   Lymphoedema in childhood   293
Sahar Mansour and Michael Sharland

19   Lymphoedema of the head and neck   306
Simon Withey, Paul Pracy and Peter Rhys-Evans

20   Breast lymphoedema   321
Marilyn Kirshbaum

21   Male genital lymphoedema   331
Neil Haldar and David Cranston

22 Oedema in advanced cancer 338

  Vaughan Keeley

23 Lymphoedema in cancer: an Indian perspective 359

  MR Rajagopal

Index 364

Foreword

This book is very welcome. The scene is set by the opening chapter written by a patient. There follows chapters by the medical, nursing and physiotherapy professions.

I have a copy of a popular arts and science encyclopaedia, dated 1806, in which the function and structure of the lymphatics is well-described and one may assume that, even at that time, a large lay readership was well-informed. Even so, the lymphatic system remains neglected. Some of us have struggled to get the health professionals more interested in a system which removes all excess water, unwanted macromolecules and inflammatory cells and provides essential communication for the immunological system. It also controls the resilience and elasticity of the organs drained.

The few people who are members of the International Society of Lymphology get together about every two years and ask the question 'How can we make the lymphatics more popular?' In dermatology, the neglect is so great that it is impossible to have it as a title for a workshop or seminar at an international or world congress because the scientific committee responsible for the programme knows that no-one would want to attend. From this state of paranoia, it is a pleasure to write a foreword to a book which is easy to read and may even be read.

When the skin fails, as a consequence of lymphatic failure, all the functions of the skin are impaired. The skin as an organ of communication – love at first sight, colour prejudice, 'thick skinned' and so on, is not displayed. It cannot thermoregulate or perceive so efficiently. It no longer protects against a threatening environment and, consequently, it is traumatised, irritated and a state of chronic inflammation persists.

More than a decade ago, Robert Twycross, Claud Regnard, Peter Mortimer, Caroline Badger and I, among others, responded to appeals from persons in the UK who had been subjected to surgery or radiotherapy of the lymph glands of the upper limb because of breast cancer and we set up the British Lymphology Interest Group. Initially, much of the discussion was about how little help or interest from the medical profession was available to those who had swollen limbs. In the UK there was, of course, the distinguished St Thomas's group, led by John Kinmonth, who had contributed so much by developing lympho-angiography and who had brought surgical skills to the problems of those most severely affected. The gold standards for conservative therapy – bandaging, massage, exercises – were to be found in the Földi

Clinic in Bavaria. Other leaders could be found elsewhere in Brazil, such as Professor Mayall, whose surgical skills were formidable. John Casley-Smith and his wife Judith, in Australia, were putting all their energies into exploration of the structure of the lymphatic system and the development of management in that continent. Charles and Marlys Witte in Arizona were giving leadership and bringing people together to make consensus statements.

However, specialist treatment was available only to a few, and some of us questioned why the expertise was not being made available to all. Thus, in the UK, the British Lymphology Interest Group (now the British Lymphology Society) began to forge partnerships and to disseminate its knowledge widely. The fact is that, in most of the world, self-help is the most that can be afforded. It is enormously undervalued and also technically quite difficult because of the need for painstaking transmission of information and the adoption of a rather tedious attention to detail. Concordance with such a programme is difficult to achieve without the encouragement and teaching of a professional with an answer to all the problems experienced by patients with lymphoedema. Some skills take months of practice through specialist training but simple massages can be learned in a few hours. As stated so clearly in this book, neither surgery nor conservative therapy, for which there are gold standards, is affordable or available or even appropriate for everyone.

What we need is a book such as this, which carefully explains what it is the lymphatics do and provides basic information to help the practitioner become expert. There is an additional skill which can only be learned by dealing with patients and that is how to transmit this knowledge and put it into practice on a daily basis. The position over the past decade has improved in the UK. More help is available and this book is one consequence of the distillation of the knowledge acquired. It meets a great need and the constant cry for help.

Terence Ryan
March 2000

Preface

Lymphoedema is a multiprofessional attempt to bring together current knowledge about lymphoedema in an accessible form for those involved in its management. It is clearly a British book and reflects current British biases. It is, however, considerably enhanced by contributions from Belgium, India and Israel. Although a basic grasp of medical jargon is assumed, we have tried to restrict (or explain) the more obscure terms. Even so, a medical dictionary may be a necessary companion for those readers who are not steeped in the burgeoning lymphoedema culture.

Lymphoedema is for all those who want or need an overview of the subject. It will appeal to those most commonly involved in the care of patients afflicted by lymphoedema – specialist nurses and physiotherapists – as well as those doctors who provide medical back-up for the increasing number of nurse- and physiotherapist-led lymphoedema clinics. *Lymphoedema* will also appeal to health care students wanting to understand more about the lymphatic system in both health and disease.

Inevitably there are gaps in the content of a book of this nature. Even so, we believe it will become a valuable resource for those interested in and concerned about lymphoedema. However, *the book is not a do-it-yourself manual.* Although it describes various forms of management, this cannot replace the need for proper training and supervised practice. Details of courses about lymphoedema management can be obtained from the British Lymphology Society.

The editors are grateful to all the contributors for adding writing to their already busy schedules. We should like to record our thanks to all patients whose pictures appear in the book. Thanks also to Karen Allen for her diligence and determination in typing and retyping – sometimes seemingly endlessly – the 23 chapters. Finally, thanks to Susan Brown for her work as copy-editor – helping to bring further clarity to a complex subject.

Robert Twycross
Karen Jenns
Jacquelyne Todd
March 2000

List of contributors

Justine Barrett Macmillan Lymphoedema Clinical Nurse Specialist, Leeds Cancer Centre, St James's University Hospital NHS Trust, Beckett Street, Leeds LS9 7TF

Sarah Bellhouse MLD Therapist and Vodder Accredited Teacher, 8 Wittenham Lane, Dorchester on Thames, Oxon OX10 7JW

Michaela Bercovitch Research and Information Coordinator, Tel HaShomer's Hospice, The Chaim Sheba Medical Center, Tel-HaShomer 52621, Israel

Tracey Bray Macmillan Lymphoedema Nurse Specialist, Jayne Garforth Cancer Support Centre, Calderdale Healthcare NHS Trust, Halifax HX3 0PW

Kevin Burnand Professor of Vascular Surgery, Academic Department of Surgery, St Thomas' Hospital, Lambeth Palace Road, London SE1 7EH

Thomas Carrell Lecturer in Surgery, St Thomas' Hospital, Lambeth Palace Road, London SE1 7EH

David Cranston Consultant Urologist, Urology Department, Churchill Hospital, Oxford OX3 7LJ

Neil Haldar Clinical Research Fellow, Nuffield Department of Surgery, John Radcliffe Hospital, Oxford OX3 9DU

Karen Hughes Senior Chartered Physiotherapist, Lymphoedema Service, Sir Michael Sobell House, Churchill Hospital, Oxford OX3 7LJ

Karen Jenns Clinical Nurse Specialist, Lymphoedema Service, Sir Michael Sobell House, Churchill Hospital, Oxford OX3 7LJ

Vaughan Keeley Consultant in Palliative Medicine, Nightingale Macmillan Unit, Derbyshire Royal Infirmary, 117A London Road, Derby DE1 2QS

Marilyn Kirshbaum Research Associate, Macmillan Practice Development Unit, University of Manchester, School of Nursing, Midwifery and Health Visitors, Gateway House, Piccadilly South, Manchester M60 7LP

Albert Leduc Professor Emeritus Honorarius and Professor Extraordinarius, Service de Kinesitherapie et de Readaptation, Université Libre de Bruxelles, 28 Avenue Paul Heger, CP 168, 1050 Bruxelles, Belgium

Olivier Leduc Doctorandus in Physical Therapy, Service de Kinesitherapie et de Readaptation, Université Libre de Bruxelles, 28 Avenue Paul Heger, CP 168, 1050 Bruxelles, Belgium

Nina Linnitt former Lymphoedema Sister, Lymphoedema Service, Sir Michael Sobell House, Churchill Hospital, Oxford OX3 7LJ

Sahar Mansour Specialist Registrar, Department of Clinical Genetics, St George's Hospital, Blackshaw Road, London SW17 0QT

Peter Mortimer Reader in Dermatology, University of London, Consultant Skin Physician at St George's and Royal Marsden Hospitals; St George's Hospital, Cranmer Terrace, London SW17 0RE

Paul Pracy Senior Registrar, Head and Neck Unit, Royal Marsden Hospital, Fulham Road, London SW3 6JJ

MR Rajagopal Professor of Anaesthetics, Department of Anaesthetics, The Medical College, Calicut 673 008, Kerala, India

Peter Rhys-Evans Consultant, Head and Neck Unit, Royal Marsden Hospital, Fulham Road, London SW3 6JJ

Madeleine Robertson Squire former Chairman, Lymphoedema Support Network, 9 The Green, Brampton, Cambridgeshire PE18 8RD

Terence Ryan Emeritus Professor of Dermatology, Oxford Centre for Health Care Research and Development, 44 London Road, Headington, Oxford OX3 7PD

Michael Sharland Consultant, Paediatric Infectious Diseases Unit, St George's Hospital, Blackshaw Road, London SW17 0QT

Anthony Stanton Research Fellow, Division of Physiological Medicine (Dermatology), St George's Hospital Medical School, Cranmer Terrace, London SW17 0RE

Jacquelyne Todd Lymphoedema Specialist, Ardenlea Marie Curie Centre, Queens Drive, Ilkley, West Yorkshire LS29 9QR

Robert Twycross Macmillan Clinical Reader in Palliative Medicine, Oxford University and Consultant Physician, Sir Michael Sobell House, Churchill Hospital, Oxford OX3 7LJ

Alexander Waller Hospice Director, Tel HaShomer's Hospice, The Chaim Sheba Medical Center, Tel HaShomer 52621, Israel

Simon Withey Senior Registrar, Head and Neck Unit, Royal Marsden Hospital, Fulham Road, London SW3 6JJ

Mary Woods Senior Clinical Nurse Specialist, Lymphoedema Services, Royal Marsden Hospital, Downs Road, Sutton, Surrey SM2 5PT

Medical abbreviations

AIE	acute inflammatory episode(s)
CDT	complex decongestive therapy
CT	computed tomography
DLT	decongestive lymphoedema therapy
DVT	deep vein thrombosis
MLD	manual lymphatic drainage
MLLB	multilayer lymphoedema bandaging
MRI	magnetic resonance imaging
PCT	pneumatic compression therapy
SLD	simple lymphatic drainage
TENS	transcutaneous electrical nerve stimulation

Useful addresses

British Lymphology Society
Administration Centre
P O Box 1059
Caterham
CR3 6ZU
Tel: 01883 330 253
Fax: 01883 330 254
Email: helensnoad@blsac.demon.co.uk

International Society of Lymphology
Professor M Witte
General Secretary
University of Arizona
College Medical Department of Surgery
P O Box 245063
1501 North Campbell Avenue
Tucson
Arizona 85724 – 5063
USA
Tel: 001 502 626 6118
Email: lymph@ccit.arizona.edu

Lymphoedema Support Network
St. Luke's Crypt
Sydney Street
London
SW3 6NH
Tel: 020 7351 4480
Fax: 020 7349 9809

I   The patient's perspective

Madeleine Robertson Squire

Madeleine Robertson Squire has primary lymphoedema and is the former chairman of the Lymphoedema Support Network, the first and only national organisation in the UK dedicated to providing advice and support to people with lymphoedema.

Lymphoedema can affect anybody anywhere at any time

In the UK, about 2% of the population are affected by lymphoedema to varying degrees.[1] With the growing realisation that it is for life, the onset of lymphoedema is generally a major shock.

Lymphoedema is often devastating, debilitating, stressful and painful. It can cause immense heartache and embarrassment to the patient in front of family and friends, and can reduce activity in the workplace. The frequent feeling of isolation experienced by the lymphoedema sufferer is very real, and too often compounded by a disturbing lack of understanding from health professionals and limited access, if any, to treatment.

It seems that there is still a widespread belief among doctors that there is little to lymphoedema other than possible discomfort caused by the size of the affected part of the body. Indeed, doctors often say that it is just a cosmetic problem for which little can be done, that it is 'bad luck' or that it is caused by being overweight.

Typical cases from the files of the Lymphoedema Support Network

You are a new parent and your baby has been born with swollen legs and feet and a swollen arm. A number of tests are carried out and lymphoedema is eventually diagnosed, probably some months later. What happens next?

You are 14 years old. One morning you notice that your ankles and left lower leg are swollen. For some time, you have been aware of your shoes feeling tighter and recently at the end of the day you have noticed that your clothes have felt tight too. You have taken little notice. Now you do! Panic sets in. Your parents panic too. Will your doctor be able to sort it out?

You are an adult in your 40s and have been diagnosed with breast cancer. After surgery you are informed that some lymph nodes have been removed. Mentally, you are trying to come to terms with the operation but your arm is giving you some problems – it is painful and swollen in the armpit. You are advised that there is nothing to worry about but that you might just have a little difficulty with the arm for a while. You must follow the instructions about postmastectomy exercises, keep in touch with your breast care nurse and everything will be fine. It is! Ten months later you are helping to lift a heavy box and there is a sudden burning sensation in your arm. The pain becomes excruciating and swelling occurs almost immediately in the arm, hand and the fingers. You hope your breast care nurse will sort this out!

You are in your 50s, in good health and one day when you are out walking, you slip and twist your ankle. Several weeks later, you don't understand why your ankle and lower leg are still swollen. Perhaps your doctor can help?

In many cases, people struggle to find information, obtain a full medical evaluation and identify a treatment centre. Too often, because of professional ignorance, appropriate treatment is denied to them.

The impact of lymphoedema

Lymphoedema is a source of major morbidity. The quality of life for a person with lymphoedema may be severely diminished. There is the initial lack of knowledge and understanding. Questions arise such as 'Why me?', 'How do I cope?', 'What can I do?' and 'Where do I go?'

Living with lymphoedema

The person begins to realise that from now on normal life may be a struggle. Women often cope well with the diagnosis of breast cancer and radical treatment but, for many, the onset of lymphoedema is almost unbearable. Simple daily tasks become mountains to climb when you have lymphoedema. Even when it is mild and uncomplicated, there may be a fluctuating ability to carry out normal tasks. Lymphoedema makes you realise just how much most of us take for granted. You now have to think in advance before carrying out even ordinary tasks such as washing, bathing, finding clothes and shoes which fit, getting dressed, driving, peeling vegetables, opening bottles, writing, holding a newspaper, putting on make-up, combing hair, standing about or sitting for any length of time at a desk, in the theatre or on public transport.

The embarrassment of a large swollen limb goes in tandem with constant dis-comfort and reduced mobility. Literally dragging a large limb around creates immense stress. Depression can persist from the very early stages if treatment is not offered. Some people become reclusive, particularly those with primary lymphoedema. Concomitant symptoms are common (Box 1.A), with the continuing threat of dangerous and debilitating infections (*see* p.130).

Box 1.A   Concomitant symptoms in lymphoedema

An extreme bursting sensation of the limb and body.

A feeling of heat and severe irritation in the swollen area.

A constant dull ache or severe pain in the affected region.

A burning sensation and pressure in the joints, particularly the digits.

Backache.

Cramp.

Migraine.

'Pins and needles'.

A loss of feeling as the limb becomes solid.

Spontaneous blisters and ulcers in the affected area.

Skin dehydration with flaking and skin breakdown.

Muscle wasting.

Constant exhaustion.

Increasing intolerance to changes in temperature.

Obesity.

Athlete's foot (tinea pedis).

Recurrent infections, often with the need for long-term prophylactic antibiotics.

Inadequate treatment provision

Lymphoedema is not curable and is not going to go away. Continuing support by health professionals is needed. Treatment availability is clouded by the dichotomy of offering treatment in cancer centres to cancer patients but not providing treatment for non-cancer patients. The inequality in treatment goes further with some centres offering treatment only for arm lymphoedema, for example Breast Care Clinics. Inadequate treatment results in major long-term health costs. If treatment is not provided early enough, it will result eventually in a greater need for social welfare funds.

Self-management carries on the work of the lymphoedema therapist. It is the maintenance strategy for everyday life and is worked out jointly by the afflicted person and the therapist. Self-management should not be considered a budget-saver. Regular monitoring by a suitably trained health professional is essential *for life*. The typical interval of 6 months between appointments should not be set in stone; individuals have widely varying needs. Intervals between appointments should depend on the ongoing state of that person's lymph-oedema. Lymphoedema is a condition which fluctuates as a result of various factors. Sometimes, a minor event can lead to rapid deterioration and cause great distress. Such incidents should not be interpreted as evidence of non-adherence to the agreed treatment regimen.

The relationship between patient and health professional

It is important that a person should not become a victim to lymphoedema. They need much help from health professionals to understand the condition and why it has happened, together with the assurance that with treatment they can learn to live a near normal life.[2] It is essential to evaluate a person's health problems within the social context of their everyday lives – any threat to this must be assessed and care plans drawn up accordingly.

Lymphoedema disfigurement has an insidious effect on a person's psyche, and must be considered in relation to the whole of that person's lifestyle. Only when the health professional understands the 'language of disability' – that the person may not be able to walk far, may not be able to use a hand, feels ostracised and finds the treatment too much – can appropriate individual treatment be provided and, more importantly, understood. When the health professional understands that the effect of lymphoedema is much more than just swelling, then the afflicted person can be helped to start on the road to successful long-term rehabilitation.[3]

The importance of listening to the patient

Over the last 150 years, the emergence of hospital and of scientific medicine has reduced the patient to being seen as a mere object by doctors, not need-ing to be consulted about their health problems. Once clinical tests became the method to determine what was wrong, so the patient's opinion was dis-regarded as unnecessary information and inaccurate in the face of all-conquering science. This led to a turnaround in the patient–doctor relationship. Historically, the patient had been centre stage:

'Disease was always defined in terms of the subjective feelings of the patient: the patient's lifestyle and general functioning was the norm. The focus was to what extent did the patient deviate from the norm and how could they be restored to normality.'[4]

Since the 1970s, we have seen the beginnings of a second turnaround with patients once again seeking to lead the requirement for good health and an acceptable quality of life. Alternative therapies, support groups and self-help groups have become major sources of relief, particularly for the chronically ill who have been disappointed with the offerings of mainstream medicine.

Particularly in the last decade, there have been moves to establish a partnership between patient, doctor and other health professionals so as to achieve the best outcome in any disorder. Patients want health professionals to *listen* and to work in a team with them. This is crucial when deciding the best way to rehabilitate someone with lymphoedema.

Patient guidance

People with any chronic illness need professional guidance about living with their condition. They need to learn how to cope long-term. This starts with dialogue between the individual and the doctor or other health professional, enabling the latter to discover what problems that particular person is experiencing.

It is a frequent complaint of lymphoedema patients that, at their 6-monthly check-ups, the same questions are met by the same old (unsatisfactory) answers. Bob Price, medical adviser to the LSN, states:

'Lymphoedema patients have much in common with many other patients who face a chronic illness and multiple contacts with health professionals. They learn rapidly that there is a lot of difference between disease and illness. The medical profession tries to solve disease problems whilst the patient lives with illness, and the approach to treating the problem comes from two different directions. The patient is trying to become an instant expert in the physiology of lymphoedema, the disease and its treatment while the professionals have a considerable amount to learn about being ill. Only when these two factors eventually meet will progress in treating lymphoedema and bringing relief to so many people be tangible.'[5]

Listen, think, plan care and *adapt* – these are essential rules for health professionals when treating lymphoedema. Lymphoedema is a precarious condition; no two days are alike. What one does one day may not be possible or may be more difficult the next. Lymphoedema is very visible and health professionals need to accept that the mental and physical pain of altered body image can be all-encompassing. Early in life, children with lymphoedema will often have problems at school if they are seen as different and are treated separately and specially. Children may also have difficulty in explaining just how they feel and describing the discomfort and disability they experience. Disability so early in life may deny them many opportunities and experiences which would otherwise form part of their life's foundation.

Access to treatment

Awareness of lymphoedema and its effects on a person's life has grown in recent years. However, the simple questions, 'What can I do and where can I go for treatment?' are still not easily answered because there are still few dedicated clinics. Rehabilitation is the key in long-standing lymphoedema but, for those experiencing secondary lymphoedema following cancer treatment, early diagnosis and prevention is paramount. Early diagnosis, education, practical advice and treatment at an early stage may prevent:

* years of suffering

* reliance on social services

* major functional impairment, possibly leading to wheelchair dependency later in life.

Those afflicted know that, although there is no cure for the condition, successful management exists in the form of conservative therapy and should be available to all patients. Lymphoedema is not just the unfortunate knock-on effect of surgery, radiotherapy, an accident or birth defects with which one has to live; *lymphoedema should be regarded as an illness in its own right and managed as such.*

People often contact the Lymphoedema Support Network (LSN) because there is no treatment available locally. They are advised to ask their general practitioner to refer them to a clinic in another area. Problems can emerge along the referral route and it is not unusual to experience a delay of many months before being seen. During this waiting period, irreversible damage may occur from general complications and infections.

The lack of understanding by a doctor of the long-term problems of lymphoedema creates a barrier to communication, and the person is made to feel that the doctor's time is being wasted. Some people just give up hope of ever receiving any treatment. Lymphoedema patients do not need confrontation when merely seeking relief from increasing disability.

In the UK, decongestive lymphoedema therapy (DLT) is still funded mainly by cancer charities. It is extremely fortunate if one happens to live within reach of a lymphoedema centre, either at a hospital or palliative care unit. There are, however, only a few specialist clinics which offer truly comprehensive care. For many patients, their geographical location deprives them of any treatment at all. There can be no substitute for expert professional evaluation and consistent individualised treatment. Anyone with lymphoedema should be entitled to:

- an explanation as to why they have lymphoedema and what it is likely to mean for them
- information about the body's lymphatic system
- guidance on skin hygiene and the prevention of infection
- appropriate exercise instruction
- manual lymphatic drainage (MLD)
- multilayer lymphoedema bandaging (MLLB)
- compression garments
- advice on diet
- access to support services.

It is generally essential for people with lymphoedema to wear lymphoedema-grade compression garments. These must be well-measured and properly fitted. They must be regularly replaced in line with the manufacturer's specifications, and certainly no longer than every 6 months.

People should be given guidance and training on how to self-manage between treatments or consultations. They then have the opportunity to learn how to regain some normality in their lives. Advice is needed on adapting to life with a swollen limb. Limitations when undertaking everyday activities will thereby become more acceptable, and people will learn new ways of coping rather than needlessly compromising the benefits of treatment. For example, they will learn not to overdo things and how to prevent exacerbating their condition.

The role of the support organisation

A national support organisation can highlight the lack of resources to treat a condition and point to any benchmark centres which are leading the way.

A national support organisation is also in a position to focus on the national picture, to identify the size of the problem and to be a reference point for those affected, doctors and other health professionals.

Support organisations

Until the late 1980s, The Patients' Association and local Community Health Councils almost solely represented patients' interests in the UK. The climate began to change following parliamentary and public debates generated by the National Health Service reforms of 1991. The introduction of the Patient's Charter encouraged embryonic patient groups to take on a much higher profile.[6] Patient organisations have recognised that the immense work involved in protecting and promoting the care of their members is a common requirement across the health sector. These organisations have a mutual cause and benefit from inter-relationship.

The Long-term Medical Conditions Alliance

Organisations united in a common stance make an impact on government departments. In 1989 an umbrella organisation, the Long-term Medical Conditions Alliance (LMCA), was formed as a result of public debate on NHS reforms. This organisation now embraces over 100 patient groups. The principles of the LMCA include:

- the recognition of affected people as individuals with a long-term medical condition
- a social model of care
- an appreciation that people have real expertise about their condition and their needs.

The LMCA states that long-term illness is likely to affect the majority of people in the UK, either directly through family and friends or as employers. Its incidence is growing. A government survey indicated that over 35% of the population in the UK have a long-standing illness and about 25% say this limits their lives.[7] This represents a large proportion of the population needing some form of long-term care.

The Lymphoedema Support Network

The LSN is a member of the LMCA. It was formed in 1991 in response to patients' distress at the prevalence of untreated lymphoedema and to help them adjust to living with lymphoedema. It gained charitable status in 1992 and since then has become the national patient organisation for lymphoedema. The aims of the LSN are:

- to offer advice to people with lymphoedema
- to work for better awareness of lymphoedema by NHS policy makers and by health professionals
- to lobby for the provision of appropriate and comprehensive standards of care for everyone with lymphoedema
- to promote early diagnosis, evaluation and access to the appropriate treatment.

The formation of local lymphoedema support groups is encouraged. These can play a vital role in highlighting local needs. Those with lymphoedema turn to the LSN and to local support groups for various reasons:

- they may be finding it difficult to have their condition recognised or evaluated
- they may find treatment elusive
- they may wish to benefit from the company and advice of others in a similar position.

The LSN has an important role in lobbying for adequate resources for all lymphoedema patients, and provides information to members, general enquirers, doctors and other health professionals. Sally Harrison, founder chairman of the LSN, maintains that:

> *'Sharing information saves the professional's time. Therapists are not always able to spend sufficient time with patients telling them what to do on a daily basis – the LSN fulfils this very necessary role.'*

Conclusion

The following support will give the person with lymphoedema the opportunity to lead a more normal life:

- a doctor's understanding
- careful management by a suitably trained therapist
- treatment understanding and adherence by the patient
- individualised treatment.

Self-management is crucial to success. It builds on the benefits of periodic treatments and long-term monitoring by a therapist. With the full understanding and co-operation of everyone involved, lymphoedema can be controlled. Health achieved in partnership is of long-term benefit to both individuals and the health services. Such a social approach to health care can only enhance the general wellbeing of the whole community.

References

1   The Lymphoedema Support Network UK. General leaflet.
2   Casley-Smith JR (1998) Newsletter. The Lymphoedema Association of Australia Inc.
3   Ryan TJ (1995) Skin failure and lymphoedema. *Lymphology*. **28**:171–3.
4   Extract (1997) from Down the Centuries. In: *The Patient's Network*, Vol 2, No 2, Pharmaceutical Partners for Better Healthcare.
5   Price B (1995) *Illness Careers: The Chronic Illness Experience.* Conference of the British Lymphology Interest Group (now the British Lymphology Society), Oxford Brookes University. Unpublished.
6   Lumley P (1996) The growth of self-help groups and the role of the patient. Agenda for Health Report. ABPI.
7   Living in Britain (1996) General Household Survey. HMSO.

Further reading

Casley-Smith JR (1997) *Modern Treatment for Lymphoedema*, 5th edn. The Lymphoedema Association of Australia Inc.
Swirsky J and Sackett ND (1998) *Coping with Lymphoedema*. Avery Publishing Group, New York.

2 How does tissue swelling occur? The physiology and pathophysiology of interstitial fluid formation

Anthony Stanton

The interstitial compartment of the tissues of the body is the space outside the capillaries and between the cells (*L. interstitialis*, set between). It is this which expands in oedema as a result of an increase in hydration. In swelling of longstanding, other substances are also found in excess, notably fat and fibrous tissue. Before the pathological mechanisms which lead to tissue swelling can be understood, the nature of the interstitium and the physiological processes governing interstitial fluid formation must be considered.

The nature of the interstitial compartment of tissues

The interstitium comprises approximately 50% of the wet weight of skin, 10% of skeletal muscle weight, and 16% of the total body weight. The entire interstitial compartment of the body contains 10–12 litres of fluid compared with a plasma volume of 3 litres (Figure 2.1). It consists of a framework of collagen and other fibrous molecules called glycosaminoglycans (GAG), which are long-chain amino-sugar polymers. The most abundant GAG in the interstitium of the skin is hyaluronan, which has a molecular weight of several million. The interstitial fluid occupies the minute spaces between these molecules. It consists mainly of water, plus small ions and gases in solution, and plasma proteins which leak very slowly from the microcirculation.

Interstitial 'fluid' is really a gel, and the water cannot flow easily through the fibrous framework, i.e. the hydraulic conductivity of the interstitium is normally very low. A consequence of the low mobility of interstitial water is that it does not normally flow from one part of the body to another, for instance, under the effect of gravity. In oedema, interstitial hydraulic conductivity is greatly increased.[1] The structure of the interstitium is not static; the structural macromolecules undergo turnover and are removed in the lymph. An increase in interstitial flux, and hence lymph flow, is associated with an increased mobilisation and turnover of hyaluronan.[2]

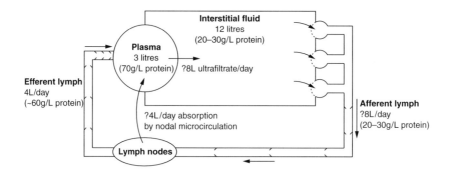

Figure 2.1 Scheme of the extracellular fluid circulation in a 65kg man. From Levick (1995)[2] with permission.

The Starling principle of fluid exchange

Interstitial fluid originates from the plasma in the microcirculation (capillaries and venules). The walls of microvessels are leaky; small molecules like water cross without hindrance but large molecules like proteins can cross only slowly. Fluid crosses the walls of microvessels at a rate determined by pressures on either side of the wall. Flux can be in either direction (filtration or resorption) but a small net loss of fluid from the circulation into the tissues is evident from the continuous flow of lymph, i.e. interstitial fluid which has entered the lymphatic system. Interstitial fluid is thus continuously produced and drained away from the tissues by the lymphatic system, ultimately to return to the blood via the connection between the systems at the base of the neck.

The pressures which operate across the capillary wall, and other factors accounting for the degree of leakiness of the wall to water and protein, are contained in Starling's principle of fluid exchange:

$$J_v = L_p A \left([P_c - P_i] - \sigma[\pi_p - \pi_i] \right).$$

J_v is the *filtration rate*, L_p denotes the *hydraulic conductance* (how leaky the capillary wall is to water), A is the *wall area*, and the product $L_p A$ is called the *capillary filtration capacity*. P_c is the *hydrostatic pressure* of the blood in the capillary and P_i is the hydrostatic pressure of the interstitial fluid on the other side of the capillary wall. P_c depends on the ratio of pre- to post-capillary resistance. The symbol π denotes the *colloid osmotic pressure* of the plasma (subscript 'p') and interstitial fluid (subscript 'i'). This pressure can be thought of as a 'suction' pressure that is exerted by the protein molecules in each space. Full colloid osmotic pressure is only exerted by molecules that are *unable* to cross the capillary wall. Because proteins can pass very slowly, the effective colloid osmotic pressure is slightly less than $\pi_p - \pi_i$. This slight

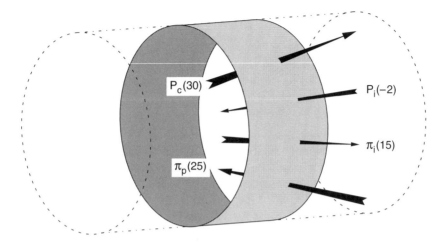

Figure 2.2 Starling pressures operating across the capillary wall at heart level. The four pressures that govern filtration rate across the capillary wall are shown. P_c, capillary hydrostatic pressure; P_i, interstitial hydrostatic pressure; π_p, plasma colloid osmotic pressure; π_i, interstitial colloid osmotic pressure. Values (in mmHg) are those typically found in the skin at heart level. By convention, these pressures are relative to atmospheric pressure (760mmHg). Thus, the 'negative' P_i (-2) represents an inward pressure of 758mmHg.

leakiness to protein is accounted for by σ (sigma), the *reflection coefficient* for plasma proteins. The pressure terms are shown in Figure 2.2, together with their typical values in humans at heart level. The *hydrostatic pressure difference* $(P_c - P_i)$ tends to cause fluid flux from capillary to interstitium, whereas the effective *colloid osmotic pressure difference* $(\sigma[\pi_p - \pi_i])$ tends to hold fluid within the circulation.

Lymph drainage

The lymphatic system can be thought of as an anatomical and physiological extension of the interstitial space. Water, protein, electrolytes, fat/chyle (in the intestines), cell debris, antigens and particulate matter enter the initial lymphatic vessels freely. Pre-nodal lymph therefore has a similar composition to interstitial fluid. Filling of lymphatic vessels depends in part on the action of fibres that tether the initial lymphatics to the surrounding tissue. The presence of an extracellular matrix closely investing the initial lymphatics, comprising a network of fine filaments and sparse ground substance, provides the functional link between the tethering fibres and the lymphatic endothelium.[3] With local expansion of the interstitium, increased traction by these fibres results in lymphatic dilation (and prevention of collapse) and the opening of junctions between endothelial cells. Fluid then enters by a mechanism which probably relies on a hydrostatic pressure gradient, although the precise nature of this is unclear.[4,5] Some of the water in lymph is removed as it flows through the lymph nodes. Capillary hydrostatic pressure is assumed to be less than the plasma colloid osmotic pressure in lymph nodes, thereby permitting the absorption of water. Post-nodal lymph consequently has a higher protein concentration and smaller volume than pre-nodal lymph.

All but the smallest lymphatic vessels (the initial lymphatics) are contractile, and there is much evidence to support the importance of active contraction of vessel walls to propel lymph. Propulsion of lymph from the initial lymphatics to the first valvular contractile vessels probably relies on external compression by tissue movements or blood vessel pulsation. Beyond this point, lymphatic vessels behave like miniature hearts and pump their contents rhythmically along from one 'chamber' to the next with a cycle of contraction and re-laxation. The interval between two valves is called a lymphangion. The rate and force of the contractions depend on the filling pressure and outflow resistance.[6]

Passive and active limb movements increase lymph flow, as does skin massage. When walking, lymph production and flow rise markedly in the feet. Obstruc-tion of lymphatics downstream, as in secondary lymphoedema, causes the vessels to pump harder, and distension and valvular incompetence may ensue, rendering intrinsic propulsion less effective. In these circumstances external compression can still propel lymph away from the swollen region.

Mechanisms of oedema formation

Homeostasis of interstitial fluid volume and the safety margin against oedema

The mechanisms that control interstitial fluid volume probably operate at a local level in each body compartment.[4] Changes in capillary and interstitial hydrostatic pressures, capillary surface area, colloid osmotic pressures and lymph flow all influence interstitial fluid volume. Three mechanisms in particular operate to provide a margin of safety against oedema:

1 *Rise in interstitial fluid pressure (P$_i$)* – in healthy tissues, a small rise in interstitial fluid volume causes a marked rise in P$_i$, which will reduce the net hydrostatic driving pressure across the capillary wall.

2 *Fall in interstitial colloid osmotic pressure (π$_i$)* – an inverse relationship exists between filtration rate (J$_v$) and interstitial fluid protein concentration, i.e. the interstitial protein concentration falls as the filtration rate rises. As

π_i falls, the effective suction pressure rises in the capillaries and venules. Both a rise in P_i and a fall in π_i attenuate a rise in J_v.

3   *Increased lymph flow* – lymph flow is almost zero in the resting limb but rises to high levels during exercise. The capacity for lymph flow to increase in response to increased interstitial fluid pressure and volume provides a further safety margin against oedema.

Together, these safety mechanisms can cope with an increase in hydrostatic pressure of capillary blood (P_c) or a decrease in colloid osmotic pressure of plasma (π_p) of 15mmHg.[7,8]

When interstitial volume progressively increases, tissue swelling is not at first clinically evident. The stretchability (*compliance*) of normal interstitium is relatively low and small changes in volume produce large changes in interstitial pressure.[7] Thus, with increasing hydration of the interstitium, interstitial fluid pressure (P_i) initially rises steeply towards zero (i.e. atmospheric pressure). At this point, stretchability suddenly increases and enables large volumes of fluid to accumulate; P_i then rising more gently to just above zero. Swelling becomes clinically evident when the interstitial volume has more than doubled. The relationship between interstitial fluid pressure and increase in volume of the arm in postmastectomy oedema is shown in Figure 2.3.[9]

Excessive interstitial fluid formation

A consideration of the terms in the Starling equation enables an understanding of some of the mechanisms of excessive interstitial fluid formation. An increase in capillary pressure (P_c), the largest and most labile of the four pressures (Figure 2.2), will increase filtration rate, as will a decrease in the colloid osmotic pressure exerted by the plasma proteins (π_p) within the circulation. These pressure changes will lead to hyperfiltration. An increase in hydraulic conductance of the capillary wall (as in inflammation) or of surface area available for exchange will also increase the filtration rate, independent of the net filtration pressure. An alternative mechanism leading to oedema is reduction in lymph flow (J_L). A change in volume of the tissues will result from a sustained imbalance between microvascular filtration rate (J_v) and lymph flow (J_L). Thus: $\Delta V/\Delta t = J_v - J_L$, where $\Delta V/\Delta t$ represents the change in tissue volume with time – this assumes that vascular volume remains constant, and included in J_L are possible fluid shifts along tissue planes.

Increased capillary pressure

A sustained increase in venous pressure is the commonest cause of increased capillary pressure. For example, the effect of gravity on the column of venous

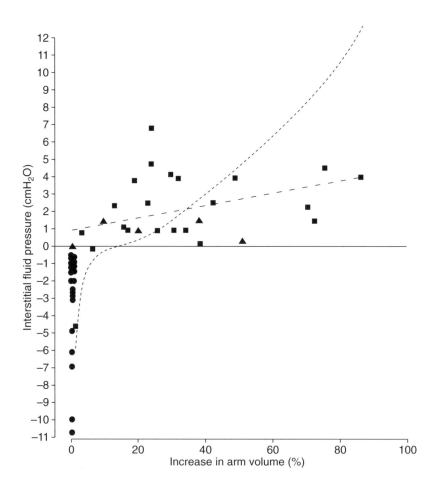

Figure 2.3 Interstitial fluid pressure plotted as a function of increase in arm volume in postmastectomy oedema. ■, swollen arms treated with compression garments; ▲, swollen arms not treated with compression garments; ●, normal arm. Short-dashed line, regression line through results for swollen arms. Long-dashed line, curve from Guyton (1965)[7] for acute experimental oedema in the dog hindlimb. From Bates et al. (1992)[9] with permission.

blood between the heart and the feet elevates venous pressure in the lower extremities during prolonged standing. The resulting capillary pressure, which is much higher than that found at heart level, raises the filtration rate per unit surface area of capillary. The increase in capillary pressure when standing is somewhat less than expected because of the veni-arteriolar response. Local arteriolar constriction occurs in response to the increased venous pressure and this raises the pre- to postcapillary resistance ratio, thus limiting the rise in capillary pressure.[10] Filtration rate is *increased*, however, and eventually overwhelms the lymphatic system leading to covert (and sometimes frank) swelling of the feet (low-protein oedema).

Restoration of the normal interstitial fluid volume occurs after a period of recumbency. Measurements of foot volume during inactive standing indicate that the swelling rate declines over a 20-minute period. Also, with the subject sitting and the feet dependent (hanging down), a lower swelling rate occurs in the afternoon than in the morning.[11,12] One of several possible explanations for these findings is that 'maximum' lymph flow is not fixed and can increase above the level at which it is initially overwhelmed.

Evidence for an anatomical adaptation of the lymphatic system in dependent tissues to cope with the greater fluid load is suggested by a greater skin lymphatic vessel density in the lower leg than in the forearm, a less dependent region (Figure 2.4).[13] Following intradermal injection of dextran labelled with a fluorescent dye, the initial lymphatic network in the skin can be visualised. The difference in density of vessels in the forearm (A) and lower leg (B) is evident. Thus, lymph transport capacity may be higher in leg skin.

Venous hypertension and tissue swelling also result from venous disease in a limb, and from cardiac failure. In cardiac failure, interstitial fluid typically accumulates in the subcutaneous tissue plane of the ankles and in the lungs (pulmonary oedema) due to raised pressure in the systemic and pulmonary veins.

Decreased colloid osmotic pressure

Loss of plasma proteins from the body or failure to synthesise them will result in hypoproteinaemia and hence a decreased plasma colloid osmotic pressure. Starvation is another cause. Abnormal loss of protein can occur in renal and bowel disease, and the resulting hypoproteinaemic oedema may be severe and widespread. Liver disease may be complicated by hypoproteinaemia because of failure to synthesise protein or because of loss due to haemorrhage, and as a result free fluid may accumulate in the peritoneal cavity (ascites) in addition to lower limb oedema.

Ascites can occur with hypoproteinaemia of any cause and with malignant infiltration of the peritoneum. Another common cause of ascites is portal hypertension, as in cirrhosis. Lymphatics on the underside of the diaphragm are important in the removal of free fluid from the peritoneal cavity but, in cancer, these may become obstructed by subphrenic metastases. As with interstitial oedema, the volume of ascites depends on the relative rates of formation and re-absorption.[14]

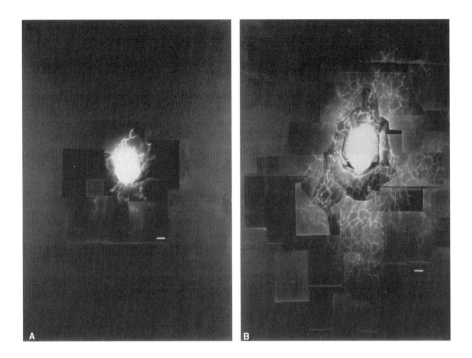

Figure 2.4 Fluorescence lymphangiograms from the forearm (A) and lower leg (shin) (B) of a healthy young man. Ten microlitres of fluorescein isothiocyanate-dextran (molecular weight 150kDa) have been injected intradermally to produce a depot at the two sites (centre of each image). The injected material has been taken up by the initial lymphatic vessels. Vessel density and spread are clearly greater in leg skin. Magnification × 23. Bars, 1mm. From Stanton et al. (1999)[13] with permission.

Increased capillary surface area

Angiogenesis increases the capillary surface area available for fluid flux and may be a contributory factor in postmastectomy lymphoedema of the arm.[15]

Oedema of inflammation

In inflammation, arteriolar dilation causes capillary pressure to rise. The hydraulic conductance of the capillary wall and its permeability to protein also increase (reduced protein reflection coefficient) which facilitates the passage of fluid and protein into the tissues. A further contributory change in the terms of the Starling equation, at least in animal models of in-flammation, is reduced (i.e. more negative) interstitial fluid pressure in the first 15–20 minutes.[4] These changes combine to increase capillary filtra-tion rate substantially, thereby causing oedema. Similar changes occur in burns.

Defective drainage

A reduction in lymph flow can also lead to oedema. Whereas no method exists to measure lymph flow in absolute units in humans, it is assumed that lymph flow is reduced, for instance, in lymphoedema of a limb following cancer surgery and radiotherapy. In postmastectomy lymphoedema, the filtration rate *per unit volume of soft tissue* in the swollen forearm (measured with the arm in the dependent position) is 47% lower than in the opposite unaffected arm. *Total* filtration rate in the swollen forearm is similar to that in the unaffected arm.[16] This suggests that total lymph flow from this segment of swollen limb is also similar to the unaffected arm because the arms were in the steady-state, i.e. the change in tissue volume with time ($\Delta V/\Delta t$) = zero, and capillary filtration rate (J_v) = lymph flow (J_L). When the limb is getting larger, J_v must exceed J_L. Capillary filtration capacity is not significantly altered in the swollen arm. These observations were made using venous occlusion plethysmography, which does not distinguish between filtration rates of the different compartments of the arm (skin, subcutis, muscle).

Lymphoedema has been traditionally classed as a 'high-protein oedema', with protein accumulating because of impaired lymph drainage. Whereas the protein concentration is indeed high in comparison with that in the oedema fluid of hyperfiltration states,[17] comparison of oedema fluid with normal in-terstitial fluid indicates that the concentration in oedema fluid is unchanged,[18,19] or even reduced (the oedema fluid therefore having a reduced interstitial colloid osmotic pressure).[20,21] The hyaluronan concentration in oedema fluid is seven times higher than in thoracic duct lymph,[19] but this is still lower than that in normal skin.[22]

In longstanding lymphoedema, material other than fluid contributes to the increased bulk of the tissue. Swelling due to increased interstitial fluid volume alone (early lymphoedema and in conditions of hyperfiltration) can be termed simple oedema. Tissues of this type are easily indentable by finger pressure (pitting oedema), indicating the increased mobility of the interstitial fluid. In contrast, longstanding lymphoedema is associated with excessive fibrous tissue and fat, and the physical properties of the tissue are con-sequently changed, becoming brawny (firm or hard) in nature.[23-25] Fibrosis of chronically oedematous tissue is well-known, for instance, in lung and heart disease.[26]

Conclusion

This chapter considers the physiological mechanisms governing interstitial fluid formation and drainage, and how disturbance of these mechanisms leads to oedema. The complexity of these mechanisms and their interplay is evident, and a full understanding is hampered by technical difficulties in measuring some of the components of the Starling equation (e.g. capillary pressure at a site other than the nail fold) and by the lack of a means to measure lymph flow. There are notable gaps in our knowledge, such as the means by which interstitial fluid enters the initial lymphatics. Recent advances in our understanding of the physiology and ultrastructure of the lymphatic system are encouraging, however, and will inspire continued investigation.

Acknowledgements

The author is supported by the Medical Research Council. Professor Rodney Levick is thanked for his helpful suggestions for the manuscript and for providing Figure 2.2.

References

1 Guyton AC *et al.* (1966) Interstitial fluid pressure. III. Its effect on resistance to tissue fluid mobility. *Circulation Research.* **19**:412–9.
2 Levick JR (1995) Circulation of fluid between plasma, interstitium and lymph. In: *An Introduction to Cardiovascular Physiology*, Butterworth-Heinemann Ltd, Oxford, pp 158–87.
3 Castenholz A (1998) Functional microanatomy of interstitial lymphatics with special consideration of the extracellular matrix. *Lymphology.* **31**:101–18.
4 Aukland K and Reed RK (1993) Interstitial-lymphatic mechanisms in the control of extracellular fluid volume. *Physiological Reviews.* **73**:1–78.
5 Schmid-Schönbein GW and Zweifach BW (1994) Fluid pump mechanics in initial lymphatics. *News in Physiological Sciences.* **9**:67–71.
6 Roddie IC (1990) Lymph transport mechanisms in peripheral lymphatics. *News in Physiological Sciences.* **5**:85–9.
7 Guyton AC (1965) Interstitial fluid pressure. II. Pressure–volume curves of interstitial space. *Circulation Research.* **16**:452–60.
8 Taylor AE and Townsley MI (1987) Evaluation of the Starling fluid flux equation. *News in Physiological Sciences.* **2**:48–52.
9 Bates DO *et al.* (1992) Subcutaneous interstitial fluid pressure and arm volume in lymphoedema. *International Journal of Microcirculation.* **11**:359–73.
10 Levick JR and Michel CC (1978) The effects of position and skin temperature on the capillary pressures in the fingers and toes. *Journal of Physiology.* **274**: 97–109.

11 Stick C *et al.* (1985) On physiological edema in man's lower extremity. *European Journal of Applied Physiology.* **54**:442–9.

12 Winkel J and Jørgensen K (1986) Swelling of the foot, its vascular volume and systemic hemoconcentration during long-term constrained sitting. *European Journal of Applied Physiology.* **55**:162–6.

13 Stanton AWB *et al.* (1999) Increased skin lymphatic vessel density in the leg compared with the arm. *Microvascular Research.* **57**:320–8.

14 Arroyo V *et al.* (1999) Pathogenesis, diagnosis, and treatment of ascites in cirrhosis. In: J Bircher *et al.* (eds) *Oxford Textbook of Clinical Hepatology, section 8.1.* Oxford University Press, Oxford, pp 697–731.

15 Roberts CC *et al.* (1994) Skin microvascular architecture and perfusion studied in human postmastectomy oedema by intravital video-capillaroscopy. *International Journal of Microcirculation.* **14**:327–34.

16 Stanton AWB *et al.* (1999) Comparison of microvascular filtration in human arms with and without postmastectomy oedema. *Experimental Physiology.* **84**:405–19.

17 Stanton AWB *et al.* (1996) Current puzzles presented by postmastectomy oedema (breast cancer related lymphoedema). *Vascular Medicine.* **1**:213–25.

18 Olszewski WL (1991) Chemistry of lymph. In: WL Olszewski (ed) *Lymph Stasis: Pathophysiology, Diagnosis and Treatment.* CRC Press, Boca Raton, Florida, pp 235–58.

19 Liu N-F and Zhang L-R (1998) Changes of tissue fluid hyaluronan (hyaluronic acid) in peripheral lymphoedema. *Lymphology.* **31**:173–9.

20 Bates DO *et al.* (1993) Change in macromolecular composition of interstitial fluid from swollen arms after breast cancer treatment, and its implications. *Clinical Science.* **86**:737–46.

21 Bates DO *et al.* (1994) Starling pressures in the human arm and their alteration in postmastectomy oedema. *Journal of Physiology.* **477**:355–63.

22 Fraser JRE and Laurent TC (1989) Turnover and metabolism of hyaluronan. In: *The Biology of Hyaluronan.* Ciba Foundation Symposium 143. John Wiley and Sons, Chichester, pp 41–59.

23 Mortimer PS (1990) Investigation and management of lymphoedema. *Vascular Medicine Review.* **1**:1–20.

24 Pflug JJ and Schirger A (1993) Chronic peripheral lymphedema. In: DL Clement and JT Shepherd (eds) *Vascular Diseases in the Limbs.* Mosby Year Book Inc., St Louis, Missouri, pp 221–38.

25 Daróczy J (1995) Pathology of lymphedema. *Clinics in Dermatology.* **13**:433–44.

26 Szidon JP (1989) Pathophysiology of the congested lung. *Cardiology Clinics.* **7**:39–48.

3 Classification of lymphoedema

Vaughan Keeley

The principal cause of lymphoedema is a low output failure of the lymphatic system, i.e. lymph transport is reduced.[1] This leads to the accumulation of relatively protein-rich interstitial fluid in the tissues. High output failure of the lymphatic circulation occurs when there is an increased capillary filtrate which overwhelms the transport capacity of intact lymphatic vessels, and results in oedema of lower protein content. This is seen in various clinical circumstances, for example chronic venous insufficiency in the leg, liver cirrhosis and nephrotic syndrome, and should be distinguished from pure lymphoedema.

If high output failure of the lymphatic system persists, a gradual deterioration of the functioning of the lymphatic vessels may occur. Thus, lymphatic output becomes reduced in the face of increased capillary filtration, producing a mixed form of lymphoedema. This may be found, for example, when there have been superimposed repeated infections. This chapter will focus mainly on lymphoedema of the limbs due to low output failure with some discussion of lymphoedema of mixed pathogenesis.

The classification into primary and secondary lymphoedema was introduced in the 1930s.[2] The term *secondary* was used for lymphoedema with a well-recognised acquired cause, for example treatment for cancer, and *primary* was used to describe lymphoedema with an obscure cause (previously called *idiopathic* or *spontaneous*). It was suggested that primary lymphoedema was caused by a congenital underdevelopment of the lymph vessels.

This broad division continues to be generally accepted (Box 3.A). Many uncertainties remain, however, including details of the pathogenesis of different conditions within primary lymphoedema. There has been a proposal recently to develop an international consensus on more precise definitions

---

Box 3.A International Society of Lymphology (ISL) definitions[1]

Primary lymphoedema

Lymphoedema due to a congenital lymphatic dysplasia.

Secondary lymphoedema

Lymphoedema due to the anatomical obliteration of the lymphatic system caused by an extrinsic process (e.g. surgery or repeated infections) or as a consequence of functional deficiency (e.g. valvular insufficiency).

for the classification and staging of lymphoedema.[3] The current situation in relation to primary lymphoedema is particularly unclear and several classifications exist. Clinically, however, arm lymphoedema is mostly secondary, particularly after treatment for breast cancer. In contrast leg lymphoedema is more common than arm and is mostly due to causes other than cancer or its treatment.[4]

Primary lymphoedema

Because the features of all primary lymphoedemas are not the same, a clinical classification based on the different ages of onset of the swelling was proposed:

- *lymphoedema congenita* present at birth or within 2 years

- *lymphoedema praecox* develops between 2 and 35 years of age

- *lymphoedema tarda* develops after 35 years of age.[2]

However, this does not take the pathogenesis into account and therefore has limited value, particularly when considering management options. In order to have a classification based on morphology, Kinmonth used lymphography in the legs of patients with primary lymphoedema. A radio-opaque substance was injected into a peripheral lymphatic in the foot previously made visible by the SC injection of patent blue dye. A series of radiographs was then taken to follow the flow of the substance proximally through the lymph trunks to the lymph nodes. Based on these studies he described three radiological appearances.[5]

- hypoplasia

- aplasia

- hyperplasia.

In hypoplasia there were smaller or fewer lymph vessels and the lymph nodes were often smaller; this was the most common pattern. In some patients there was associated 'dermal backflow' of the radio-opaque substance indicating reflux of lymph from the deeper hypoplastic vessels into the dermal plexus. In other patients there was hypoplasia at the root of a limb with an obstructive picture distal to it, for example dermal backflow with relatively normal trunks or grossly distended tortuous vessels like those seen in secondary obstructive lymphoedema.

In aplasia, there were no formed lymph trunks whereas, in contrast, in hyperplasia, the patients had large tortuous incompetent lymphatics, usually

Table 3.1 Clinical manifestations of chylous reflux

Site	Clinical features
Limb	Cutaneous vesicles containing milky fluid in proximal part of lymphoedematous limb
Peritoneum	Chylous ascites
Pleura	Chylothorax
Kidneys	Chyluria
Uterus and vagina	Chylometrorrhagia

involving only one limb, with no evidence of proximal obstruction. Valves could not be demonstrated in the affected areas and retrograde flow of the radio-opaque material was frequently seen. Some patients had chylous reflux, i.e. chyle (intestinal lymph) flowed down through incompetent lymphatics from the cisterna chyli to the perineum or leg.

The cisterna chyli is a dilated portion of the thoracic duct at its origin in the lumbar region. It receives lymphatic vessels from the legs, pelvic viscera, intestines, liver, pancreas, spleen and the lower part of the thorax. Chyle is milky in appearance because of the presence of emulsified fat taken up by the lacteals (the central lymphatics in intestinal villi). The clinical picture of chylous reflux will depend upon the site of the incompetent lymphatics (Table 3.1).

It has subsequently been argued that some of these appearances may have been artefactual.[6] For example, pedal lymphography may not demonstrate existing vessels in the thigh, iliac region or even iliac nodes when there are no vessels found in the distal part of the leg. In addition, lymphographic appearances may change over time, for example because of the 'die-back' phenomenon, when proximal damage to lymph vessels is followed by progressive obliteration of vessels distally. Thus, lymphography alone may not accurately reflect the clinical abnormalities. In order to address this, Browse and Stewart developed a clinical classification which took into account the lymphographic findings and subdivided primary lymphoedema into congenital and acquired (Box 3.B).[6] Browse later elaborated on three common varieties of primary lymphoedema (Table 3.2).[7]

Distal obliteration of lymph vessels is the commonest and typically presents as mild oedema of the ankles and lower legs in women at around puberty with no history of injury. Even so, there is likely to be an acquired component of some kind. Lymphography in these patients shows hypoplasia or aplasia as

---

Box 3.B Browse and Stewart's classification of primary lymphoedema[6]

Congenital

1 Congenital aplasia or hypoplasia of peripheral lymphatics. (Lymphographic abnormality and/or oedema present at or appearing within 2 years of birth.)

2 Congenital abnormalities of the abdominal or thoracic lymph trunks (sometimes with chylous reflux).

3 Congenital valvular incompetence. This is always associated with 'megalymphatics' (dilated incompetent vessels on lymphangiography) and often with chylous reflux.

Acquired

1 Intraluminal or intramural lymphangio-obstructive oedema:
   - distal – acquired obliteration of the distal limb lymphatics, cause unknown
   - proximal – acquired obliteration of the lymphatics in the proximal part of the limb generally associated with distal dilation, cause unknown
   - combined – acquired obliteration of all the lymphatics of the limb.

2 Obstruction by the lymph nodes. Obliteration of the lymph conducting pathways through the node by hilar fibrosis. This may cause lymphangio-obstructive oedema and acquired valvular incompetence.

Table 3.2 Common types of primary lymphoedema[7]

	Distal obliteration	Proximal obliteration	Congenital hyperplasia
Proportion	80%	10%	10%
Preponderance	Mainly female	Male + female	Male + female
Family history	+	–	+
Onset			
Time	Puberty	Any age	Congenital
Location	Ankle	Whole leg/thigh	Whole leg
	Bilateral	Unilateral	Uni- or bilateral
Progression	Slow	Rapid	Progressive

defined by Kinmonth.[5] However, it is not generally clear whether the patient is born with a reduced number of vessels which 'fail' in later life (for example following episodes of inflammation) causing oedema or whether this represents an acquired occlusion due to damage of normal lymph vessels.

The second common variety presents as a unilateral lymphoedema at any age which progresses rapidly in just a few weeks or months. It is often preceded by a minor event, for example a joint strain, insect bite or skin infection. Lymphography shows normal or dilated vessels in the foot, lower limb and thigh but reduced vessels and nodes in the inguinal and iliac regions; the lymph nodes are small and fibrotic and collateral vessels may be present.

The most likely cause is an acquired fibrotic proximal obliteration within the lymph nodes complicated by the 'die-back' phenomenon. This is believed to be a result of the dilation of lymphatics leading to the obstruction causing valvular incompetence and subsequent spread of this vascular distension down the limb. The distended vessels become damaged and occluded by endothelial proliferation or fibrin thrombus.

The third common variety is true congenital oedema and presents at or soon after birth. It may occur with several other congenital abnormalities including faint pink angiomas of the skin. There may be chylous reflux. Lymphography shows dilated hyperplastic incompetent lymphatic vessels (megalymphatics) throughout the limb and trunk (Kinmonth's hyperplasia).[5]

Olszewski[8] has described a further classification of lymphoedema based upon clinical examination, lymphoscintigraphy, lymphangiography, venography and histology (Box 3.C). He argues that there is no evidence of 'hypodevelopment'

Box 3.C   Olszewski's classification of lymphoedema[8]

Idiopathic hyperplastic (varicose) lymphoedema:
- develops at a young age (most likely present at birth)
- dilated tortuous lymphatics with incompetent valves.

Idiopathic acquired praecox or tarda (primary) lymphoedema:
- type A – peripheral swelling, distal stasis, small inguinal nodes
- type B – similar to A but swelling up to and including the calf
- type C – more advanced; entire limb swollen; obstructive changes in inguinal nodes; seen in older patient with deep vein abnormalities.

Postsurgical lymphoedema:
- leg – after inguinal or iliac node removal and radiotherapy for malignancy
- arm – typically after mastectomy.

Postinflammatory lymphoedema – mainly affects legs after acute infection of the skin.

Postinflammatory lymph stasis associated with chronic varicose ulcers – mixed lymphatic and venous pathology.

Lipoedema – not true lymphoedema.

of the lymphatics and, therefore, there is likely to be an as yet undefined acquired cause for this type of so-called primary lymphoedema.

Congenital syndromes involving the lymphatic system

Congenital lymphatic malformations are rare. Some may relate to chromosomal abnormalities whereas others may relate to single gene abnormalities or exposure to teratogens. Some are sporadic and of unknown cause.[9]

Milroy's disease

Also known as *hereditary lymphoedema type 1* or *Nonne-Milroy type hereditary lymphoedema*. It comprises brawny oedema of the legs, particularly distally, and is present from birth or before puberty (Figure 3.1). It may involve swelling of the genitalia, arms and face.[10] Lymphoscintigraphic studies of families with Milroy's disease show a wide range of lymphatic abnormalities including:

* absence or paucity of lymphatic trunks

* abnormal distribution of collectors

* lymphatic reflux and incompetence

* variable uptake by lymph nodes

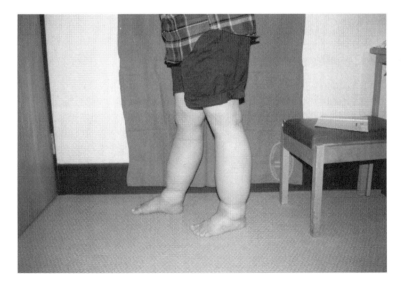

Figure 3.1   Milroy's disease.

- mixed lymphatic and blood vascular disturbances, e.g. combined lymphatic and venous dysplasia/reflux.

There may even be structural and functional lymphatic abnormalities in non-swollen limbs.[10] Fluorescence microlymphography has shown aplasia or extreme hypoplasia of both lymphatic capillaries and collectors in the oedematous limb.[11]

Milroy's disease occurs in 1 in 6000 births. Inheritance is probably autosomal dominant with incomplete penetrance (about 50%). Mutations in the gene for flt4 (fms-like tyrosine kinase 4), the receptor on lymphatic endothelial cells for vascular endothelial growth factor (VEGF-C), have been identified in some affected and at risk individuals. This gene is localised on the distal region of the long arm of chromosome 5 (5q34–35).[10] It has been suggested that the genetic mechanisms may be more complex with other gene abnormalities involved.[10] Genetic complexity may, therefore, be responsible for the wide variety of clinical findings present in families considered to have Milroy's disease. For example, associated abnormalities such as microcephaly, distichiasis (*see* pp 295 and 299), intestinal lymphangiectasia and extradural cysts have been described.[12] However, another recent study of families with Milroy's disease genetically mapped to the 5q35.3 region revealed only lymphatic abnormalities and no other dysmorphic features in its group of patients.[13] In the same study, the inheritance was also dominant with an estimated penetrance ratio of 0.84. It is therefore possible that true Milroy's disease is a relatively pure lymphatic abnormality and that other examples of primary congenital lymphoedema with associated abnormalities represent other conditions with different genotypes.

Klippel–Trenaunay–Weber syndrome

This is also known as *angio-osteohypertrophy syndrome*. The characteristic features include hemihypertrophy, varicose veins and cutaneous haemangiomas, as well as arteriovenous fistulae in some individuals (Figure 3.2).[14] Lymphography of patients with Klippel syndrome has revealed a tendency towards underdevelopment and insufficiency of the lymphatics of the affected limb.[15]

Chromosomal aneuploidy

Aneuploidy means an abnormality in the number of chromosomes.

Turner's syndrome

Women with Turner's syndrome (XO karyotype) may have cystic hygromas, hydrops foetalis and peripheral oedema. It is suggested that lymph channels become distended during embryonic development as a result of delayed or

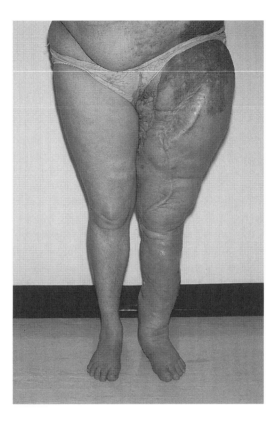

Figure 3.2 Klippel-Trenaunay-Weber syndrome. Characterised by proximal cutaneous haemangioma and increased limb length. This case shows lymphatic changes with swelling and cutaneous lymphangioma.

failed emptying of jugular lymph sacs into central veins. It may be that the webbed neck characteristic of Turner's syndrome is due to redundant skin which was once stretched by distended underlying lymphatics and then later relieved by the delayed joining of truncal lymphatics to the venous system. Finally, distended lymphatics in the thoracic cage may lead to the 'shield chest' and widely spaced nipples seen in this syndrome.

Klinefelter syndrome
Men with this syndrome (XXY karyotype) may occasionally present with lymphoedema.

Down's syndrome
People with trisomy 21 may occasionally develop cystic hygromas and lymphoedema.

Noonan's syndrome

People with Noonan's syndrome have similar physical features to Turner's syndrome, including peripheral lymphoedema, hypoplastic nails and shield chest. They may also have intestinal lymphangiectasia and lymphangiomas resulting from long-standing lymphoedema.

Meige's syndrome

This is also known as *hereditary lymphoedema II* or *Letessier-Meige syndrome*. It is generally similar to Milroy's disease but the peripheral oedema appears at a later age (i.e. from puberty to 50 years). It mainly affects the lower limbs (one or both) but may involve the upper limbs. It has been reported as being associated with cleft palate and possibly dystrophic yellow nails. Most cases are sporadic but some have an autosomal dominant pattern of inheritance. There may be aplasia or hypoplasia of peripheral lymphatics with dilation of lymphatic trunks.[16]

Yellow nail syndrome

Yellow nail syndrome is an uncommon disorder which has sometimes been classified as part of hereditary lymphoedema II.[16] It has been suggested that the basic defect is hypoplasia or obstruction of the lymphatic system, although more recent evidence indicates that impaired lymphatic drainage is a secondary functional effect rather than a primary structural deficit.[17] The three main clinical features are:

- thickened dystrophic yellow nails which are excessively curved from side to side (100%, i.e. an absolute requirement for the diagnosis)[18]
- lymphoedema of the lower limbs (80%)
- exudative pleural effusions (36%).

There may also be sinusitis and bronchiectasis.[19] The three main features may develop at different times and it is thought that lymphoedema and pleural effusions may occur in some patients only when the lymphatic system is stressed by infection. In some patients, the syndrome is sometimes associated with other disorders, for example thyroiditis, rheumatoid arthritis, nephrotic syndrome, malignant disease. Yellow nail syndrome may sometimes resolve spontaneously and it has been suggested that treatment of the concurrent disease may be associated with improvement, although there is no definite evidence for this.[20]

Lymphoedema-distichiasis

Lymphoedema-distichiasis is a rare autosomal dominant inherited syndrome with the onset of lymphoedema at or just after puberty.[21] Most individuals have distichiasis (see pp 295 and 299) from birth. Associated features include congenital heart defects, vertebral anomalies, extradural cysts, ptosis and cleft palate. A recent study has mapped the gene for this condition to chromosome 16q24.3 and suggested that the abnormal gene may be the N-proteinase for type 3 collagen or a cell matrix adhesion regulator.[21]

Miscellaneous syndromes

Primary lymphoedema can also occur as part of a number of other syndromes, for example neurofibromatosis type I (Von Recklinghausen syndrome)[9] and the extremely rare cholestasis–lymphoedema syndrome (Aagenaes syndrome)[22] and lymphoedema–hypoparathyroidism.[23]

Current position

The classification of primary lymphoedemas based upon pathogenesis will inevitably evolve as more is understood about the different clinical manifestations described above. Many cases of lymphoedema praecox and tarda which were previously considered as primary hypoplastic lymphatic disorders may be more accurately seen as acquired obstructive processes arising in regional lymph nodes, i.e. examples of secondary lymphoedema.[24]

Techniques such as fluorescence microlymphography are helping to elucidate structural and functional abnormalities in the superficial lymphatics. For example, it has been shown that the number of lymphatic capillaries is not reduced and the structure of the lymphatic capillary network is not damaged in patients with hypoplasia of the lymphatic collectors.[25] With a similar technique, the flow velocity of lymph in cutaneous microlymphatics has been measured.[26] In patients with primary lymphoedema this demonstrated rhythmic cutaneous backflow caused by the contraction of lymphatic collectors and retrograde pumping of lymph through incompetent valves.

The importance of a better understanding of primary lymphoedemas is also important in the development of more effective treatments.

At present, terms describing different types are often used loosely; for example, patients may be labelled as having Milroy's disease when there is no firm clinical basis for this diagnosis. As described above, genetic markers have recently been identified for Milroy's disease[13] and lymphoedema–distichiasis.[21] In the future, therefore, a better understanding of the genetics of primary lymphoedema is likely to aid accurate diagnosis and refine the classification. For the time being, however, a simple clinical classification is recommended[27] with the definition of primary lymphoedema as lymph-oedema in which no external cause has been identified (Box 3.D).

Box 3.D   Clinical classification of primary lymphoedema[27]

Congenital

Milroy's disease (familial).
Congenital vascular malformations with lymphangioma, e.g. Klippel-Trenaunay-Weber syndrome.
Chylous lymphoedema.

Congenitally-determined late onset

Meige's syndrome (familial).
Distal hypoplasia (bilateral leg oedema).
Proximal obstructive nodal disease (unilateral whole leg swelling).
Megalymphatics (bilateral whole leg swelling).

Secondary lymphoedema

Secondary lymphoedema arises from anatomical obliteration or a functional deficiency of lymphatic vessels, caused by an identifiable process external to the lymphatic system.[1] It is more common than primary lymphoedema and may result from a combination of factors. The causes can be divided into four main groups:

- cancer-related
- infection
- inflammation
- trauma.

Cancer-related lymphoedema

This is the most common form of lymphoedema in the UK and may be caused by the malignant disease itself and/or its treatment.[4] Cancer may occasionally present as limb oedema, particularly if there is venous compression or thrombosis in addition to lymph node infiltration. Lymphoedema occurs more frequently, however, as the aftermath of surgical excision of lymph nodes and radiotherapy. The following specific situations will be considered:

- breast cancer
- gynaecological cancer
- prostate cancer
- groin dissection
- Kaposi's sarcoma.

Breast cancer

The prevalence of lymphoedema in women treated for breast cancer is about 25–30%,[28] although some reports put the figure as low as 6% (Figure 3.3).[29] The source of patients, length of follow-up, measurement techniques and definition of lymphoedema vary in different reports. In general, lower incidences of lymphoedema are recorded in studies with shorter follow-up. This is consistent with the well-recognised pattern of delay in the onset of swelling, which may occur in the absence of recurrence of the cancer several years after the primary treatment. Damage to the lymphatics by axillary surgery and radiotherapy seems to be the main cause of the oedema but other factors may contribute (see p.321). Investigation of potential risk factors, however, has led to unclear and conflicting results which makes it difficult to draw firm conclusions (Table 3.3).

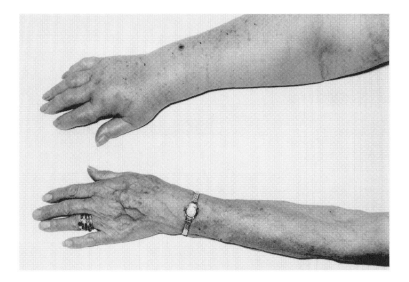

Figure 3.3   Breast cancer-associated arm oedema.

In one study, the incidence of lymphoedema (patient plus observer impression) after treatment for breast cancer was found to be similar after axillary radiotherapy alone (8%), axillary sampling plus radiotherapy (9%) and axillary clearance alone (7%).[30] However, after axillary clearance plus radiotherapy, the incidence was 38%.

Seroma formation refers to the accumulation of fluid close to the surgical wound which requires repeated drainage. In a retrospective study of 49 consecutive patients who underwent modified radical mastectomies but no radiotherapy, the development of seromas in > 50% and ipsilateral lymphoedema of the arm in 10% was associated with high volumes of postoperative wound drainage.[37] This presumably reflected the extent of interruption of the lymphatics at surgery. The seromas were found to contain lymph rather than serum as judged by the protein concentration.

In a prospective study, patients undergoing modified radical mastectomy for breast cancer were randomised to receive physiotherapy commencing on postoperative day 1 or day 7. There was a higher incidence of seromas in the group which started physiotherapy on day 1 (38%) compared with the group starting on day 7 (22%). There was no difference in shoulder function in the two groups. Other studies, however, have suggested that delaying physiotherapy has no effect on seroma formation.[38]

'Cording' is the development of tender cord-like structures either on the chest wall, in the axilla or down the inner aspect of the arm. Stretching of these cords

Table 3.3 Risk factors for the development of breast cancer-related lymphoedema[30–36]

Definitely	Possible	No risk
Extent of breast surgery (mastectomy → wide local excision)	Wound infection	Age
	Seroma formation	Menopausal status
	Cording	Handedness
Extent of axillary surgery	Congentital predisposition	Total dose of
Axillary radiotherapy (and time since radiotherapy)	Concomitant venous abnormalities	radiation
		Drug therapy
Radiotherapy to breast	Early lymphoedema (in first 2 months)	
Nodal disease status at diagnosis	Minor trauma of 'at risk' limb, e.g. venepuncture, blood pressure measurement	
Tumour T stage at diagnosis	Air travel	
Axillary recurrence		
Obesity		
An oblique surgical incision		
Hypertension		
History of infection in the affected arm		

across the axilla on arm abduction can be painful and can cau: of shoulder movement. The cords are thought to result from lym, lymphatic thrombosis.[32]

The prevalence of lymphoedema increases with time after postoperative radiotherapy. Lymphoedema is twice as common in women who have had a mastectomy compared with those who have had a wide local excision.[37] It has also been suggested that there may be a pre-existing congenitally-determined lymphatic insufficiency which predisposes some women to develop oedema after treatment for breast cancer. This is based on the observation that, in women with bilateral breast disease, the tendency to develop oedema in one arm is not independent of the tendency in the other.

Modifications to surgery and radiotherapy so as to reduce morbidity, including lymphoedema, have been the subject of recent debate. Some advocate axillary clearance without subsequent radiotherapy[39] whereas, at the other extreme, sentinel node biopsy is proposed.[40] The latter aims to biopsy the node to which lymph from the region of the breast tumour preferentially drains. The nodes can be identified pre-operatively using a radio-active tracer. If the sentinel node does not contain metastatic tumour, further axillary surgery can be avoided. The technique and its outcome, however, are still being investigated and it is not yet routine clinical practice (see p.325). Axillary node sampling of three to four nodes remains the usual routine staging procedure.

The following factors should reduce the incidence of breast cancer-related lymphoedema:

- wide local excision rather than mastectomy
- earlier detection by breast screening facilitating wide local excision
- avoidance of axillary radiotherapy following axillary clearance
- modification of radiotherapy techniques
- avoidance of arm infections/inflammation.[41]

Gynaecological cancer

In a study of patients following total hysterectomy, excision of pelvic lymph nodes and radiotherapy for cancer of the uterine cervix, about 40% of women had a unilateral increase in leg volume of $\geq 5\%$.[42] Of these, 70% had slight (5–9.9% volume increase), 15% had moderate (10–14.9%) and 15% had severe swelling ($\geq 15\%$ volume increase) (Figure 3.4). Over half had lymphoedema severe enough to cause symptoms. In this study, surprisingly, no cases of bilateral lymphoedema were identified. Radical vulvectomy with bilateral groin lymph node dissection for cancer of the vulva is associated with an incidence of lower limb lymphoedema of up to 70%.[43]

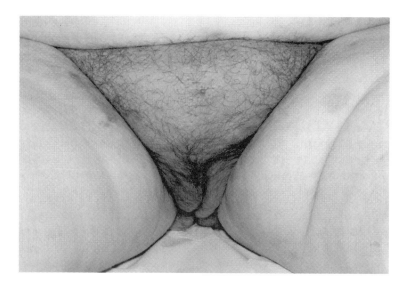

Figure 3.4 Gynaecological cancer-related oedema.

Prostate cancer

Lymphoedema of the lower limbs and genitalia can occur after treatment for prostate cancer with risk factors similar to those in breast cancer.[44]

Groin dissection

In a study of 40 patients who had undergone superficial groin dissection and 27 who had had radical ilio-inguinal dissections (without radiotherapy) for malignant melanoma, soft tissue sarcoma and squamous cell cancer, the overall incidence of mild–moderate lymphoedema (determined by difference of leg circumference and symptoms) was 21%.[45] Lymphoedema was more common in patients with primary lesions in the leg (26%) compared with those with lower trunk lesions (6%). Using different definitions and surgical techniques, another study found measurable lymphoedema in > 80% after 5 years.[46]

Kaposi's sarcoma

The prevalence of Kaposi's sarcoma has increased in recent years as a result of human immunodeficiency virus/acquired immune deficiency syndrome (HIV/AIDS). The progenitor cell line for Kaposi's sarcoma is lymphatic epithelium and in consequence this tumour may cause obstructive lymphoedema.[47]

Infection

Theoretically, infection may cause damage to lymphatic vessels as a result of lymphangitis, perilymphadenitis and lymphangiothrombosis. The most important of these are:

- bacterial cellulitis and erysipelas
- filariasis
- tuberculosis.

Of these, the former is the most common in the UK but worldwide filariasis is the major cause with about 90 million people affected.[4] Less common infective causes of lymphoedema include tuberculous lymphogranuloma inguinale in the tropics.[4]

Bacterial cellulitis and erysipelas

Bacterial infection may cause cellulitis and erysipelas.[48] Erysipelas involves the more superficial layers of the skin and cutaneous lymphatics, whereas cellulitis extends more deeply into the subcutaneous tissues. Clinically, however, differentiation between the two is not always clear. Both cause local signs of inflammation and often a fever and leucocytosis.

Lymphangitis and lymphadenitis may occur and episodes may be recurrent, probably because the lymphatic system becomes damaged. In erysipelas the area of inflammation may be raised above the surrounding skin and there may be a distinct demarcation between the infected skin and the surrounding normal skin. The infecting organism in most cases of classic erysipelas is the β-haemolytic Streptococcus (typically group A); in cellulitis some cases are caused by *Staphylococcus aureus* and other bacteria, e.g. *Streptococcus pneumoniae* and *Haemophilus influenzae*.[48]

The question has been raised as to whether cellulitis/erysipelas leads to lymphoedema in a previously normal limb or whether there may be an underlying primary lymphatic abnormality without oedema which predisposes to infection, leading to lymphatic damage and subsequent lymphoedema. In a study of patients who had had erysipelas of the legs, using indirect lymphography, abnormalities of the initial lymphatics and collectors were found not only in most of the affected limbs but also in about half of the apparently healthy unaffected limbs.[49] This suggests that there may indeed be a previously unrecognised, asymptomatic lymphatic abnormality in many patients who then develop cellulitis or erysipelas.

Filariasis

Lymphatic filariasis is caused by parasitic tissue-dwelling filarial nematode worms which are endemic to the tropics.[50] The infection is transmitted by mosquitoes. The infecting organisms are:

- *Wuchereria bancrofti*
- *Brugia malayi*
- *Brugia timori.*

Acute clinical features may occur and include:

- fever
- headache
- malaise
- lymphadenitis of inguinal and axillary nodes
- retrograde lymphangitis of the limb(s)
- cellulitis, abscess formation and ulceration
- funiculo-epididymo-orchitis leading to hydrocoele.

Chronic clinical features follow prolonged exposure or repeated acute attacks and include:

- hydrocoele
- lymphoedema, particularly of the legs but sometimes in the arm or breast
- abdominal lymphatic varices which may burst into the urinary tract and cause chyluria or lymphuria.

Inflammation

Several chronic inflammatory processes may lead to the development of lymphoedema of the limbs, such as:

- inflammatory arthritis
- contact dermatitis
- endemic elephantiasis (podoconiosis)
- pretibial myxoedema

- tenosynovitis

- retroperitoneal fibrosis.

Inflammatory arthritis

Over a 25-year period, arm oedema (bilateral in about half) has been reported in 29 patients with rheumatoid or psoriatic arthritis.[51] Oedema was equally frequent in men and women and presented a mean of 6.5 years after the arthritis. Clinical evidence of underlying synovitis was seen in half of the patients. Four cases of arm oedema associated with marked wrist and carpal psoriatic arthropathy have also been described.[51] Lymphoscintigraphy was abnormal in 3 cases and oedema progression was accompanied by radiographic progression of the arthritis.

Similarly, a lymphoscintigraphic study of patients with lymphoedema associated with rheumatoid arthritis revealed severely impaired lymphatic drainage of the affected limb.[52] It has been suggested that inflammatory products from the synovium are deposited in adjacent lymphatics, causing lymphangitis and subcutaneous lymphatic obstruction. Disease-modifying treatment can lead to the resolution of the lymphoedema.

Contact dermatitis

Persistent oedema of the hands has been described as a complication of allergic contact dermatitis of the hands.[53] Infection seems to have contributed to the clinical picture but no specific tests of lymphatic function were described.

Endemic elephantiasis (podoconiosis)

Endemic elephantiasis of the legs is a common condition in the tropics. It is estimated that the number of cases in Africa exceeds 500 000.[54] It can develop in childhood and is found where fertile clay soils from alkaline volcanic rocks are cultivated by bare-footed people. Examination reveals total destruction of the peripheral lymphatics and of the macrophages by silica from the soil. Particles of silica and silicates are found in the macrophages in the lymph nodes which receive afferent lymphatics from the affected parts. Early symptoms include a burning and itching sensation of the foot and lower leg. Plantar oedema develops under the metatarsal heads with swelling of the forefoot; swelling then spreads proximally.

Pretibial myxoedema

Pretibial myxoedema in its most extreme form clinically resembles lymphoedema. Fluorescence microlymphography has demonstrated collapse or obliteration of the initial lymphatics and lymphoscintigraphy has shown reduced lymphatic drainage of the affected limb.[55] It has been suggested that mucin deposition in the dermis may cause compression/occlusion of the dermal lymphatics and subsequent oedema.

Tenosynovitis

MRI in a case of peroneus longus tenosynovitis with localised swelling showed a characteristic honeycomb pattern typical of lymphoedema in the subcutaneous tissues.[56] The authors suggested that localised lymphoedema could be due to tenosynovitis. However, no lymphoscintigraphic studies were reported.

Retroperitoneal fibrosis

A case of lymphoedema associated with retroperitoneal fibrosis has been described.[57] However, the diagnosis was made on the basis of clinical appearance of the oedema (evenly distributed, firm, pale and cool to the touch) and no investigations of lymphatic or venous function were reported.

Trauma

Traumatic damage of the lymphatics can be responsible for the subsequent development of lymphoedema. This can take the form of accidental injury (e.g. extensive burns, particularly with circumferential skin loss) or may result from surgical excision (e.g. of lymph nodes). Oedema may even follow apparently limited surgery, such as after femoropopliteal artery by-pass. In patients who had undergone this operation, lymphangiograms showed severely disrupted inguinal lymphatics[58] and the severity and duration of the oedema was correlated to the magnitude of this disruption. Venograms were generally normal. Modification of the surgical technique to minimise inguinal lymphatic damage was recommended.

Factitious lymphoedema has also been described.[8] Patients, generally with psychiatric illnesses, deliberately injure themselves, for example with tourniquets or blows to the back of the hand. This leads to swelling. There is often a proximal circumferential discoloured constriction ring. Lymphangiography shows dilated lymphatics and multiple blowouts.

References

1 Consensus Document of the International Society of Lymphology Executive Committee (1995) The diagnosis and treatment of peripheral lymphoedema. *Lymphology.* **28**:113–7.

2 Kinmonth JB *et al.* (1957) Primary lymphoedema. *British Journal of Surgery.* **45**:1–10.

3 Witte MH *et al.* (1998) ISL Consensus Document revisited: suggested modifications. *Lymphology.* **31**:138–40.

4 Harwood CA and Mortimer PS (1995) Causes and clinical manifestations of lymphatic failure. *Clinics in Dermatology.* **13**:459–71.

5 Kinmonth JB (1969) Primary lymphoedema. *Journal of Cardiovascular Surgery.* Special No. for XVIIth Congress of European Society of Cardiovascular Surgery 65–77.

6 Browse NL and Stewart G (1985) Lymphoedema: pathophysiology and classification. *Journal of Cardiovascular Surgery.* **26**:91–105.

7 Browse NL (1986) The diagnosis and management of primary lymphoedema. *Journal of Vascular Surgery.* **3**:181–4.

8 Olszewski WL (1991) Clinical picture of lymphoedema. In: WL Olszewski (ed) *Lymph Stasis: Pathophysiology, Diagnosis and Treatment.* CRC Press, Boca Raton, Florida, pp 347–77.

9 Greenlee R *et al.* (1993) Developmental disorders of the lymphatic system. *Lymphology.* **26**:156–68.

10 Witte MH *et al.* (1998) Phenotypic and genotypic heterogeneity in familial Milroy lymphoedema. *Lymphology.* **31**:145–55.

11 Bollinger A *et al.* (1983) Aplasia of superficial lymphatic capillaries in hereditary and connatal lymphoedema (Milroy's disease). *Lymphology.* **16**:27–30.

12 Shanklin DR and Esterly JR (1990) Lymphedema I. In: ML Buyse (ed) *Birth Defects Encyclopedia.* Blackwell Scientific Publications, Oxford, pp 1087–8.

13 Evans AL *et al.* (1999) Mapping of primary congenital lymphoedema to the 5q35.3 region. *American Journal of Human Genetics.* **64**:547–55.

14 Viljoen DL (1990) Angio-osteohypertrophy syndrome. In: ML Buyse (ed) *Birth Defects Encyclopedia.* Blackwell Scientific Publications, Oxford, pp 141–2.

15 Kinmonth JB *et al.* (1976) Mixed vascular deformities of the lower limbs, with particular reference to lymphography and surgical treatment. *British Journal of Surgery.* **63**:899–906.

16 Goodman RM (1990) Lymphoedema II. In: ML Buyse (ed) *Birth Defects Encyclopedia.* Blackwell Scientific Publications, Oxford, pp 109–10.

17 Bull RH *et al.* (1996) Lymphatic function in the yellow nail syndrome. *British Journal of Dermatology.* **134**:307–12.

18 Nordkild P *et al.* (1986) Yellow nail syndrome – the triad of yellow nails, lymphedema and pleural effusions. *Acta Medica Scandinavica.* **219**:221–7.

19 Varney VA *et al.* (1994) Rhinitis, sinusitis and the yellow nail syndrome: a review of symptoms and response to treatment in 17 patients. *Clinical Otolaryngology.* **19**:237–40.

20 Pavlidakey GP *et al.* (1984) Yellow nail syndrome. *Journal of the American Academy of Dermatology.* **11**:509–12.

21 Mangion J *et al.* (1999) A gene for lymphoedema-distichiasis maps to 16q24.3. *American Journal of Human Genetics.* **65**:427–32.

22 Aagenaes O (1998) Hereditary cholestasis with lymphoedema (Aagenaes Syndrome, Cholestasis – Lymphoedema Syndrome). *Scandinavian Journal of Gastroenterology.* **33**:335–45.

23   Toriello HV (1990) Lymphoedema–hypoparathyroidism. In: ML Buyse (ed) *Birth Defects Encyclopedia*. Blackwell Scientific Publications, Oxford, p 1089.

24   Witte MH and Witte CL (1995) Epilogue: Beyond the sphere of knowledge in lymphology. *Clinics in Dermatology*. **13**:511–4.

25   Jäger K *et al.* (1983) Fluorescence microlymphography in patients with lymphoedema and chronic venous incompetence. *International Angiology*. **2**:129–36.

26   Fischer M *et al.* (1997) Flow velocity of cutaneous lymphatic capillaries in patients with primary lymphoedema. *International Journal of Microcirculation*. **17**:143–9.

27   Mortimer PS (1995) Managing lymphoedema. *Clinical and Experimental Dermatology*. **20**:98–106.

28   Logan V (1995) Incidence and prevalence of lymphoedema: a literature review. *Journal of Clinical Nursing*. **4**:213–9.

29   Petrek JA and Heelan MC (1998) Incidence of breast carcinoma-related lymphoedema. *Cancer*. **83**:2776–81.

30   Kissin MW *et al.* (1986) Risk of lymphoedema following the treatment of breast cancer. *British Journal of Surgery*. **73**:580–4.

31   Segerström K *et al.* (1992) Factors that influence the incidence of brachial oedema after treatment of breast cancer. *Scandinavian Journal of Plastic and Reconstructive Hand Surgery*. **26**:223–7.

32   Stanton AWB *et al.* (1996) Current puzzles presented by post-mastectomy oedema (breast cancer related lymphoedema). *Vascular Medicine*. **1**:213–25.

33   Rockson SG (1998) Precipitating factors in lymphoedema: myths and realities. *Cancer*. **83**:2814–16.

34   Mozes M *et al.* (1982) The role of infection in postmastectomy lymphoedema. *Surgery Annual*. **14**:73–83.

35   Mortimer PS *et al.* (1996) The prevalence of arm oedema following treatment for breast cancer. *Quarterly Journal of Medicine*. **89**:377–80.

36   Witte CL and Witte MH (1998) Consensus and dogma. *Lymphology*. **31**:98–100.

37   Tadych K and Donegan WL (1987) Post-mastectomy seromas and wound drainage. *Surgery, Gynecology and Obstetrics*. **165**:483–7.

38   Schultz V *et al.* (1997) Delayed shoulder exercises in reducing seroma frequency after modified radical mastectomy: a prospective randomised study. *Annals of Surgical Oncology*. **4**:293–7.

39   Robinson DS *et al.* (1992) Role and extent of lymphadenectomy for early breast cancer. *Seminars in Surgical Oncology*. **8**:78–82.

40   Pressman PI (1998) Surgical treatment and lymphoedema. *Cancer*. **83**:2782–7.

41   Meek AG (1998) Breast radiotherapy and lymphoedema. *Cancer*. **83**:2788–97.

42   Werngren-Elgström M and Lidman D (1994) Lymphoedema of the lower extremities after surgery and radiotherapy for cancer of the cervix. *Scandinavian Journal of Plastic Reconstructive and Hand Surgery*. **28**:289–93.

43   Stehman FB *et al.* (1992) Groin dissection versus groin radiation in carcinoma of the vulva: a gynaecologic oncology group study. *International Journal of Radiation, Oncology, Biology and Physics*. **24**:389–96.

44   Anonymous (1998) Lymphoedema following prostatectomy and radiation therapy. *Cancer Practice*. **6**:73–6.

45   Karakousis CP *et al.* (1983) Lymphoedema after groin dissection. *American Journal of Surgery*. **145**:205–8.

46 Papachristou D and Fortner JG (1997) Comparison of lymphoedema follow-ing incontinuity and discontinuity groin dissection. *Annals of Surgery.* **185**: 13–16.

47 Allen PJ *et al.* (1995) Lower extremity lymphoedema caused by acquired immune deficiency syndrome-related Kaposi's sarcoma: Case report and review of literature. *Journal of Vascular Surgery.* **22**:178–81.

48 Bisno AL and Stevens DL (1996) Streptococcal infections of skin and soft tissues. *New England Journal of Medicine.* **334**:240–5.

49 Stöberl C and Partsch H (1987) Erysipel und Lymphödem – Ei oder Henne? *Zeitschrift Für Hautkrankheiten.* **62**:56–62.

50 Duke BOL (1997) Filarial infections and diseases. *Medicine.* **25**:72–6.

51 Mulherin DM *et al.* (1993) Lymphoedema of the upper limb in patients with psoriatic arthritis. *Seminars in Arthritis and Rheumatism.* **22**:350–6.

52 Sant SM *et al.* (1995) Lymphatic obstruction in rheumatoid arthritis. *Clinical Rheumatology.* **14**:445–50.

53 Lynde CW and Mitchell JC (1982) Unusual complication of allergic contact dermatitis of the hands – recurrent lymphangitis and persistent lymphoedema. *Contact Dermatitis.* **8**:279–80.

54 Price EW (1987) Endemic elephantiasis as a paediatric problem in the tropics. *Annals of Tropical Paediatrics.* **7**:77–81.

55 Bull RH *et al.* (1993) Pretibial myxoedema: a manifestation of lymphoedema? *Lancet.* **341**:403–4.

56 Hanmoudeh M *et al.* (1994) Localised lymphoedema due to tenosynovitis. *British Journal of Rheumatology.* **33**:891–2.

57 Mahoney EM and Edwards EA (1962) Spontaneous regression of leg oedema and hydronephrosis following idiopathic retroperitoneal fibrosis. *American Journal of Surgery.* **103**:514–7.

58 Porter JM *et al.* (1972) Leg oedema following femoropopliteal autogenous vein bypass. *Archives of Surgery.* **105**:883–8.

4 Clinical features of lymphoedema

Vaughan Keeley

The focus in this chapter is limb oedema. Features specific to lymphoedema affecting the genitalia, for example, are dealt with elsewhere (*see* p.331). In both primary and secondary lymphoedema there may be associated truncal swelling.

Nature of oedema

Lymphoedema is often described as 'brawny' and non-pitting oedema. However, in its early stages, the swelling may often be soft and pit easily on digital pressure. At this stage some reduction of the oedema after elevation of the affected limb may also occur. However, as time goes by, the high-protein oedema is compounded by fibrosis within the subcutaneous tissues. The oedema then becomes firmer and does not pit so readily. Swelling which does not go down significantly after overnight elevation is likely to be due to lymph stasis.[1]

Using the International Society of Lymphology's grading classification (Box 4.A), Casley-Smith measured pretreatment volumes and grades of lymphoedema in 408 patients with unilateral lymphoedema and related them to the duration of swelling before treatment in an attempt to document changes in untreated lymphoedema over time.[2,3] He found that lymphoedema volume and grade increased with time. Primary lymphoedema progressed more slowly through the grades than secondary lymphoedema. Postmastectomy lymphoedema took about the same time to reach each grade as secondary leg oedema, whereas primary leg oedema took three times as long. In primary lymphoedema the volume increased more for each grade compared with secondary lymphoedema, suggesting that primary lymphoedema causes relatively less fibrosis.

Skin changes

The typical skin changes which develop in lymphoedema are important diagnostic features. Initially, however, the skin may be normal with only mild postural oedema and is of no diagnostic value. With time the skin texture changes, although the rate of change varies widely:

- the thickness of the skin increases

- there is a build-up of horny scale on the surface (hyperkeratosis)

Box 4.A   Clinical classification of lymphoedema (International Society of Lymphology)

Grade 1

No or minimal fibrosis, i.e. oedema pits on pressure and reduces with limb elevation.

Grade 2

Substantial fibrosis clinically, i.e. oedema does not pit and does not reduce with limb elevation.

Grade 3

Grade 2 plus elephantine (trophic) changes.

- skin creases deepen, e.g. around the ankle and the bases of the toes

- in time, worsening hyperkeratosis can produce a warty appearance to the skin

- it is difficult to pick up a skin fold between the fingers.

The inability to pick up a fold of skin at the base of the second toe (Stemmer's sign) is said to be diagnostic of lymphoedema (Plate 4.1).[4] Further progression leads to a picture of 'elephantiasis' with severe hyperkeratosis and papillomatosis, i.e. papules or nodules protruding from the skin surface (Figure 4.1). The latter are dilated skin lymphatics surrounded by rigid fibrous tissue; they leak lymph if damaged. The severe changes of elephantiasis in the foot can lead to the appearance known as 'mossy foot'. At this advanced stage there may be little oedema as such, the swelling being largely due to fibrosis and fatty tissue. In the later stages in particular, recurrent acute inflammatory episodes (AIE) also contribute to the clinical picture.[5] Other skin features include:

- lymphangiomas

- chylous reflux

- *lymphoedema ab igne.*

Lymphangiomas

Acquired cutaneous lymphangiomas can occur as a result of damage to deeper lymphatic vessels (Figure 4.2).[6] A lymphangioma consists of extremely dilated lymphatic vessels in the superficial dermis which bulge on the skin

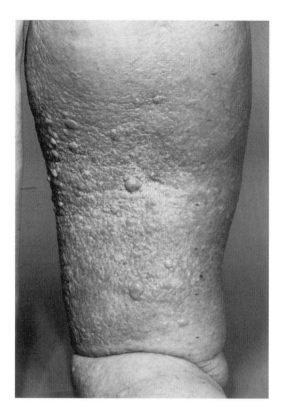

Figure 4.1 Skin changes including papillomatosis in chronic leg lymphoedema.

surface giving the appearance of a blister. It generally contains clear fluid but sometimes is blood-stained.[6] Lymphangiomas may burst causing localised wetness or even profuse leakage (lymphorrhoea). They therefore act as a significant portal for infection in the swollen limb. With tissue organisation they may gradually change to form firm skin nodules.

Radiotherapy for various cancers, for example of the breast and cervix uteri, may result in fibrosis and obstruction of the deep collecting lymphatics and so lead to lymphangiomas. They may develop with or without more widespread lymphoedema. They also occur after surgery alone, for example radical mastectomy.

When severe, multiple lymphangiomas give a clinical appearance which resembles frog spawn. If limited to an area of skin < 5cm across, it is often called *lymphangioma circumscriptum*.[7] The thin-walled vesicles generally contain clear fluid but sometimes it is blood-stained. They may occur at any age, particularly at birth or early childhood, and are often found in the

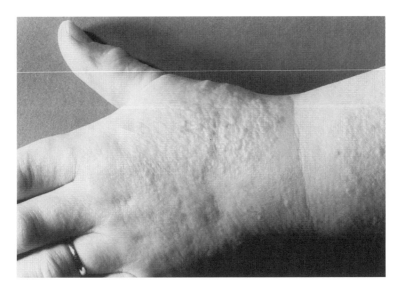

Figure 4.2   Acquired lymphangiomas (lymph blisters) in lymphoedema of the arm.

axillary folds, shoulders, neck, proximal limbs, perineum, tongue and buccal mucous membrane.[1]

The condition is probably caused by abnormal lymphatic cisterns deep to the dermis which do not connect to deeper lymphatics and therefore form a closed system with vessels running superficially towards the skin surface. These vessels dilate as fluid enters the superficial dermal plexus and is unable to pass out through the deeper system in the normal way. If the lesions are more widespread the term *lymphangioma diffusum* is used.

Chylous reflux

This most commonly occurs in the perineum and thigh. It comprises reflux of chyle (intestinal lymph) to the skin as a result of valvular incompetence in the main lymphatic trunks. Various skin lesions can occur:

- vesicles which rupture and form fistulae

- white vesicles which discharge when damaged

- solid and semisolid cream or yellow warty plaques.

Lymphoedema ab igne

A reticulate pattern of prominent compressible ridges of tissue situated predominantly on the upper part of the lower legs in 8 elderly immobile women with dependency oedema ('armchair legs') has been described recently.[8] The authors compared the site and clinical pattern of the abnormality with that of *erythema ab igne* but, on the basis of histological findings, suggested that the underlying abnormality was lymphatic rather than vascular. They coined the term *lymphoedema ab igne* to describe this.

Miscellaneous conditions

Several skin conditions occur more commonly in lymphoedema, including:

- xanthomatous deposits
- atypical pemphigoid
- toxic epidermal necrolysis
- atypical neutrophilic dermatosis (Sweet's syndrome).[1]

Pain

Lymphoedema may be associated with various pains and discomforts (*see* p.68).[9]

Physical disabilities

Impaired limb function and reduced mobility can be a major consequence of lymphoedema (*see* p.140).

Psychosocial consequences

Significant psychological morbidity is associated with lymphoedema. Issues of altered body image, disability and fear of cancer recurrence are all contributory (*see* p.89).[10]

Complications of lymphoedema

The complications arising in a lymphoedematous limb include:

- AIE
- lymphorrhoea

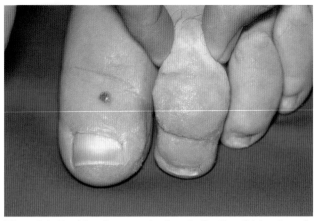

Plate 4.1 Positive Stemmer's sign, indicating thickening of the skin at the base of the second toe.

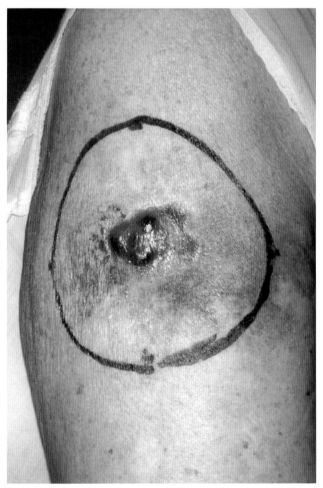

Plate 4.2 Lymphangiosarcoma.

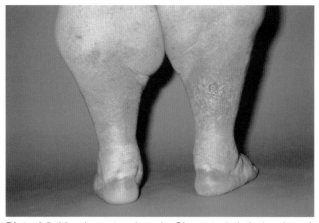

Plate 4.3 Lipodermatosclerosis. Characteristic indrawing of skin over gaiter area due to subcutaneous induration. Pitting oedema above and below lipodermatosclerotic region.

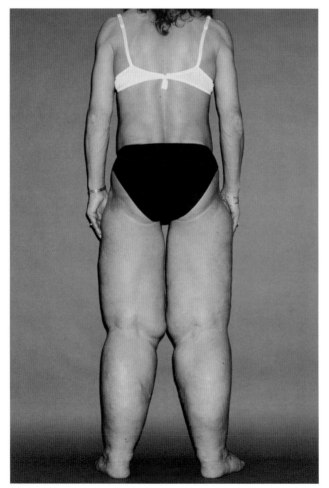

Plate 4.4 Lipoedema. Swelling of legs due to abnormal deposition of fat between ankle and hip.

- deep vein thrombosis (DVT)

- malignant disease.

The first and last of these are probably associated with altered local immune responses.

Altered local immune responses

The lymphatics are an important part of the immune response to allergens and are the pathway for the passage of immune complexes, T lymphocytes, Langerhans cells and macrophages to the regional lymph nodes. A study using dinitrochlorobenzene to test the afferent (sensitisation) and efferent (elicitation or recall) loops of the allergic contact response confirmed that there is a suppression of immune competence in postmastectomy arm lymph-oedema.[11] Sensitisation was particularly affected with a quarter of the swollen arms failing to sensitise compared with none of the controls. There also appeared to be an alteration in the elicitation response, although this was less conclusive. The exact mechanism of these changes is not clear but may be related to the disruption of lymph flow from the skin to regional lymph nodes which are intimately involved in the normal response.

Acute inflammatory episodes

AIE are common complications of lymphoedema, with an increased susceptibility to bacterial and fungal infections (*see* p.130).

Lymphorrhoea

Lymphorrhoea is the leakage of lymph through the skin. It may occur through lacerations and abrasions of the altered dry skin of chronic oedema or via rupture of lymphangiomas. Lymphorrhoea predisposes to the development of infection, the break in the skin acting as a portal for bacteria.

Deep vein thrombosis

Lymphoedema is a risk factor for developing a DVT in the affected limb. This may relate to several factors:

- immobility from the heavy oedematous limb

- reduced venous flow as part of a mixed lymphovenous oedema

- altered venous flow due to treatment for malignant disease, e.g. surgery and radiotherapy[12]

- active malignant disease, e.g. by extrinsic venous compression by tumour, perhaps exacerbated by increased coagulability of blood.

DVT can occur even when a patient is wearing a compression garment.

Malignancy

Although rare, new malignancies may occur in lymphoedematous limbs:

- lymphangiosarcoma

- Kaposi's sarcoma

- squamous cell cancer

- liposarcoma

- malignant melanoma

- malignant fibrous histiocytoma

- basal cell cancer

- lymphoma.

The relationship with lymphoedema has not been fully established for most of these, although it is certain for lymphangiosarcoma.

Lymphangiosarcoma

This is an uncommon malignant disease arising from lymphatic endothelial tissue (Plate 4.2). It occurs most frequently in a chronic lymphoedematous limb.[13] The term *Stewart-Treves syndrome* refers specifically to its occurrence in postmastectomy lymphoedema but it may occur in congenital,[14] post-traumatic,[15] dependency[16] or filarial lymphoedema.[17] The incidence of post-mastectomy lymphangiosarcoma of the arm is $< 0.45\%$.[18] The mean time of onset in postmastectomy lymphoedema is about 10 years; in other types of lymphoedema it is about 20 years. Clinical features are:

- single or multiple bluish/red nodules in the skin or subcutaneous tissues

- rapid spread in concentric, distal or proximal directions, forming satellite lesions which may become confluent and ulcerate.

The diagnosis is made by skin biopsy. The prognosis is poor with a median survival of < 3 years. Prognosis is worse in postmastectomy lymphoedema. Spread tends to be rapid both locally and with early pulmonary metastases. In the absence of distant spread, amputation offers the best chance of cure. Radiotherapy and chemotherapy are generally not very effective. There is debate about the exact cell type of origin, whether blood capillary or lymphatic. Some authors suggest the term angiosarcoma is preferable.[15]

Kaposi's sarcoma

Kaposi's sarcoma has been described in chronic oedematous limbs and there is some evidence of a localised immunological deficiency associated with this.[19]

Squamous cell cancer

There have been several reports of squamous cell cancer arising in lymph-oedematous limbs.[20] Although it may occur because of altered immune responses, reports are few and it is possible that there is not a causal relationship.

Liposarcoma

Wyatt et al.[21] described a liposarcoma in a patient with lipodystrophy and primary lymphoedema of the lower limbs. However, liposarcoma is the second most common soft tissue tumour in adults and a causal relationship with lymphoedema has not been established.

Malignant melanoma

Cases of malignant melanoma in lymphoedematous arms 10 years after mastectomy have been described.[22] Malignant melanoma has also been described as a second primary cancer in patients already suffering from breast cancer, not necessarily associated with lymphoedema.

Malignant fibrous histiocytoma

A metastasising malignant fibrous histiocytoma originating in the lower limb of a patient with primary lymphoedema has been described.[23]

Differential diagnosis

There are many causes of oedema which form the differential diagnosis of a swollen limb. Some may reflect a more systemic pathology, for example cardiac failure, whereas others may be very localised, for example angioedema. A useful classification based upon the type of disturbance of the lymphatic system is:[24]

- low output failure (= lymphoedema) where the lymphatic transport is reduced

- high output failure where a normal or increased transport capacity of intact lymphatics is overwhelmed by an excessive burden of capillary filtrate; may be local (e.g. post-thrombotic syndrome) or general (e.g. cardiac failure).

As discussed above, where there is longstanding high output failure, there may be a gradual deterioration of lymphatic function resulting in a combination of high and low output failure, for example recurrent infections, burns and repeated allergic reactions.

The diagnosis of lymphoedema is generally made on the basis of the medical history and clinical examination, particularly of the skin and subcutaneous tissues, taking into account the features described above. Lymphoedema is usually localised but may be exacerbated by concurrent factors which tend to be more generalised such as fluid-retaining drugs (e.g. NSAIDs and corticosteroids) or cyclic idiopathic oedema in women. These should be considered in the initial diagnostic evaluation. The enlargement of the limb may not be due to oedema but caused by, for example, lipoedema or limb hypertrophy (Box 4.B). Early lymphoedema may pose some diagnostic difficulty when there is only minimal swelling.

Box 4.B   Causes of localised swelling and/or enlargement

Lipoedema.

Tumours:
- neurofibromas
- lipomas
- lymphangiomas
- haemangiomas.

Popliteal cysts.

Limb hypertrophy:
- arteriovenous anastomoses
- hemihypertrophy
- Proteus syndrome.

Proteus syndrome consists of congenital lipomas, occasionally with elements of lymphangioma and haemangioma. These are found predominantly subcutaneously on the cranium and intracranially. There may be associated central nervous system malformations, for example mega-encephaly, and partial gigantism with hypertrophy of soft and bony tissues of the feet and hands.

Diagnosis of lymphoedema after breast cancer treatment

The patient's awareness of symptoms and physical changes should be evaluated because these may precede any objective evidence of lymphoedema.[25] These may include a sensation of fullness, tightness or heaviness of the arm, shoulder or chest and altered mobility of the shoulder. An early diagnosis enables health professionals to provide appropriate advice and information about care of the arm. Clinical features include:

- detectable swelling or enlargement of arm or trunk with or without pitting
- an increase in the thickness of skin folds, in the axilla or arm
- change in texture of the skin
- asymmetric increase in the adiposity of subcutaneous tissues.

Other causes of these symptoms and signs need to be considered and appropriate investigations carried out (see p.58):

- DVT
- recurrence of breast cancer.

The development of symptoms in, say, the first 3 months after treatment, may represent transient changes which resolve as healing occurs. It is not clear if these changes will predispose to the subsequent development of lymphoedema.[25]

With recurrence of breast cancer, the axillary nodes may enlarge and exacerbate the lymphoedema. Recurrent disease may also involve the brachial plexus, giving rise to neuropathic pain, altered sensation and weakness of the arm. The development of metastatic skin nodules in the chest wall (cancer en cuirass) or upper arm causes further reduction in lymphatic drainage and can result in severe lymphoedema which is difficult to manage. Evidence of cancer recurrence should be sought in patients with worsening oedema, pain and neurological symptoms. Treatment specifically aimed at the cancer, for example chemotherapy or hormone therapy, may improve the lymphoedema in these situations.

Chronic venous disease

Chronic venous disease may be classified as:

- congenital – present since birth

- primary – of undetermined cause

- secondary – associated with known cause (e.g. post-thrombotic, post-traumatic).[26]

Oedema can be a significant feature of this condition. Other aspects may include venous dilation, skin changes and ulceration (Box 4.C). The venous and lymphatic systems are inextricably linked and the chronic failure of the former will ultimately lead to failure of the latter.

Box 4.C   Clinical features of chronic venous disease[26]

Venous dilation:

- submalleolar venous flare
- telangiectasia ⎱
- reticular veins ⎬ more severe disease.
- varicose veins ⎰

Oedema in more advanced disease.

Skin changes:

- pigmentation
- venous eczema
- lipodermatosclerosis.

Ulceration.

Chronic lipodermatosclerosis consists of thickening and induration of the skin and subcutaneous tissue of the lower leg associated with chronic venous insufficiency resulting in the 'inverted champagne bottle' appearance; the skin is brown, shiny and fixed to hard subcutaneous tissue (Plate 4.3).

Bollinger *et al.*[27] using fluorescence microlymphography, found that in severe chronic venous incompetence leading to trophic changes in the skin, there was evidence of lymphatic micro-angiopathy in the medial aspect of the ankle. This took the form of obliteration of parts of the superficial lymphatic capillary network, cutaneous reflux and increased permeability of capillary fragments. They suggested that trophic changes in this situation are of mixed venous and lymphatic origin.

In a study using quantitative lymphoscintigraphy, Bull et al.[28] found that lymphatic drainage was significantly lower in the legs of patients with chronic venous hypertension than in the control patients, whether or not the leg was ulcerated. Lymphatic function was also reduced in patients with superficial varicosities and deep venous incompetence before any trophic skin change had developed.

Conversely, in true lymphoedema, it has been suggested that the excess tissue fluid gradually impedes venous return which in turn aggravates the underlying lymphoedema.[29] This proposal was based on measurements of venous dynamics by air plethysmography (ambulatory venous pressure, venous volume, venous filling index and ejection fraction). Thus, it seems that abnormalities of lymphatic and venous function are often inextricably linked.

Post-thrombotic syndrome

Post-thrombotic syndrome can follow DVT of the leg. DVT may destroy valves in the veins leading to incompetence and flow of blood from the deep venous system to the superficial via the perforating veins, particularly on muscular activity or standing. This together with any residual chronic occlusion from the thrombus itself results in increased venous and capillary pressure. This causes oedema and rupture of small superficial veins in the vicinity of the perforating veins, for example in the region of the medial malleolus. This subcutaneous haemorrhage can lead to the deposition of haemosiderin (stasis pigmentation), subcutaneous fibrosis and cutaneous atrophy (lipodermato-sclerosis) and stasis ulceration. Patients report dull diffuse pain provoked by dependency and generally relieved by elevation.

Prandoni et al.[30] found the cumulative incidence of post-thrombotic syndrome to be 23% after 2 years, 28% after 5 years and 29% after 8 years. Severe post-thrombotic manifestations were present in < 10% after 8 years. The incidence is lower than in other studies, possibly because patients were instructed to wear graduated compression stockings (providing 40mmHg of pressure at the ankle) for at least 2 years. This has been shown to halve the incidence of post-thrombotic syndrome.[31] The risk of developing post-thrombotic syndrome was significantly higher if there had been recurrence of the DVT in the affected limb. Interestingly, there was no significant association between the occurrence of post-thrombotic syndrome and the extent of the thrombosis.

Chronic leg oedema associated with immobility

This is also known as *armchair legs* or *lymphostasis verrucosis* (Figure 4.3).[1] It is a common condition in immobile patients who spend most of the day

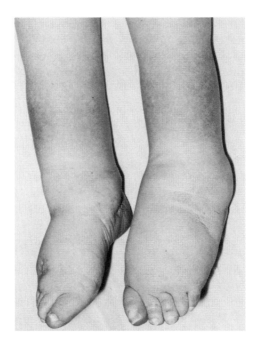

Figure 4.3 'Armchair legs'.

(and sometimes night) sitting in a chair. The immobility may be caused by various conditions, including chronic arthritis, chronic respiratory conditions, neurological disabilities (e.g. post-stroke) and psychiatric disorders. The immobility and dependency of the legs in this type of lifestyle cause a reduction in both lymphatic and venous flow because both depend upon muscular activity for efficient function (*see* p.140). The clinical features are those of lymphoedema. It may occur unilaterally in a paralysed limb.

Lipoedema

This condition is also known as a *lipodystrophy, painful fat syndrome, massive obesity of the lower legs* and *adipositas spongiosa* (Plate 4.4).[32] *Erythrocyanosis frigida* (cold reddish-blueness of the legs of girls and chillblains) is sometimes misnamed lipoedema because it is commonly associated with an abnormally large amount of fat above the ankles.

The term was originally coined in 1940 and a detailed account was reported in the 1950s.[33] It occurs almost exclusively in women and consists of bilateral and symmetrical enlargement of the legs and lower half of the body due to an abnormal deposition of fat. Generalised obesity is present in up to 80% of patients.[32,34] Characteristically the feet are not involved, thereby producing an 'inverse shouldering' effect at the malleoli. There may be no pitting oedema or mild oedema may develop with time. There may be associated pain in the lower leg, tenderness over the shin and a tendency to bruise easily. An unusual tingling or burning discomfort in the plantar surface of the foot has been described.[35] Lipoedema does not respond to elevation or weight loss. Although dieting may lead to a reduction in fat elsewhere in the body, it does not have a major effect on the abnormally fatty limbs.

Other features include a family history in about 50% of cases,[33,34] superficial varicose veins in about 60%[32,34] and a tendency to develop genu valgum, talipes planus and osteo-arthrosis of the knees.[34] Psychological morbidity can be severe, particularly in younger women, mainly because of the altered body image.

Studies of venous function have shown variable results. One investigation found only minor changes in 2 out of 10 patients using photoplesthysmography.[32] Isotope and contrast studies in 39 patients showed that about 30% of patients had incompetent venous valves due to post-thrombotic changes and > 50% had varicose veins, which may be hidden by the subcutaneous fat when evaluated clinically.[34] Venous disease mainly affects the lower leg and may explain the heaviness and discomfort felt.

Disturbed lymphatic function has also been reported in > 50% of 35 patients examined by isotope lymphoscintigraphy. Contrast lymphography in 25 patients revealed 'dermal backflow' and reduced numbers of lymphatics in about 30%, whereas in 50% there were changes in inguinal and pelvic nodes consistent with an inflammatory reaction and early fibrosis. Some of the patients had had varicose vein surgery before lymphangiography which may well have damaged the lymphatics and resulted in a disproportionately high incidence of abnormal lymphatic function.[34] A study of 10 patients with quantitative lymphoscintigraphy, however, showed only a 'sluggish lymphatic system'.[32]

In lipoedema, oedema may occur due to overloading of the functional capacity of an otherwise normal lymphatic system (high output failure).[32] It has been proposed that the reduced interstitial resistance of the surrounding fatty tissue results in a raised capillary filtration rate and that a reduction in the transmission of intermittent 'massaging' pressures through the fatty tissue leads to inefficient lymph drainage.

The underlying cause of lipoedema is not known but histological studies of skin and subcutaneous tissue showed minimal perivascular fibrotic change in the subcutaneous tissue, no dermal thickening and no histological abnormality of the excessive subcutaneous tissue.[35] A comparison of the clinical features of lymphoedema and lipoedema is given in Table 4.1.

Table 4.1   Comparison of the clinical features of lymphoedema and lipoedema[32–34]

Clinical features	Lymphoedema	Lipoedema
Gender	Male and female	Female[a]
Age of onset	Any age	60–70% around puberty
Family history	20%	16–50%
Obesity	Variable	40–85%
Distribution	Distal leg initially	Entire leg
Symmetry	Often asymmetrical	Always bilateral
Involvement of feet	Generally	Never
Skin consistency	Thicker/firmer	Normal
Pitting	Some in early stages	Minimal[b]
Easy bruising	–	40%
Pain/discomfort	Infrequent	30–40% (particularly legs)
Tenderness	Infrequent	50%
Stemmer's sign	Generally positive	Negative in 100%
Varicosities	Variable	20–60%[c]
Pattern of elevation	Reduction in early stages	No effect in 70%
Weight loss	Both from trunk and legs	No loss from legs in 90%
History of AIE	Common	Absent

a   one male described[33]
b   pretibial oedema in 60% in one study but many patients had had varicose vein surgery[34]
c   one study suggested that some varicose veins were hidden by fatty tissue.[34]

Investigation of lymphoedema

The diagnosis of lymphoedema is generally made on the basis of the medical history and clinical examination. However, in the early stages of limb swelling, particularly if there is no clear cause, investigations may be appropriate. The aims of the investigations are:

- confirmation of diagnosis

- detection of the site of lymphatic malfunction
- detection of lymphatic malignant disease
- detection of venous abnormalities, including DVT
- pre-operative planning if surgery is an option.

Several techniques may be employed such as:

- direct lymphangiography
- indirect lymphography
- lymphoscintigraphy
- CT
- MRI
- ultrasound
- fluorescence lymphangiography.

Direct lymphangiography

Direct lymphangiography and lymphography show the lymphatic vessels and nodes respectively. It involves the injection of a contrast medium into a peripheral lymphatic vessel and subsequent radiographic visualisation of the vessels and nodes. It remains the 'gold standard' for showing structural abnormalities of larger lymph vessels[36] but can be technically difficult and may cause further damage to the lymphatics.[3] It has largely become obsolete as a routine method of investigation. It may, however, still have a place in the investigation of complicated lymphoedemas such as those associated with chylous reflux.[3]

Indirect lymphography

This involves the injection of a water-soluble non-ionic radiographic contrast medium intradermally, i.e. *not* directly into a lymph vessel.[37] Dermal and subcutaneous collecting lymphatics within 10–30cm of the site of the injection can be shown by radiographic imaging. Characteristic patterns are produced depending upon the underlying abnormality, for example lymphatic capillaries can be shown in conditions where there are incompetent valves in larger lymphatics and dermal backflow. The technique is not useful for examining larger lymph vessels and nodes. It has played a role in developing the understanding of the physical abnormalities underlying lymphoedema[37] but has little role in the routine investigation of the swollen limb.

Lymphoscintigraphy

This technique, also called *isotope lymphangiography/lymphangioscintigraphy*, has largely replaced direct radiographic lymphography as the main diagnostic tool for the investigation of lymphoedema and the visualisation of peripheral lymphatics (Figure 4.4).[24] It is based on the principle that one of the essential functions of the lymphatic system is the transport of large molecules from the interstitial space back to the vascular compartment. The injection of a radioactive-labelled (e.g. ^{99}Tc^m) protein or colloid into the tissue, followed by its detection in the initial lymphatics, large collectors and regional lymph nodes using an external gamma camera provides a measure of lymphatic function rather than anatomical detail.[37]

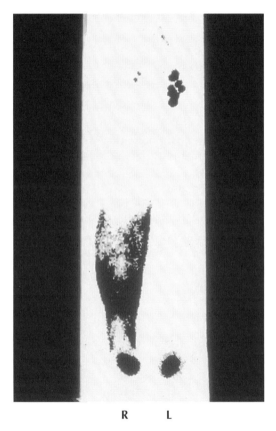

R   L

Figure 4.4 Lymphoscintigraphy. Subcutaneous injection of radio-labelled colloid in the web-space of each foot. Normal drainage to the ilio-inguinal lymph nodes in the left leg. Very little uptake in the right ilio-inguinal lymph nodes and extensive dermal backflow in the right calf.

Qualitative lymphoscintigraphy provides static images following the injection of a radioactive tracer. These can show:

- lymph vessels and nodes
- dilation of lymphatic vessels
- existence of collateral vessels
- presence of dermal backflow.

With this method, the diagnosis of lymphoedema can be established in 70% of cases.[38] However, quantitative measures based upon the clearance of the tracer from the distal limb to the regional nodes can detect abnormal lymphatic function in all cases where present.[38]

Qualitative lymphoscintigraphy can also be used to select patients for micro-surgical procedures such as lymphovenous anastomosis and to confirm patency of vessels following such procedures.[39] Lymphoscintigraphic techniques are not standardised among different centres.[1] Variables include:

- different tracers
- different injected volumes and radioactivity
- intracutaneous *v* subcutaneous injection
- SC *v* IM injection
- one or more injections
- at rest or under different protocols of physical activity
- varied imaging times.

These variables make comparison difficult. Lymph transport is significantly affected by muscular activity and, therefore, a standardised protocol for physical exercise is essential for the provision of a quantitative measure of this, and the definition of normal and abnormal results. For example, for the routine evaluation of subcutaneous lymph transport, a standard technique of a subcutaneous injection of tracer with subsequent measurement of lymph node uptake following an exercise regimen of 15 minutes walking on a horizontal treadmill at a speed of 3.2km/h, is recommended.[37]

Nonetheless, the method can provide valuable images of the lymphatics and lymph nodes (qualitative) as well as data on lymph transport (quantitative). It is able to confirm or rule out the diagnosis of lymphoedema and can often show preclinical defects of lymph drainage.[37] It has also contributed to our understanding of various conditions by, for example, showing abnormalities of lymphatic function in patients with chronic venous leg ulcers.[28]

Recent developments of the technique include two-compartment lympho-scintigraphy, which has been reported to be valuable in the evaluation of leg oedema.[40] In this technique the subcutaneous and muscle compartments are examined separately by SC and IM injections of the tracer respectively. It has been shown that in post-thrombotic syndrome, for example, muscle lymph transport is markedly reduced whereas subcutaneous lymph transport is increased. This method can thus contribute to the understanding of the patho-genesis of oedema and may help in establishing the diagnosis when this is uncertain.

Computed tomography

CT of a lymphoedematous limb reveals a coarse, non-enhancing, reticular pattern in an enlarged subcutaneous compartment (Figure 4.5).[41] The use of a single axial CT slice through the mid-calf has been advocated as a useful tool in the differential diagnosis of a swollen leg.[42] The following findings are reported:

- increased cross-sectional area of the muscle compartment in venous obstruction

- subcutaneous fat layer increased in obesity and lipoedema

- prominent interstitial spaces with a honeycomb pattern due to fibrosis in chronic lymphoedema

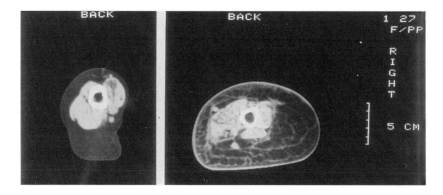

Figure 4.5   CT section of both upper arms of a patient with unilateral post-mastectomy oedema.

- fluid collections between muscle planes in popliteal cyst extensions

- intramuscular areas of high attenuation in haematomas of the calf muscles.

CT has also been used to monitor the therapeutic response to compression therapy in lymphoedema, by measuring changes in cross-sectional area.[43] Compression significantly reduced the cross-sectional area of the sub-cutaneous compartment. CT of appropriate areas of the body may be valuable in confirming or excluding malignant disease as the cause of secondary lymphoedema.

Magnetic resonance imaging

MRI can demonstrate a number of characteristic features in lymphoedema:

- in the subcutis – diffuse oedema or a honeycomb or reticular pattern and 'lakes of fluid' surrounded by fibrotic tissue

- in patients with lymphatic hyperplasia – dilated lymphatic trunks parallel to the long axis of the limb

- in chylous reflux syndromes – dilated lymphatic collectors

- central (retroperitoneal) lymphatics – lumbar lymphangiectasia.[44]

Some of these features may not be easily shown by lymphoscintigraphy, for example retroperitoneal lymphatics. In addition, MRI is valuable in the diagnosis of peripheral cavernous lymphangiomatosis which may be mistaken for congenital lymphoedema. The MRI features of this condition are prominent lattice-like signals in the fatty tissue with notable thickness of the subcutis. In patients with venous oedema, MRI shows increased fluid within muscle and subcutaneous fat,[45] whereas in lipoedema there is a diffuse homogeneous increase in the subcutaneous fat and skin thickness with a normal diameter of muscle mass.[46]

Ultrasound

The use of ultrasound scanning (with a 7.5MHz transducer) in the investigation of lower limb lymphoedema and lipoedema has been reported.[46] In lymphoedema there was:

- increased skin thickness

- increased subcutaneous tissue thickness

- absence of echogenic band beneath the subcutaneous tissue
- a 'stone-paved' pattern.

In lipoedema there was:

- normal skin thickness
- increased subcutaneous tissue thickness.

This method can also detect other abnormalities in swollen limbs such as a popliteal cyst.[47]

High-frequency ultrasound (with a 20MHz transducer) is at present a research tool which has been used to study cutaneous water content. It has helped in the understanding of the pathogenesis of oedemas. For example, it has shown that fluid is localised in different parts of the dermis in different oedemas:

- subepidermal in lipodermatosclerosis
- deep dermal in heart failure
- uniformly in lymphoedema.[48]

In the future there may be practical applications for this technique, for example in the monitoring of the results of treatment.

Colour Doppler ultrasound

Colour Doppler ultrasound and real time imaging is used to evaluate accurately venous abnormalities of the limb including DVT, venous incompetence, perforating veins and reflux. It has a role therefore, in the evaluation of the swollen limb.[49] The introduction of this technique has reduced the need for venography.

Fluorescence lymphangiography

This technique involves the subepidermal injection of a fluorescent material (generally FITC-dextran) and subsequent visualisation by videomicroscopy of the superficial dermal network of lymphatic capillaries by which the dye is taken up. So for it has been a useful research tool which shows abnormalities in these vessels in various conditions, for example in chronic venous insufficiency in areas of trophic skin changes.[50] At present, however, this technique does not have a role in the routine diagnosis of lymphoedema.

Who to investigate?

In some, multiple causal factors may be responsible for the limb swelling. The combined use of qualitative lymphoscintigraphy and colour Doppler ultrasound has been proposed for the evaluation of patients with unexplained leg oedema.[49] With this approach it was possible to establish the cause of the oedema in > 80% of the patients. Only 16% of the patients had abnormalities on both lymphoscintigraphy and Doppler ultrasound; in one case this was due to obstruction of both veins and lymphatics by a pelvic mass. The authors suggest that, if this is not diagnostic, then CT or MRI may be helpful.

References

1 Harwood CA and Mortimer PS (1995) Causes and clinical manifestations of lymphatic failure. *Clinics in Dermatology.* **13**:459–71.

2 Casley-Smith JR (1995) Alterations of untreated lymphoedema and its grades over time. *Lymphology.* **28**:174–85.

3 Casley-Smith JR *et al.* (1985) Summary of the 10th International Congress of Lymphology Working Group Discussions and Recommendations. *Lymphology.* **18**:175–80.

4 Stemmer R (1976) Ein klinisches Zeichen zur Früh-und Differential-diagnose des Lymphödems. VASA – *Journal for Vascular Diseases.* **5**:261–2.

5 Ryan TJ and DeBerker D (1995) The interstitium, the connective tissue environment of the lymphatics and angiogenesis in human skin. *Clinics in Dermatology.* **13**:451–8.

6 Mallett RB *et al.* (1992) Acquired lymphangioma: report of four cases and a discussion of the pathogenesis. *British Journal of Dermatology.* **126**:380–2.

7 Leshin B *et al.* (1986) Lymphangioma circumscriptum following mastectomy and radiation therapy. *Journal of American Academy of Dermatology.* **15**:1117–9.

8 Cox NH *et al.* (1996) A reticulate vascular abnormality in patients with lymphoedema: observations in eight patients. *British Journal of Dermatology.* **135**:92–7.

9 Badger CMA *et al.* (1998) Pain in the chronically swollen limb. *Progress in Lymphology.* **11**:243–6.

10 Tobin MB *et al.* (1993) The psychological morbidity of breast cancer related arm swelling. *Cancer.* **72**:3248–52.

11 Mallon E *et al.* (1997) Evidence for altered cell-mediated immunity in post-mastectomy lymphoedema. *British Journal of Dermatology.* **137**:928–33.

12 Svensson WE *et al.* (1994) Colour Doppler demonstrates venous flow abnormalities in breast cancer patients with chronic arm swelling. *European Journal of Cancer.* **30A**:657–60.

13 Mulvenna PM *et al.* (1995) Lymphangiosarcomata – experience in a lymphoedema clinic. *Palliative Medicine.* **9**:55–9.

14 Offori TW *et al.* (1993) Sarcoma in congenital hereditary lymphoedema (Milroy's disease) – diagnostic beacons and a review of the literature. *Clinical and Experimental Dermatology.* **18**:174–7.

15 Trattner A et al. (1996) Stewart-Treves angiosarcoma of arm and ipsilateral breast in post-traumatic lymphoedema. *Lymphology.* **29**:57–9.

16 Sinclair SA et al. (1998) Angiosarcoma arising in a chronically lymphoedematous leg. *British Journal of Dermatology.* **138**:692–4.

17 Muller R et al. (1987) Lymphangiosarcoma associated with chronic filarial lymphoedema. *Cancer.* **59**:179–83.

18 Janse AJ et al. (1995) Lymphoedema-induced lymphangiosarcoma. *European Journal of Surgical Oncology.* **21**:155–8.

19 Ruocco V et al. (1984) Kaposi's sarcoma on a lymphoedematous immuno-compromised limb. *International Journal of Dermatology.* **23**:56–60.

20 Lister RK et al. (1997) Squamous cell carcinoma arising in chronic lymphoedema. *British Journal of Dermatology.* **136**:384–7.

21 Wyatt LE et al. (1996) Well-differentiated liposarcoma (atypical lipoma) of the lower extremity in a patient with bilateral leg lipodystrophy and lymphoedema. *Plastic and Reconstructive Surgery.* **98**:1076–9.

22 Bartal AH and Pinsky CM (1985) Malignant melanoma appearing in a post-mastectomy lymphoedematous arm: a novel association of double primary tumours. *Journal of Surgical Oncology.* **30**:16–8.

23 Fergusson CM et al. (1985) Unusual sarcoma arising lymphoedema. *Journal of the Royal Society of Medicine.* **78**:497–8.

24 Consensus Document of the International Society of Lymphology Executive Committee (1995) The diagnosis and treatment of peripheral lymphoedema. *Lymphology.* **28**:113–7.

25 Rockson SG et al. (1998) Diagnosis and management of lymphoedema. *Cancer.* **83**:2882–5.

26 Porter JM et al. (1995) Reporting standards in venous disease: an update. *Journal of Vascular Surgery.* **21**:635–45.

27 Bollinger A et al. (1982) Lymphatic microangiopathy: a complication of severe chronic venous incompetence (CVI). *Lymphology.* **15**:60–5.

28 Bull RH et al. (1993) Abnormal lymph drainage in patients with chronic venous leg ulcers. *Journal of American Academy of Dermatology.* **28**:585–90.

29 Kim DI et al. (1999) Venous dynamics in leg lymphoedema. *Lymphology.* **32**:11–14.

30 Prandoni P et al. (1996) The long-term clinical course of acute deep vein thrombosis. *Annals of Internal Medicine.* **125**:1–7.

31 Brandjes DPM et al. (1997) Randomised trial of effect of compression stockings in patients with symptomatic proximal-vein thrombosis. *Lancet.* **349**: 759–62.

32 Harwood CA et al. (1996) Lymphatic and venous function in lipoedema. *British Journal of Dermatology.* **134**:1–6.

33 Wold LE et al. (1951) Lipoedema of the legs: a syndrome characterised by fat legs and oedema. *Annals of Internal Medicine.* **34**:1243–50.

34 Ketterings C (1998) Lipodystrophy and its treatment. *Annals of Plastic Surgery.* **21**:536–43.

35 Rudkin GH and Miller TA (1994) Lipoedema: a clinical entity distinct from lymphoedema. *Plastic and Reconstructive Surgery.* **94**:841–7.

36 Mortimer PS (1990) Investigation and management of lymphoedema. *Vascular Medicine Review.* **1**:1–20.

37 Partsch H (1995) Assessment of abnormal lymph drainage for the diagnosis of lymphoedema by isotopic lymphangiography and by indirect lymphography. *Clinics in Dermatology.* **13**:445–50.

38 Weissleder H and Weissleder R (1988) Lymphoedema: evaluation of qualitative and quantitative lymphoscintigraphy in 238 patients. *Radiology.* **167**:729–35.

39 Vaqueiro M *et al.* (1986) Lymphoscintigraphy in lymphoedema: an aid to microsurgery. *Journal of Nuclear Medicine.* **27**:1125–30.

40 Bräutigam P *et al.* (1998) Analysis of lymphatic drainage in various forms of leg oedema using two compartment lymphoscintigraphy. *Lymphology.* **31**:43–55.

41 Gamba JL *et al.* (1983) Primary lower extremity lymphoedema: CT diagnosis. *Radiology.* **149**:218.

42 Vaughan BF (1990) CT of swollen legs. *Clinical Radiology.* **41**:24–30.

43 Collins CD *et al.* (1995) Computed tomography in the assessment of response to limb compression in unilateral lymphoedema. *Clinical Radiology.* **50**:541–4.

44 Liu N-F and Wang C-G (1998) The role of magnetic resonance imaging in diagnosis of peripheral lymphatic disorders. *Lymphology.* **31**:119–27.

45 Duewell S *et al.* (1992) Swollen lower extremity: role of MR Imaging. *Radiology.* **184**:227–31.

46 Dimakakos PB *et al.* (1997) MRI and ultrasonographic findings in the investigation of lymphoedema and lipoedema. *International Surgery.* **82**:411–6.

47 Swett HA *et al.* (1975) Popliteal cysts: presentation as thrombophlebitis. *Radiology.* **115**:613–5.

48 Gniadecka M (1996) Localisation of dermal oedema in lipodermatosclerosis, lymphoedema and cardiac insufficiency. *Journal of the American Academy of Dermatology.* **35**:37–41.

49 Wheatley DC *et al.* (1996) Lymphoscintigraphy and colour Doppler sonography in the assessment of leg oedema of unknown cause. *British Journal of Radiology.* **69**:1117–24.

50 Jäger K *et al.* (1983) Fluorescence microlymphography in patients with lymphoedema and chronic venous incompetence. *International Angiology.* **2**:129–36.

5 Pain in lymphoedema

Robert Twycross

The reported incidence of pain in lymphoedema varies from 9–63%.[1–8] At a specialist lymphoedema clinic, the incidence when first seen was 57% (Table 5.1).

Table 5.1   Incidence of tightness and pain in 100 lymphoedema patients[6]

Group	Number of patients	Tightness (%)	Pain (%)
Overall	100	32	57
Non-cancer	22	23	64
Active cancer	46	43[a]	67[a]
Inactive cancer	32	21	37

a   compared with patients with inactive cancer, the incidence of tightness and pain were significantly greater in those with active cancer, $p < 0.05$ and $p < 0.01$, comparison of two proportions.[9]

Characteristics of pain in lymphoedema

In a study of 22 women with postmastectomy lymphoedema, the 10 most common descriptive words chosen from the McGill Pain Questionnaire were *tight, tiring, throbbing, heavy, nagging, aching, shooting, tingling, hot and annoying*.[10] Although the causes of the pain were not given, the following characteristics of pain associated with lymphoedema were listed:

- the affected arm feels heavy, tight and aches

- swelling and pain worsen as the day progresses and during hot weather

- use of the affected limb commonly exacerbates pain

- analgesic drugs are not always effective but resting the arm in a supported position generally gives relief

- patients have difficulty sleeping if a comfortable position cannot be found and maintained.

Analgesics were used by only half the women and most were taken 'as needed', not regularly round-the-clock. Only nonopioids were used – but no details about drugs, doses and timing were given. Even so, 2 women obtained complete relief, 1 good relief and 3 moderate relief with their analgesics (6/11), whereas the other 5 obtained only slight relief. Thus, the limited data available indicate that half the patients were helped considerably by nonopioid drugs.

After 3 months of conservative lymphoedema management, the swelling in the affected arms had decreased almost by half and pain was much reduced (Table 5.2). This supports the oft-repeated statement that the best treatment for lymphoedema-related pain is to reduce the swelling. In another study, skin care was associated with reduced pain,[11] possibly the result of fewer acute inflammatory episodes (AIE).

Table 5.2   Average pain intensity in women with postmastectomy lymphoedema[10]

	Initial evaluation	After 3 months[a]
None	–	12
Mild	7	7
Moderate	12	3
Severe	3	–
Total	22	22

a   a significant reduction in pain was recorded at the 3-month evaluation (none + mild *v* moderate + severe), Chi-squared test = 4.46 (p < 0.5).

In patients with breast cancer and *en cuirass* disease extending onto the upper arm, the likelihood of reducing the swelling is remote. The arm may well become even more swollen and more painful, and use may become even more limited because of an associated progressive brachial plexopathy. The pain of nerve damage is typically neurodermatomal in distribution and superficial and burning in character with associated allodynia (i.e. light touch and other non-noxious stimuli cause pain). There may also be spontaneous stabbing pain, i.e. unrelated to movement. A different strategy is often necessary to manage the pain in these circumstances (*see* p.85).

Neuropathic pain, however, is not always an indication of recurrence/ progressive disease.[6,8] One woman with severe lymphoedema developed diffuse brachial plexopathy manifesting with persistent pain, sensory changes and weakness.[8] CT showed entrapment of the brachial plexus in the

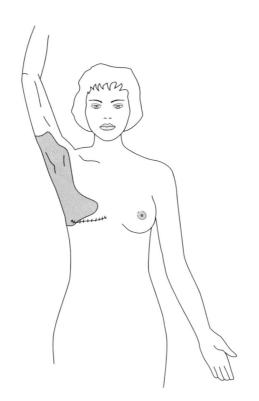

Figure 5.1   The intercostobrachial nerve can be injured during breast surgery. The nerve has a variable distribution to the skin of the axilla and anterolateral chest wall (shaded area).

supraclavicular area. Because of her general good physical health, a diagnosis of plexus entrapment secondary to lymphoedema and scar tissue was made.

Some patients with breast cancer and lymphoedema may have concurrent postmastectomy intercostal neuralgia. The pain in this condition is superficial and burning in character, with associated numbness (Figure 5.1). The area affected is the inner aspect of the upper arm and a band around the adjacent chest wall at the level of the axilla. There may also be intermittent stabbing pains, which occasionally are the dominant feature. Postmastectomy inter-costal neuralgia accounts for up to 20% of cases of arm pain in breast cancer (Table 5.3).

Occasionally a patient presents with pain maintained by excessive regional sympathetic neural activity. The essential features are:

• pain (often burning)

Table 5.3 Causes of ipsilateral arm pain in 38 patients with breast cancer[8]

Cause	Number of patients	
Lesions of the brachial plexus	17	
tumour infiltration		8
radiation-induced fibrosis		5
fibrous entrapment/lymphoedema		1
transient neuritis		3
Cervical radiculopathy	4	
vertebral metastasis		
Carpal tunnel syndrome	4	
with lymphoedema		2
without lymphoedema		2
Postsurgical pain	8	
postmastectomy neuralgia		7
postsurgical neuroma		1
Adhesive capsulitis of shoulder	5	

- a sensory disorder

- a poor response to nonopioids and opioids; and often also to adjuvant analgesics

- relief after a regional sympathetic nerve block.

Differentiation between nerve injury burning pain and sympathetically-maintained burning pain may be difficult because clinical features overlap. Sympathetic nerves travel with the arterial system, however, and the distribution of sympathetically-maintained pain is vasotopographic rather than neurodermatomal – but this may not be clinically obvious. There may also be radiographic evidence of osteoporosis and of hot spots on isotope bone scans which may be mistaken for osteolytic metastases.

If sympathetically-maintained pain is suspected in a cancer patient, a diagnostic sympathetic block should be performed with local anaesthetic. This serves not only to confirm the diagnosis but may also give relief which outlasts the duration of the local anaesthetic effect.

Evaluation of pain

It is of crucial importance to appreciate that pain is a somatopsychic experience – not merely a sensation.[12] All pain is modified, for better or for worse, by a person's mood and morale, and the meaning of the pain for them. This means that pain evaluation must extend beyond the physical and embrace psychological, social and spiritual aspects of suffering as well.

As always, evaluation must precede treatment, and is based on *probability* and *pattern recognition* (Table 5.4). The list of potential causes includes:

- myofascial trigger points
- adhesive capsulitis ('frozen shoulder')
- arthritis
- bursitis
- tendinitis
- deep vein thrombosis (DVT).[13]

Myofascial pains occur particularly around the pectoral girdle and in the neck.

Neuropathic pain may be caused by:

- postmastectomy intercostal neuralgia
- radiation-induced fibrosis
- recurrence (axillary, supraclavicular, cervical, spinal)
- chemotherapy
- cervical spondylosis.

Table 5.4 Causes of pain at initial evaluation of lymphoedema[6,a]

Type	Number of patients
None	43
Tissue distension	25
Myoligamentous strain	15
Neuropathy	12[b]
AIE or infection	5

a   although some patients had more than one pain, they were categorised according to the dominant one

b   all cancer patients, including 10 with active disease; in 3 patients the pain was thought to be caused by cervical spondylosis but the possibility of neuropathy secondary to post-radiation fibrosis was not excluded.

Two distinct brachial plexus syndromes have been described:

- radiation plexopathy
- plexopathy associated with supraclavicular disease recurrence.

The latter is much more common and, in most patients, there will be clear evidence of metastatic disease, characteristically from cancer of the head and neck, breast or bronchus. But if there is no evidence of recurrence and the patient has had radiotherapy to this area in the past, the question arises as to whether the plexopathy could be caused by radiation-induced fibrosis. The distinction is important because, if metastatic, anticancer treatment (radiotherapy, hormonal manipulation or chemotherapy) may be beneficial. MRI, proceeding if necessary to gadolinium-enhanced imaging, will generally identify the presence of recurrence. The clinical features of the two conditions often differ, however, with pain more common and more severe in patients with recurrence (Table 5.5).

Lymphoedema is associated more frequently with radiation plexopathy and may not develop until several years after treatment. Patients complain of pain, sensory changes and weakness in the limb (Table 5.5). The symptoms and signs are often confined to those areas receiving innervation from the *upper*

Table 5.5   Characteristics of pain in 100 patients with brachial plexopathy[14]

	Active cancer (n = 78)	Post-radiation (n = 22)
Presenting symptom	82%	18%
Location	Shoulder, upper arm, elbow; radiates to 4th and 5th fingers	Shoulder, wrist, hand
Nature	Aching pain in shoulder; stabbing pain in elbow and ulnar aspect of hand; occasional dysaesthesia, burning, freezing sensations	Aching pain in shoulder; tightness and heaviness in arm and hand; paraesthesiae in C5, 6 distribution
Severity	Moderate–severe; 98% severe	Mild–moderate; 35% severe
Course	Progressive neurological dysfunction, atrophy and weakness C7–T1 distribution; pain persistent	Progressive weakness in C5, 6 distribution; pain stabilises or improves with appearance of weakness

brachial plexus. This includes the shoulder girdle, lateral aspect of both the upper and lower arm, and the lateral hand. The upper portion of the brachial plexus seems to be at particular risk of radiation injury, perhaps because it is not protected by bony structures.

Patients with features of lower plexus involvement should be considered to have recurrent disease until proved otherwise. The lower plexus is at risk of compression by enlarged lymph nodes or metastasis extending from the apex of the lung. Lower brachial plexopathies tend to cause weakness in the intrinsic muscles of the hand, and sensory changes in the medial hand and forearm. Horner's syndrome (ptosis, meiosis and anhydrosis) is more likely with a lower plexus lesion.

Case history

A 76 year-old woman who had had a left mastectomy for cancer nearly 40 years earlier developed pain in the left arm. It increased in intensity over 18 months and was associated with loss of function in the hand and forearm. The arm then became swollen but no masses were palpable. A presumptive diagnosis of recurrent breast cancer was made and tamoxifen prescribed. Within 3 months the swelling resolved but the neurological signs and symptoms persisted. The pain changed to a more superficial, burning discomfort with marked allodynia. She was treated with a tricyclic antidepressant and oral morphine with moderate benefit. Tamoxifen induced a prolonged remission and the patient lived at home with her husband until she died of other causes some 5 years later.

Management of pain

A multimodal approach should be adopted in pain management (Table 5.6). All patients prescribed analgesics need to be monitored in order to achieve maximum comfort with minimal adverse effects. If there are several anatomically distinct pains, relief should be evaluated in relation to each one. Re-evaluation is a continuing necessity; old pains may get worse and new ones develop. In practice, it is best to aim at progressive pain relief:

- relief at night
- relief at rest during the day
- relief on movement.

Table 5.6 A multimodal approach to pain management

Explanation to reduce psychological impact of pain	*Anticancer treatment*
	Surgery
	Radiation therapy
Analgesics	Hormone therapy
Antipyretic (nonopioid)	Chemotherapy
Opioid	
Adjuvant	*Interruption of pain pathways*
corticosteroids	Local anaesthesia
antidepressants	lidocaine (lignocaine)
anti-epileptics	bupivacaine
muscle relaxants	Neurolysis
antispasmodics	chemical (e.g. alcohol, phenol)
	cold (cryotherapy)
Non-drug methods	heat (thermocoagulation)
Physical	Neurosurgery
heat pads (*not in lymphoedema*)	cervical cordotomy
TENS	
	Modification of way of life and environment
Psychological	Avoid pain-precipitating activities
relaxation	Walking aid
cognitive-behavioural therapy	Wheelchair
psychodynamic therapy	Hoist

Non-drug measures

Professional time spent exploring a patient's worries and fears is time well spent, and relates directly to pain management. Indeed, if the patient remains very anxious and/or depressed, the pain may remain intractable.[12]

For most patients, supporting the arm on a pillow or cushion so that the weight of the limb is no longer pulling on the shoulder provides considerable relief – but only at the expense of enforced rest/inactivity. The situation may be further helped, however, by modifications to the patient's way of life and environment. This is where the input of a physiotherapist and an occupational therapist are invaluable.

With functional muscle pains (muscle cramp and myofascial pains) the correct approach is explanation, physical therapies (including muscle stretching and massage), diazepam and relaxation therapy. If necessary the trigger point(s) can be injected with local anaesthestic (e.g. bupivacaine 0.5%).

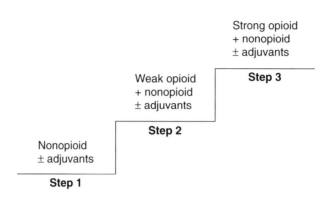

Figure 5.2 The World Health Organization analgesic ladder for cancer pain management.

Analgesics

An appropriate trial of analgesics should be undertaken (Figure 5.2). The principles governing their use can be summarised as:

- by the mouth
- by the clock
- by the ladder
- individualised dose titration
- use adjuvant drugs
- pay attention to detail.[15,16]

Particularly in end-stage cancer, regular by the clock administration is increasingly necessary, combining a nonopioid with an opioid – and titrating the dose upwards until the best balance between relief and adverse effects is achieved (Figure 5.3). Paracetamol is a good choice of nonopioid because it does not cause fluid retention. Using morphine as an analgesic-cum-night sedative may be a good idea even if, for some, daytime morphine causes a reduced attention span and unacceptable drowsiness. In other words, patients should be guaranteed pain-free sleep-full nights.

The concept behind the analgesic ladder is 'broad-spectrum analgesia', i.e. drugs from each of the three classes of analgesic are used appropriately either singly or in combination so as to maximise their analgesic impact (Figure 5.4). As a general rule, however, the benefits of the analgesic ladder should be exploited before adding or substituting an adjuvant analgesic. Adjuvant

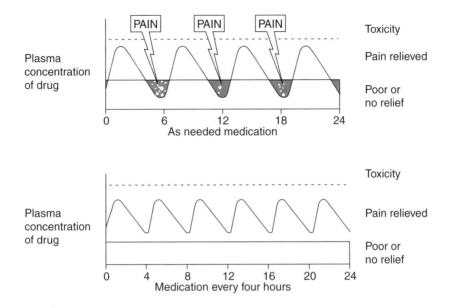

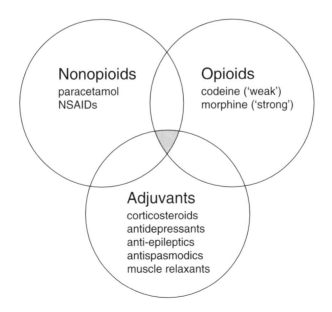

Figure 5.3   A comparison of morphine 'as needed' (p.r.n.) with regular morphine q4h.

Figure 5.4   Broad-spectrum analgesia; analgesics from different classes are used in various combinations to maximise pain relief.

analgesics are needed for the majority of patients with neuropathic pain – but not all.[17] Psychotropic medication may be necessary for highly anxious patients (an anxiolytic) and for those who are clinically depressed (an antidepressant).

Nonopioids

Nonopioids comprise the nonsteroidal anti-inflammatory drugs (NSAIDs) and paracetamol. NSAIDs are of particular benefit for pains associated with inflammation, for example soft tissue infiltration and bone metastases. Because inflammation leads to central sensitisation and increased pain, NSAIDs are sometimes of crucial importance in relieving cancer-related neuropathic pain.[18] Ibuprofen, diclofenac and naproxen are all widely used NSAIDs. Flurbiprofen is the NSAID of choice at some centres in the UK. Availability, fashion, cost, patient convenience and adverse effects profile dictate choice as much as efficacy.

NSAIDs act at several sites, both peripheral and central. The central analgesic effects of NSAIDs have not been fully elucidated and clinically important differences may emerge when more data are available. NSAIDs inhibit cyclo-oxygenase (COX), an important enzyme in the arachidonic acid cascade which results in the production of tissue and inflammatory prostaglandins (PG). Inhibition of PG synthesis does not account for the total analgesic effect of NSAIDs, although it appears to explain most of the adverse effects.[19]

In hot countries, NSAIDs are sometimes discouraged because of the risk of acute renal failure in hypovolaemic patients. Paracetamol is used instead. The main drawback with paracetamol is the frequency of administration, typically q.d.s. On the other hand, because the mechanism of action of NSAIDs and paracetamol differ, the two can be used together with an additive effect.

NSAIDs differ in their effect on platelet function. In patients undergoing chemotherapy or with thrombocytopenia from another cause, it is best to use a NSAID which has no effect on platelet function (Table 5.7). The new generation of specific COX-2 inhibitors promise to combine the benefits of traditional NSAIDs without risk of gastroduodenal damage.[20]

Weak opioids

Weak opioids used in combination with nonopioids comprise step 2. A large dose of a weak opioid is as effective as a small dose of morphine. This means that step 2 is pharmacologically unnecessary. In many countries, however, it is much easier to obtain and supply a weak opioid preparation. Codeine is about 1/10 as potent as morphine. The typical dose range for codeine is

Table 5.7 NSAIDs and platelet function

Drug	Effect on platelets	Comment
Aspirin	+	*Irreversible* platelet dysfunction (acetylation of platelet COX-1)
Nonacetylated salicylates	–	No effect at recommended doses (choline magnesium trisalicylate, diflunisal, salsalate)
Non-specific COX inhibitors	+	Reversible platelet dysfunction (includes all other long-established NSAIDs) *except diclofenac*
Preferential COX-2 inhibitors	–	Meloxicam, nimesulide (not available in UK)
Specific COX-2 inhibitors	–	Celecoxib (not yet available in UK), rofecoxib

30–60mg q4h. Much of the analgesic effect of codeine depends on biotrans-formation to morphine.[21,22] Dihydrocodeine is often used instead in the UK. Compound tablets (i.e. nonopioid + weak opioid) are also widely used, e.g. co-proxamol 32.5/325 (dextropropoxyphene 32.5mg + paracetamol 325mg).

Strong opioids

Globally, morphine remains the strong opioid of choice; other strong opioids are used mainly when morphine is not readily available or when the patient has intolerable adverse effects with morphine. Morphine is administered as tablets (normal-release 10mg, 20mg, 50mg) or aqueous solutions (10mg/5ml, 100mg/5ml). An increasing range of modified-release (m/r) preparations is available – tablets, capsules and suspensions – most of which are recom-mended for 12-hourly administration. Although there are no generic m/r morphine tablets, there is generally no problem if patients are switched from one preparation to another – certainly as far as the 12-hourly preparations are concerned.[23] Patients can be started on either an ordinary (normal-release) or an m/r preparation (Box 5.A).

The use of morphine is determined by analgesic need and by response to its use, not by the doctor's estimate of a patient's life expectancy. Some patients with non-progressive conditions take morphine with good effect for years. The correct dose of morphine is what gives adequate relief for 4 hours without

Box 5.A   Starting patients on oral morphine

Morphine is indicated in patients with pain which does not respond to the combined optimised use of a nonopioid and a weak opioid. The starting dose of morphine is calculated to give a greater analgesic effect than the medication already in use:

- if the patient was previously receiving a weak opioid, give 10mg q4h or m/r 30mg q12h by mouth
- if changing from an alternative strong opioid, a much higher dose of morphine may be needed (Table 5.8).

With frail elderly patients, however, a lower starting dose (e.g. 5mg q4h) helps to reduce initial drowsiness, confusion and unsteadiness. Upward titration of the dose of morphine stops when either the pain is relieved or intolerable adverse effects supervene. In the latter case, it is generally necessary to consider alternative measures. The aim is to have the patient free of pain and mentally alert. M/r morphine may not be satisfactory in patients troubled by frequent vomiting or those with diarrhoea or an ileostomy.

Scheme 1: ordinary (normal-release) morphine tablets or solution

- morphine given q4h 'by the clock' with p.r.n. doses of equal amount
- after 1–2 days, recalculate q4h dose based on total used in previous 24h (i.e. regular + p.r.n. use)
- continue q4h and p.r.n. doses
- increase the regular dose until treatment gives adequate relief from pain, maintaining availability of p.r.n. doses
- *a double dose at bedtime obviates the need to wake the patient for a q4h dose during the night.*

Scheme 2: ordinary (normal-release) morphine and m/r (modified-release) morphine

- begin as for scheme 1
- when the q4h dose is stable, replace with m/r morphine q12h, or o.d. if a 24h preparation is prescribed
- the q12h dose will be *three times* the previous q4h dose; an o.d. dose will be *six times* the previous q4h dose, rounded to a convenient number of tablets
- continue to provide ordinary morphine solution or tablets for p.r.n. use.

Scheme 3: m/r (modified-release) morphine when ordinary (normal-release) morphine is unavailable

(In some countries, q12h m/r morphine is available but ordinary morphine preparations are not.)

- starting dose generally m/r morphine 20–30mg b.d.
- use a weak opioid or an alternative strong opioid for p.r.n. medication
- dose of m/r morphine adjusted every 48h until adequate relief is obtained throughout each 12h period
- if of benefit, maintain the availability of p.r.n. doses of a weak opioid or an alternative strong opioid.

Table 5.8 Approximate oral analgesic equivalence to morphine

Analgesic	Potency ratio with morphine[a]	Duration of action (h)[b]
Codeine } Dihydrocodeine }	1/10	3–6
Pethidine	1/8	2–4
Tramadol	1/5[c]	4–6
Dipipanone (in Diconal UK)	1/2	4–6
Papaveretum	2/3[d]	3–5
Oxycodone	1.5–2[c]	3–4
Dextromoramide	[2][e]	2–3
Levorphanol	5	4–6
Phenazocine	5	6–8
Methadone	5–10[f]	8–12
Hydromorphone	7.5	4–5
Buprenorphine (*sublingual*)	60	6–8
Fentanyl (*transdermal*)	150	72[g]

a   multiply dose of opioid by its potency ratio to determine the equivalent dose of morphine sulphate

b   dependent in part on severity of pain and on dose; often longer lasting in very elderly and those with renal dysfunction

c   tramadol and oxycodone are both relatively more potent by mouth because of high bio-availability; parenteral potency ratios with morphine are 1/10 and 3/4 respectively

d   papaveretum (strong opium) is standardised to contain 50% morphine base; potency expressed in relation to morphine sulphate

e   dextromoramide: a single 5mg dose is equivalent to morphine 15mg in terms of peak effect but is shorter acting; overall potency ratio adjusted accordingly

f   methadone: a single 5mg dose is equivalent to morphine 7.5mg. However, its long plasma halflife and broad-spectrum of action result in a much higher than expected potency ratio when given repeatedly[24]

g   after removal of skin patch; with single dose IV, duration of action only 3–4h.

unacceptable adverse effects. Maximum recommended doses, derived mainly from postoperative parenteral single dose studies, are not applicable for patients with chronic pain taking regular oral doses.

When adjusting the dose of morphine upwards, increases are typically 33–50%. In advanced cancer, most patients never need more than 30mg q4h (m/r morphine 100mg q12h); the rest need up to 200mg q4h (m/r morphine 600mg q12h) and occasionally more. The p.r.n. dose should be the same as the q4h dose of morphine and *is increased when the regular dose is increased.* Instructions must be clear: an extra 'as needed' dose of morphine does not mean that the next dose of regular morphine is omitted.

An anti-emetic should be supplied in case of need (e.g. haloperidol 1.5mg stat, o.n. and p.r.n.) and a laxative (e.g. co-danthrusate 2 capsules o.n. initially). *Constipation may be more difficult to manage than the pain.* Suppositories and enemas continue to be necessary in about one third of patients. Patients should be warned about the possibility of initial drowsiness. If swallowing is difficult or vomiting persists, change from the oral to the subcutaneous route, preferably by infusion with a portable syringe driver. In the UK, 1/3–1/2 of the oral dose of morphine is given as diamorphine; elsewhere 1/2 of the oral dose of morphine should be given. Alternatively, morphine may be given rectally (same dose as orally) or a switch made to transdermal fentanyl.

It is pharmacological nonsense to prescribe two weak opioids or two strong opioids concurrently. It is sometimes justifiable for a patient receiving morphine to be given another opioid (weak or strong) for breakthrough pain. On the other hand, patients could perhaps more easily be advised to take an extra dose of morphine. Strong opioids generally cause the same range of adverse effects (Table 5.9), although to a varying extent. For example, trans-dermal fentanyl is less constipating than morphine.[24,25] Differences between opioids also relate to variations in receptor affinity.

Because pain is a physiological antagonist to the central depressant effects of morphine, strong opioids used correctly do not cause clinically important

Table 5.9   Adverse effects of opioid analgesics

Common initial	*Occasional*
Nausea and vomiting	Dry mouth
Drowsiness	Sweating
Unsteadiness	Pruritus
Delirium (confusion)	Hallucinations
	Myoclonus
Common ongoing	*Rare*
Constipation	Respiratory depression
Nausea and vomiting	Psychological dependence

respiratory depression in cancer patients in pain. In contrast to postoperative patients, cancer patients with pain:

- generally have already been receiving a weak opioid (i.e. are not opioid naive)
- take medication by mouth (slower absorption, lower peak concentration)
- titrate the dose upwards step by step (less likelihood of an excessive dose being given).

It is therefore extremely rare to need to use naloxone (a specific opioid antagonist) in chronic pain management. Because of the possibility of an additive sedative effect, however, care needs to be taken when strong opioids and psychotropic drugs are used concurrently.

Tolerance to strong opioids is not a practical problem.[12] The fear of patients developing psychological dependence (addiction) is unfounded and should not limit the use of strong opioids for cancer pain. Caution in this respect should be reserved for patients with a present or past history of substance abuse; even then strong opioids should be used when there is clinical need. Physical dependence does not prevent a reduction in the dose of a strong opioid if the patient's pain ameliorates, for example, as a result of radiotherapy or a nerve block.

In patients who have intolerable adverse effects with morphine, it may be necessary to substitute an alternative strong opioid (Table 5.10). The first step, however, is to reduce the dose of morphine (and possibly other drugs) and review.[26] For adverse effects such as cognitive failure, hallucinations or myoclonus, hydromorphone and oxycodone (where available) can be used. However, for patients experiencing opioid-induced hyperexcitability, methadone is preferable.[27]

Methadone is a μ-receptor agonist,[28] a NMDA-receptor-channel blocker[29] and a blocker of presynaptic serotonin re-uptake.[30] Theoretically, therefore, methadone should be a better analgesic than morphine for neuropathic pain.[27] Some patients with nociceptive pain who obtain poor relief and severe adverse effects (drowsiness, delirium, nausea and vomiting) with morphine (and a NSAID), obtain good relief and few adverse effects with a low dose of methadone (and a NSAID).[27,31]

Methadone is also useful in patients with renal failure who have developed excessive drowsiness and/or delirium with morphine because of cumulation of morphine-6-glucuronide (M6G). Methadone does not have a comparable active metabolite and its effects are therefore not altered in renal failure.

Transdermal fentanyl is increasingly used for patients because of its convenience.[32] Patches are applied every 3 days. Pethidine and dextromoramide

Table 5.10 Potential intolerable effects of morphine

Type	Effects	Initial action	Comment
Gastric stasis	Epigastric fullness, flatulence, anorexia, hiccup, persistent nausea	Metoclopramide 10–20 mg q4h; cisapride 10–20mg b.d.	If the problem persists, change to an alternative opioid
Sedation	Intolerable persistent sedation	Reduce dose of morphine; consider methylphenidate 10mg o.d.–b.d.	Sedation may be caused by other factors; stimulant rarely appropriate
Cognitive failure	Agitated delirium with hallucinations	Reduce dose of morphine and/or prescribe haloperidol 3–5mg stat and o.n.; if necessary switch to an alternative opioid	Some patients develop intractable delirium with one opioid but not with an alternative opioid
Myoclonus	Multifocal twitching ± jerking of limbs	Reduce dose of morphine but revert to former dose if pain recurs; consider a benzodiazepine	Unusual with typical oral doses; more common with high dose IV and spinal morphine
Hyperexcitability	Abdominal muscle spasms and symmetrical jerking of legs; whole-body allodynia and hyperalgesia manifesting as excruciating pain	Reduce dose of morphine; consider changing to an alternative opioid	A rare syndrome in patients receiving IT or high dose IV morphine; occasionally seen with typical PO and SC doses
Vestibular stimulation	Incapacitating movement-induced nausea and vomiting	Cyclizine or dimenhydrinate or promethazine 25–50mg q8h–q6h	Rare; try an alternative opioid or levomepromazine (methotrimeprazine)
Histamine release cutaneous	Pruritus	Oral antihistamine (e.g. chlorphenamine (chlorpheniramine) 4mg b.d.–t.d.s.)	If the pruritus does not settle in a few days, prescribe an alternative opioid
bronchial	Bronchoconstriction → dyspnoea	IV/IM antihistamine (e.g. chlorphenamine 5–10mg) and a bronchodilator	Rare; change to a chemically distinct opioid immediately; e.g. methadone or phenazocine

have short durations of action and are not recommended for regular prophylactic analgesia. Because of its rapid onset of action, however, some centres use dextromoramide for breakthrough pain in patients taking regular morphine, or as prophylactic additional analgesia before a painful dressing or other procedure. In contrast, at other centres, such procedures are timed to coincide with the peak plasma concentration after a regular or p.r.n. dose of morphine. Pentazocine should not be used; it is a weak opioid by mouth and often causes psychotomimetic effects (dysphoria, depersonalisation, frightening dreams, hallucinations). When converting from an alternative strong opioid to oral morphine, the initial dose depends on the relative potency of the two drugs (Table 5.8).

Adjuvant analgesics

These include corticosteroids, tricyclic antidepressants, anti-epileptics and muscle relaxants. Corticosteroids are important for pain associated with nerve root or nerve trunk compression, and for pain associated with spinal cord compression. Dexamethasone 4–8mg o.m. is prescribed for nerve compression pain, and 16mg or more for spinal cord compression (followed by radiotherapy).

Nerve injury pains often do not respond well to nonopioids and opioids, nor to the addition of a corticosteroid. They may well be eased, however, by an antidepressant (e.g. amitriptyline 25–75mg o.n.) or an anticonvulsant (e.g. sodium valproate 400–1000mg o.n.) or both, generally used in combination with morphine ± a nonopioid.[17] Further options include class 1 anti-arrhythmic drugs (e.g. mexiletine), NMDA-receptor-channel blockers (e.g. methadone, ketamine) and spinal analgesia (e.g. morphine + bupivacaine ± clonidine). About 3% of cancer patients referred to a specialist palliative care unit eventually need spinal analgesia.[33]

Nerve blocks

A nerve block may occasionally be necessary.[17] For example, a woman with lymphoedema secondary to breast cancer and severe arm pain which did not respond to opioids (details not available) was treated with a continuous brachial plexus block using bupivacaine, a local anaesthetic.[34] A Tuohy needle was advanced from the skin surface towards the brachial plexus with a peripheral stimulator to locate the plexus accurately. When satisfactorily positioned, an epidural catheter was introduced (and the Tuohy needle withdrawn). Relief was established with a bolus of bupivacaine and maintained with a continuous infusion. The patient remained pain-free until her death

2 weeks later. The analgesia allowed active treatment of the lymphoedema and mobilisation of the limb.

In patients with sympathetically-maintained pain, a regional sympathetic block (stellate ganglion or lumbar sympathetic chain) may be necessary.[35-37]

Conclusion

Satisfactory pain relief can be achieved in most patients with lymphoedema. The cause(s) of the pains must first be evaluated – generally on the basis of probability and pattern recognition. The doctor must determine which pains are caused by cancer and which are not, and be able to recognise functional muscle pains. It is necessary also to be familiar with the use of corti-costeroids, antidepressants and anti-epileptics in neuropathic pain. It must not be forgotten that pain is a somatopsychic experience. Finally, patients prescribed analgesics or other drugs must be closely monitored to evaluate benefit and adverse effects, and to modify treatment as necessary.

References

1   Stillwell GK (1969) Treatment of postmastectomy lymphoedema. *Modern Treatment.* **6**:369–412.
2   Markowski J *et al.* (1981) Lymphoedema incidence after specific postmastectomy therapy. *Archives of Physical Medicine and Rehabilitation.* **62**:922–6.
3   Brismar B and Ljungdahl I (1983) Postoperative lymphoedema after treatment of breast cancer. *Acta Chirurgica Scandinavica.* **149**:687–9.
4   Corneillie P *et al.* (1984) Early and late postoperative sequelae after surgery for carcinoma of the breast. *Acta Chirurgica Belgium.* **84**:227–31.
5   Kissin MW *et al.* (1986) The risk of lymphoedema following treatment of breast cancer. *British Journal of Surgery.* **73**:580–4.
6   Badger CMA *et al.* (1988) Pain in the chronically swollen limb. In: H Partsch (ed) *Progress in Lymphology XI.* Elsevier Science Publishers BV, Amsterdam, pp 243–6.
7   Alliot F *et al.* (1990) Secondary upper limb lymphoedema can be painful and disturb the quality of life. World Lvmphology Conference, Tokyo.
8   Vecht CJ (1990) Arm pain in the patient with breast cancer. *Journal of Pain and Symptom Management.* **5**:109–17.
9   Armitage P (1971) *Statistical Methods of Medical Research.* Blackwells, Oxford, p 129.
10   Carroll D and Rose K (1992) Treatment leads to significant improvement: effect of conservative treatment in pain in lymphoedema. *Professional Nurse.* **8**:32–6.
11   Sitzia J and Sobrido L (1997) Measurement of health-related quality of life of patients receiving conservative treatment for limb lymphoedema using the Nottingham Health Profile. *Quality of Life Research.* **6**:373–84.
12   Twycross RG (1994) *Pain Relief in Advanced Cancer.* Churchill Livingstone, Edinburgh.

13   Newman ML *et al.* (1996) Lymphedema complicated by pain and psychological distress: a case with complex treatment needs. *Journal of Pain and Symptom Management.* **12**:376–9.

14   Kori SH *et al.* (1981) Brachial plexus lesions in patients with cancer: 100 cases. *Neurology [NY].* **31**:45–50.

15   World Health Organization (1986) *Cancer Pain Relief.* WHO, Geneva.

16   World Health Organization (1996) *Cancer Pain Relief: With a Guide to Opioid Availability.* WHO, Geneva.

17   Grond S *et al.* (1999) Assessment and treatment of neuropathic cancer pain following WHO guidelines. *Pain.* **79**:15–20.

18   Dellemijn PL *et al.* (1994) Medical therapy of malignant nerve pain. A randomised double-blind explanatory trial with naproxen versus slow-release morphine. *European Journal of Cancer.* **30A**(9):1244–50.

19   Yaksh TL *et al.* (1998) Mechanism of action of nonsteroidal anti-inflammatory drugs. *Cancer Investigation.* **16**:509–27.

20   Berde C and Sundel R (1998) COX-2 inhibitors: a status report. *IASP Newsletter.* **Sept/Oct**:3–6.

21   Quiding H *et al.* (1993) Analgesic effect and plasma concentrations of codeine and morphine after two dose levels of codeine following oral surgery. *European Journal of Clinical Pharmacology.* **44**:319–23.

22   Clearly J *et al.* (1994) The influence of pharmacogenetics on opioid analgesia: studies with codeine and oxycodone in the Sprague-Dawley/Dark Agouti rat model. *Journal of Pharmacology and Experimental Therapeutics.* **271**: 1528–34.

23   Collins SL *et al.* (1998) Peak plasma concentrations after oral morphine: a systematic review. *Journal of Pain and Symptom Management.* **16**:388–402.

24   Grond S *et al.* (1997) Transdermal fentanyl in the long-term treatment of cancer pain: a prospective study of 50 patients with advanced cancer of the gastro-intestinal tract or the head and neck region. *Pain.* **69**:191–8.

25   Donner B *et al.* (1998) Long-term treatment of cancer pain with transdermal fentanyl. *Journal of Pain and Symptom Management.* **15**:168–75.

26   Fallon M (1997) Opioid rotation: does it have a role? *Palliative Medicine.* **11**:177–8.

27   Morley JS and Makin MK (1998) The use of methadone in cancer pain poorly responsive to other opioids. *Pain Reviews.* **5**:51–8.

28   Raynor K *et al.* (1994) Pharmacological characterization of the cloned κ, δ, and μ-opioid receptors. *Molecular Pharmacology.* **45**:330–4.

29   Gorman AL *et al.* (1997) The d-and l-isomers of methadone bind to the non-competitive site on the N-methyl-D-aspartate (NMDA) receptor in rat forebrain and spinal cord. *Neuroscience Letters.* **223**:5–8.

30   Codd EE *et al.* (1995) Serotonin and norepinephrine inhibiting activity of centrally acting analgesics: structural determinants and role in antinociception. *Journal of Pharmacology and Experimental Therapeutics.* **274**:1263–70.

31   Manfredi PL *et al.* (1997) Intravenous methadone for cancer pain unrelieved by morphine and hydromorphone: clinical observations. *Pain.* **70**:99–101.

32   Twycross RG *et al.* (1998) *Palliative Care Formulary.* Radcliffe Medical Press, Oxford.

33   Miller MG (1999) Unpublished data.

34 Fischer HBJ *et al.* (1996) Peripheral nerve catheterization in the management of terminal cancer pain. *Regional Anesthesia.* **21**:482–5.

35 Churcher MD and Ingall JRF (1987) Sympathetic dependent pain. *The Pain Clinic.* **1**:217–8.

36 Churcher MD (1988) Sympathetic dependent pain mimicking tumour spread. *The Pain Clinic.* **2**:169–71.

37 Churcher MD (1990) Cancer and sympathetic dependent pain. *Palliative Medicine.* **4**:113–6.

6 Psychosocial aspects of lymphoedema

Mary Woods

This chapter considers the psychosocial aspects of lymphoedema and how the condition can influence many areas of a person's life. Lymphoedema can compromise lifestyle and make ordinary tasks difficult. At worst, it becomes a major physical and social handicap. Self-esteem can diminish because of the stigma attached by society to a deviation from normal. Lymphoedema requires skilled psychosocial care to facilitate adaptation and encourage motivation. In this way, people can be helped to regain a sense of control over their lives. The challenge for the therapist is to empower those with lymphoedema and to help them set and achieve their own personal goals.

The needs and problems of people with lymphoedema

The experience of lymphoedema is personal and unique, emphasising needs and causing problems which stem from the individual's and society's expectations of what is normal and desirable. Human needs differ according to the person and situation but encompass the emotional, intellectual, sociocultural and physical domains.[1] These overlap and interact with each other. For the person with lymphoedema, needs will also vary according to their awareness and knowledge of the condition.

In order to find a solution to a problem, the needs of an individual have to be identified and acknowledged. The need is expressed either verbally or nonverbally through behaviour which reflects underlying unexpressed emotions and concerns.[2] The therapist, who is likely to perceive the person's needs from a professional standpoint, must develop a relationship and provide an environment in which a person can express needs and feelings. If this is achieved, the person feels understood and supported, and this leads eventually to emotional healing.

The experience of a chronic condition

Any chronic condition has an impact on an individual's life. The condition tends to produce a rupture between body, self and the world; it means that life may become permanently altered in some way.[3] When lymphoedema is related to cancer or its treatment, it reminds the person of the cancer. Indeed when the swelling first appears, the person may fear that the cancer has returned. The swelling is a visible sign to the person and others that all is not well.

Understanding the condition forms the basis for adjustment to it. The person with lymphoedema has to make sense of their situation before finding ways of integrating the experience into everyday life. This presents difficulties for some individuals; and those with mild uncomplicated swelling do not necessarily find adjustment easier. The individual's response incorporates personal, social and cultural factors into an understanding of the condition. This creates a unique experience of lymphoedema for that person.

Quality of life

In a discussion of the psychosocial aspects of lymphoedema, it is necessary to reflect on the meaning of 'quality of life'. Although linked to multiple factors, quality of life is primarily a subjective impression perceived by an individual about their own situation.[4] This perception stems from what the individual expects to be possible or views as ideal. Dimensions of quality of life include physical health, mental health, social functioning, role functioning and general wellbeing.[5] These are all areas which have implications for the person with lymphoedema.

Several instruments have been developed to measure the quality of life of cancer patients and some of these have been used in studies involving people with lymphoedema.[6] Quality of life measures provide a means of evaluation and can provide an indication of the outcome of treatment.

Body image

One of the most significant problems which occurs in lymphoedema is the visible physical change in the size and shape of a limb. The effects of the original surgery frequently remain hidden but, when visible swelling occurs, it becomes a disability which can be difficult to hide with clothing and, in cancer patients, is a constant reminder of its underlying cause.

We form our body image in both personal and social contexts. The way we feel about our body is influenced by the way our body really is, the ideal of what we think our body should look like and the way we present our body to the social world through dress, grooming, posture and function.[7] How individuals personally react to changes is as significant as how other people react.

Body image is a vulnerable part of our make-up. Our ideals are influenced by upbringing, culture and the media. Presentation is often adjusted to try to reconcile body reality with body ideal. For the person with lymphoedema, a physical imperfection highlights a discrepancy between body reality and body ideal. This can lead to a negative self-image and comparable negative effects on confidence and motivation.

In a society where the media place great emphasis upon appearance, beauty and fitness, negative feelings can be underlined and confirmed by the inability of the person with lymphoedema to achieve the high standards expected. The attitudes of society form the basis of judgements by others who measure an individual against their own personal ideal. Personal reactions to an altered body image depend upon several factors. These include:

- usual coping mechanisms
- the significance of the altered body image for the future
- the level of support received from others.[7]

Lymphoedema can be difficult to disguise. Adjusting to the change in body image demands strength, perseverance and determination from the individual, coupled with understanding and support from the therapist, family and friends. By respecting a person's grief over their changed body image and by setting short-term goals in relation to body reality, confidence can be rekindled and so permit the setting of more long-term goals. With some people, for instance, the wearing of compression garments presents a greater body image problem than the swelling itself. A short-term goal of wearing the garments at home for 2–3 hours each day may, in time, encourage the patient to aim for longer periods and so help narrow the gap between body reality and body ideal.

Body presentation

Concerns over the appearance of one's body are frequently dealt with by camouflage. Many people with lymphoedema go to great lengths to hide their swollen limb. For some, this necessitates a complete change from their preferred style of dress.[8] Dresses with large baggy sleeves, trousers with wide legs, long floaty skirts and big baggy jumpers are examples of clothing which people with lymphoedema adopt whatever their former personal preferences.

However, even garments of an alternative style may fit badly if the swelling increases. Some people reserve certain clothes for bad days and others for good days according to the degree of swelling. The size of their wardrobe then grows to accommodate the variations. There is anxiety when buying clothes because of the fear that clothing may get stuck when it is tried on.

Communal changing rooms and efficient sales assistants perpetuate feelings of being different and self-esteem can easily be knocked.

Footwear

For the person with lymphoedema, a swollen foot can make shopping for shoes time-consuming, costly and depressing. Foot swelling can be permanent or temporary and often the degree of swelling varies according to activity. The skin on the swollen foot is vulnerable to damage and footwear needs to be well-fitting, supportive and have a smooth lining.

Ill-fitting shoes can lead to a mis-shaped foot and make compression stockings difficult to fit and less effective. In addition, a pair of shoes which will accommodate the swollen foot is likely to slip off the normal foot and adversely affect safety and comfort. On the other hand, a well-fitting shoe is very beneficial in providing support and promoting shape to the foot. Carefully chosen footwear can be comfortable, stylish and affordable (Box 6.A).

Box 6.A   Choosing footwear for swollen feet

Choose:
- a qualified fitter
- natural materials
- openings which extend to the toes
- adjustable fastenings
- low cupped heels.

Avoid:
- shopping when the feet are most swollen
- seams which cause friction.

Compression garments

The benefits of wearing a compression garment are generally recognised by the person with lymphoedema but difficulties may arise in accepting the garment as part of one's self-image or body presentation. If it is considered an intrusion into oneself, the garment will be viewed as yet another reminder that all is not well.

The time required to put a garment on and the struggle which ensues in the process can create a powerful battleground of conflict between adherence and non-adherence. Education in the correct application of garments helps, but support and encouragement are vital.

A further area of concern is the comments and questions from total strangers about the swelling or the compression garment. Remarks can be particularly distressing for those who feel that their body presentation is being challenged and their deviation from normal emphasised. Control over when and where an individual chooses to disclose personal information about their condition is called into question and serves to further enhance the perceived need for camouflage in body presentation.

The effect on physical function and wellbeing

Lymphoedema is a problem which affects the daily life of many people. For some, the effect on physical wellbeing is profound and compromises their ability to undertake everyday tasks, fulfil certain roles and pursue their chosen occupation.

A person's functional ability is related to the individual's perception of how capable they are of performing tasks necessary to their daily way of life. Functional impairment can occur as a result of the weight of a grossly swollen limb which, over time, becomes increasingly difficult to move. Immobility then leads to joint stiffness which makes even simple tasks seem impossible. Swollen fingers mean that jewellery and rings have to be removed and fine movements become difficult. Brachial plexus neuropathy results in loss of sensation which in extreme cases results in the swollen arm hanging limp and lifeless beside the body.

If the dominant arm is affected, the problems are even more profound because that is the arm which is used to perform many tasks which seem impossible to complete with the other. Writing becomes arduous and using a computer or musical keyboard becomes laborious.

Although not used as extensively as the dominant arm, the non-dominant arm has a major role to play in the maintenance of personal hygiene, dressing and many other activities. It is frequently used as a 'support' for tasks undertaken by the dominant arm. When shopping, for instance, goods are picked off the shelf with the dominant arm but put into a shopping-basket carried by the non-dominant arm.

People with leg swelling find activities requiring the leg to bend particularly difficult, for example kneeling, climbing stairs or steep hills, and driving a car. With experience and adaptation, these activities are restricted but it involves planning to ensure that potential problems are minimised.

A swollen heavy leg can affect spatial body awareness. When tired or during lapses of concentration, the leg can drag, balance be lost and a fall result. Standing, sitting for long periods and walking are other common areas of difficulty. Because all are situations in which swelling can increase, adaptation is required.

Occupation

For some, the physical effects of the swelling spill over to their chosen occupation. Larger limbs result in greater physical problems and the impact is particularly distressing if financial security is put in jeopardy because employment ceases. Women with arm swelling who work outside the home have significantly larger arms than those who don't work.[9] This could be because the combined demands of family life and those of work make it difficult for sufficient attention to be paid to the control of the swelling.

Social activities

For many people with lymphoedema, the pursuit of hobbies and social activities is also affected by the swelling. Choice of an activity may be determined by previous experience of problems and discomfort, and some activities and hobbies are curtailed. On the other hand, lymphoedema can offer the opportunity to take up a new activity which can be beneficial, such as swimming, provided self-consciousness can be overcome.

A person may experience conflict because of the knowledge that previously enjoyed activities and social relationships now carry a penalty, namely increased swelling and discomfort. When an activity is no longer possible, the loss of social relationships will affect morale. Further, if the swollen limb becomes a focus for attention by others, a loss of interest in social activities may ensue. For some, in order to 'get on with life', avoidance of difficult or uncomfortable situations becomes inevitable.

Social support

The reactions of family and friends to the lymphoedema has a big impact on the affected individual. By experiencing the way others react, an individual develops their own understanding and response to the condition. A perceived lack of physical or psychological support promotes fears of rejection and causes misery. The individual feels isolated in a world which has changed because of the swelling.

Sexual relationships

A loss of self-esteem may contribute to difficulties in interpersonal and sexual relationships. The demands of coping with lymphoedema may place a strain upon relationships because it leaves little energy for others. In addition, problems with altered body image and the need for compression garments may make intimacy difficult. Understanding and support helps the individual to make sense of the experience of lymphoedema and feel emotionally more secure.

The therapist

The therapist's attitude can be highly influential in developing the individual's response to the condition. The need to maintain normality yet wanting the impact of the swelling to be acknowledged illustrates the conflict the patient brings to the therapist. Discussions concerning the most appropriate management of the condition should focus on the individual's aims and objectives. In this way the person feels supported and empowered.

People move between dependence and independence, needing the advice and support of the therapist to control the swelling while simultaneously aiming to continue the activities of normal life. The therapist has the opportunity to understand the individual's experience by encouraging feelings to be expressed within a supportive relationship. Good communication skills are essential for the therapist.[10,11]

Summary

This chapter has outlined some of the psychosocial aspects of lymphoedema. It illustrates the conflict which may be experienced as a person with a chronic condition tries to manage life normally despite limitations and, sometimes, far-reaching effects on everyday tasks and roles. The extent of the swelling is not the only factor which determines the impact lymphoedema has; personal, social and cultural factors dictate how the individual responds to the experience and incorporates it into their life.

A sense of lack of control can threaten the hope that all will be well and foster negative thoughts about the swelling. By understanding the person's unique experience and acknowledging their individuality, the therapist and their family and friends can support and empower the person with lymphoedema as they learn to live with a chronic condition, thereby restoring hope.

References

1 Bergman R (1982) Understanding the patient in all his human needs. *Journal of Advanced Nursing.* **8**:185–90.
2 McKillip J (1987) *Need Analysis. Tools for the Human Services and Education.* Sage Publications, Newbury Park.
3 Williams G (1984) The genesis of chronic illness: narrative reconstruction. *Sociology of Health and Illness.* **6**:175–99.
4 Grahn G (1996) Coping with the cancer experience. 1. Developing an education and support programme for cancer patients and their significant others. *European Journal of Cancer Care.* **5**:176–81.
5 Ware J (1987) Standards for validating health measures: definition and content. *Journal of Chronic Disability.* **40**:473–80.
6 Sitzia J and Sobrido L (1997) Measurement of health-related quality of life of patients receiving conservative treatment of limb lymphoedema using the Nottingham Health Profile. *Quality of Life Research.* **6**:373–84.
7 Price B (1990) Body Image: *Nursing Concepts and Care.* Prentice Hall, London, pp 3–16.
8 Woods M (1993) Patients perceptions of breast-cancer related lymphoedema. *European Journal of Cancer Care.* **2**:125–8.
9 Woods M (1995) Sociological factors and psychosocial implications of lymphoedema. *International Journal of Palliative Nursing.* **1**:17–20.
10 Silverman J *et al.* (1998) *Skills for Communicating with Patients.* Radcliffe Medical Press, Oxford.
11 Kurtz S *et al.* (1998) *Teaching and Learning Communication Skills in Medicine.* Radcliffe Medical Press, Oxford.

Further reading

Englund F (1996) *Living With Lymphoedema in Advanced Cancer.* Msc Thesis. University of London.
Potter S (1995) *An Investigation into the Problems and Needs of Patients with Secondary Lymphoedema of the Leg.* Msc Thesis. University of Surrey.

7 Management strategies

Karen Jenns

Conservative therapy is the most effective strategy for the management of lymphatic disorders and is the focus of this chapter.[1-4] There are many studies reporting its efficacy in reducing and controlling lymphoedema.[5-14]

A key feature is rehabilitation. Rehabilitation comes from the Latin word *rehabilitare*, meaning to re-enable. Central to the concept of rehabilitation is the development of the maximum possible level of function and independence. The aim is to transfer responsibility to the patient through a process of empowerment. Patients have the right to become experts in their own disorder, thereby enabling them to make informed choices about their own health care and lifestyle.[12-15]

The term chronic oedema is used to describe swelling of > 3 month's duration. The British Lymphology Society (BLS) divides the population with chronic oedema into four management groups:

1   At risk.

2   Mild uncomplicated.

3   Moderate to severe or complicated.

4   Advanced cancer (Table 7.1).[3]

Although the emphasis on the different elements of the treatment may vary, conservative therapy is beneficial irrespective of the cause of the lymphoedema.

Evaluation

The cause of the oedema should be established before an individual treatment plan is devised. In most cases, an experienced health professional can determine the diagnosis on the basis of an accurate history and physical examination without the need for expensive tests.[16-20] With swelling of recent onset it is important to exclude conditions such as cardiac or renal failure.

Evaluation is a cyclical process which takes into account the possibility that a person's health may change over time (Figure 7.1). A structured evaluation should be carried out initially and at each review (Boxes 7.A and 7.B). Evaluation should include the subjective aspects of the disorder and the patient's expectations.[20-22] Factors affecting the goals and outcome of treatment can

Table 7.1 Classification of chronic oedema[3]

At risk	Mild uncomplicated	Severe complicated	Advancing cancer
Those who have one or more of the following:	*Excess limb volume < 20%[a]*	*Excess limb volume > 20%[a]*	*Uncontrolled metastatic disease with shortened life expectancy*
Hereditary predisposition	No truncal/head/genital/ digit swelling	Truncal/head/genital/ digit/swelling	May be due to obstruction or dependency and compounded
Malignancy ± radiation	Subcutaneous tissue soft	Subcutaneous tissue	by renal and/or cardiac failure
Chronic venous insufficiency	and pitting	non-pitting	Hypoproteinaemia
Immobility	Normal shape	Distorted limb shape	Weeping and ulceration of skin
Filariasis	Intact healthy skin	Abnormal skin	Tension in the tissues
Trauma to lymph nodes and/or vessels	Normal arterial supply	Venous occlusion	Impaired mobility
Chronic skin disorder	No active malignant disease in area affected	Arterial insufficiency	Impaired function
		AIE	Heaviness
		Lymphorrhoea	
		Active controlled malignant disease	

a with bilateral swelling, measurement of limb volume becomes subjective.

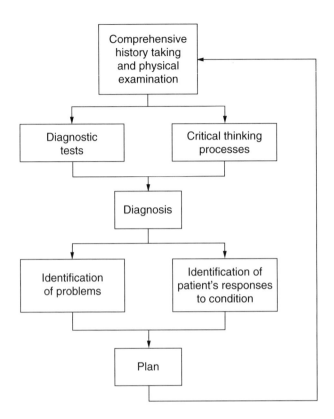

Figure 7.1   A cyclic representation of the evaluation process.

then be identified and treatment adapted accordingly (Box 7.C). The intervals between evaluations vary with individual need. Limb volume measurement is a common way of determining the response to treatment and deciding the intervals between reviews. Over time a shared understanding of the condition and its effects will develop between the patient and the professional carers. Good communication is essential for this to happen; patients need empathy and understanding.

Surveys show that patients want to take an active role in improving and maintaining their health.[21–23] A patient-centred approach should be adopted.[21–25] This requires:

- educating the patient about the disorder
- understanding the whole person
- finding common ground

Box 7.A Initial evaluation

Medical history.

Medication and allergies.

Cancer history:
- diagnosis
- treatment
- present status
- follow-up.

History of oedema:
- onset
- location
- duration
- characteristics
- associated symptoms
- exacerbating and relieving factors
- past treatment.

History of AIE:
- precipitating factors
- frequency
- treatment.

Location and extent of oedema.

Presence or absence of venous complications.

Presence or absence of arterial complications.

Skin condition, presence or absence of complications.

Underlying subcutaneous tissue, i.e. pitting, non-pitting, tissue tone.

Joint range of movement; muscle power and function.

Neurological status.

Shape, normal or distorted.

Discomfort and pain.

Weight and height → body mass index.

4cm circumferential limb volume measurements.

Diagnostic tests.

Box 7.B   Monitoring lymphoedema treatment

Sites and extent of oedema, including trunk.

Condition of the skin.

Condition of the subcutaneous tissue.

Measurement of joint range of movement.[a]

Functional evaluation.

AIE.[a]

Discomfort and pain.

Changes in cancer status or general medical condition.

Limb volume measurements.[a]

Weight and body mass index.[a]

Compression garments:
- therapeutic effect
- ease of use
- comfort.

Adherence to self-care regimen.

Review of goals.

a   objective outcome measures.

Box 7.C   Factors influencing the outcome of DLT

Adherence to self-care regimen.

Active cancer.

AIE.

Concurrent skin disorders, e.g. dermatitis, psoriasis.

Venous insufficiency.

Arterial insufficiency.

Immobility.

Obesity.

Neurological deficits.

Discomfort/pain.

Mental state.

Cognitive impairment.

Renal/cardiac failure.

- incorporating prevention and health promotion
- enhancing the relationship over time
- being realistic about the goals which are likely to be achieved.[19]

For nurses, lymphology is a relatively new area of specialisation. The first nurse-led clinic was established in Oxford in 1984. Since then there has been a steady increase in the number of nurses specialising in this area. Indeed consumerism has led to the de-medicalisation of some services in favour of nurse- and physiotherapy-led initiatives.[26,27] These services have emerged in response to changes in the expectations of society and the delivery of health care.[28,29]

Historical perspective

Von Winiwarter first described conservative therapy for lymphoedema in 1892. His regimen included bed rest, elevation, bandaging and exercises.[30] During the second world war, Vodder used massage to drain the lymphatics in patients with enlarged neck nodes as a result of infection. Winiwarter's ideas were further developed in the 1950s by Földi in his lymphology clinic in Germany. Information regarding his approach began to permeate slowly throughout Europe. Földi called his treatment complex decongestive physical therapy and described it as a 2-phase treatment (Box 7.D).[2,6] Comparable treatment has been variously called complex decongestive therapy, controlled compression therapy or complex physical therapy.[5,7-9] A consensus to use the term decongestive lymphoedema therapy (DLT) emerged during the American Cancer Society Congress in 1998. This term will be used in this book.

Lymphology is a specialty in its own right. Because lymphoedema is a chronic condition, a multiprofessional approach is desirable. Such an approach is advocated by the BLS – a multiprofessional organisation committed to encouraging education about and research into lymphatic disorders.

Prevention

Prevention is an important concept in lymphoedema management. It applies as much to those at risk of developing lymphoedema as to those already living with it. The physical and psychological manifestations of lymphoedema can be prevented or at least reduced if recognised and treated early.

Box 7.D   Elements of Földi's complex decongestive physical therapy

Phase 1: decongestion

Skin hygiene.
Multilayer lymphoedema bandaging (MLLB).
Manual lymphatic drainage (MLD).
Exercises.

Phase 2: conservation

Skin care.
Compression garments.
Regular exercise.
MLD twice weekly.

Any damage to the lymphatic pathways has the potential to cause lymph-oedema. There may well be a latent period of several years between the time of the damage and the development of lymphoedema. Health professionals have a responsibility to warn those at risk. They require information about lymphoedema, why they are at risk and what can be done to minimise the risk. People are thus able to make informed choices about how they want to manage that risk. The provision of written information and access to appropriate health professionals or support groups can reduce the anxiety of being at risk.

Should they develop lymphoedema inevitably there will be concern, particularly if there is a history of cancer. Education and access to treatment is crucial. In order for lymphoedema patients to become partners-in-care and take on responsibility for a self-care regimen, they will need to become knowledgeable about the condition. The health professional is the key person for supplying the needed information.

Decongestive lymphoedema therapy

Like its precursors, DLT comprises two phases. The first is a short intensive period of therapist-led care. The second is the maintenance phase during which the patient uses a self-care regimen to control the swelling long-term with only occasional professional intervention. Each element of care is explained further in later chapters, and summarised in Table 7.2.[3,31]

Table 7.2 Lymphoedema management

DLT maintenance phase	DLT intensive phase	Palliative therapy
Mild uncomplicated lymphoedema (BLS group 2)	*Moderate/severe complicated (BLS group 3)*	*Local recurrence of cancer affecting swelling (BLS group 4)*
Indications		
Excess volume < 20%	Swelling > 20%	Short life expectancy
Normal shape	Distorted shape	
	Digit swelling	
	Skin folds	
	Secondary skin changes	
	Lymphorrhoea	
Overall aim		
Optimal long-term control of oedema	Improve capillary filtration and absorption and flow of lymph	Improve quality of life
Rehabilitation	Reduce limb volume	Alleviate symptoms
Psychological adjustment to chronic condition	Improve limb shape	Maintain function and mobility
Prevention of disability e.g. AIE, restricted mobility/movement	Reduce fibrosis	

continued

Table 7.2 *continued*

	DLT maintenance phase	DLT intensive phase	Palliative therapy
Skin care			
Aim	Maintain or improve hydration of skin Prevent skin problems/AIE	Optimal management of skin problems Rehydration of skin Promotion of healthy skin and upper tissues	Rehydration of skin Prevention of lymphorrhoea
Strategy	Daily skin hygiene Daily moisturising with an emollient General advice and education about infection risk and preventive measures	Daily skin hygiene Daily moisturising with appropriate oil/cream Management of skin complications Multiprofessional approach – dermatologist, podiatrist etc	Daily skin hygiene Daily moisturising with appropriate oil/cream Advice regarding prevention of infection and trauma Check for lymphorrhoea
Lymphatic drainage massage			
Aim	Stimulate lymph drainage Prevent congestion at the proximal end of limb	Stimulate contraction of lymphangions and movement of lymph Promote lymph drainage from congested truncal areas Clear pathways for lymph to drain	Move fluid around the limb Prevent fibrosis and tissue tightness Promote comfort and wellbeing Clear congested truncal areas

continued

Table 7.2 *continued*

DLT maintenance phase	DLT intensive phase	Palliative therapy
Lymphatic drainage massage (*cont*)		
Strategy		
Daily simple lymphatic drainage (SLD) massage	Manual lymphatic drainage (MLD) Daily SLD by patient	Daily SLD Massage of affected limb and adjacent truncal areas (*avoid areas of cutaneous tumour*) Involve partners/family/friends as appropriate
Compression		
Aim		
Encourage venous and lymphatic flow Provide support for muscles	Reduce excess volume Reshape limb(s) Encourage lymphatic flow	Provide support and comfort Prevent tissue tightness Prevent accumulation of fluid
Strategy		
Continental compression garments (classes 2–4) Choice of styles and colours Worn daily Replace garments according to manufacturer's recommendations	Daily multilayer lymphoedema bandaging of affected limbs: cotton under-layer digit bandage foam padding soft padding use of pressure pads where appropriate short-stretch compression bandages	Realistic approach Light support compression garments if comfortable, i.e. class 1 Shaped Tubigrip if comfortable (*not tubular*) Support bandaging offering light compression applied daily with soft padding

continued

Table 7.2 *continued*

DLT maintenance phase	DLT intensive phase	Palliative therapy
Exercise		
Aim		
Prevent joint stiffness	Promote lymph and venous drainage	Prevent joint stiffness
Enhance lymph and venous flow	Increase limb movement	Increase limb mobility (if appropriate)
	Improve limb function	Promote good posture
	Encourage good posture	Familiarise patient with relaxation techniques
Strategy		
Encourage normal use	Refer to physiotherapist for specific exercise programme	Gentle active and passive movements
Regular gentle exercise	Exercise programme daily after bandaging	Support heavy limb when resting
Elevation with good support when resting	Short periods of exercise and then rest	Use of broad arm sling when mobilising
Avoid overexercise and static exercise	Rest in horizontal elevation	Encourage normal use as far as possible

Adapted with permission from Twycross (1997).[31]

The intensive phase (complex decongestive therapy (CDT))

This phase of DLT comprises skin care, manual lymphatic drainage (MLD), multilayer lymphoedema bandaging (MLLB) and exercises. The main aims of this treatment are to enhance capillary filtration and improve lymphatic flow. Treatment goals are mutually agreed between patient and therapist. Potential problems about adherence to the self-care regimen after intensive therapy need to be identified at this stage and addressed.

The indications for intensive therapy are given in Table 7.2. The length of treatment is dependent on the severity of the lymphoedema and the goals of treatment, and typically is 2–4 weeks (Figure 7.2). Once the goals of treatment have been achieved, the patient proceeds to the maintenance phase.

Skin care

Lymphoedema predisposes to various skin problems. The aim of skin care is to maintain skin hydration and to reduce the risk of AIE.[32,33] During intensive therapy, the skin in an affected area should be inspected daily, any abnormality treated (e.g. fungal infections) and skin hygiene attended to (see p.118).

Manual lymphatic drainage

The aim of MLD is to encourage protein resorption and stimulate contraction of the lymphangions, thereby increasing the movement of lymph from the superficial vessels into the deep lymphatics.[5,34–36] The sequence and direction of the massage is designed to stimulate lymphatic flow and drainage away from congested areas. In the UK there are various schools of MLD therapy, for example Vodder, Leduc, Földi, Casley-Smith. The different schools use different hand movements. For example, Vodder uses stationary circles and pump techniques, whereas Leduc uses resorption and inciting techniques.[5,15,34–35] Despite these differences, the approach in terms of the sequence, direction of the movements and the gentleness of the pressure applied are the same.[5,15,34–36] The absence of research comparing the effectiveness of the different methods of MLD has probably limited its application in the UK. However, functional changes have been shown to occur in the lymphatics after massage as the result of changes in local tissue pressure.[15]

Ideally, MLD should be performed daily during CDT. The patient, partner or friend should be encouraged to perform a modified form of MLD, called simple lymphatic drainage (SLD), twice daily for one week before CDT, daily during CDT and for two weeks afterwards. Helping the patient to perfect the skills of SLD, during intensive therapy, will help the patient become skilled and motivated enough to carry on daily massage as part of the maintenance programme.

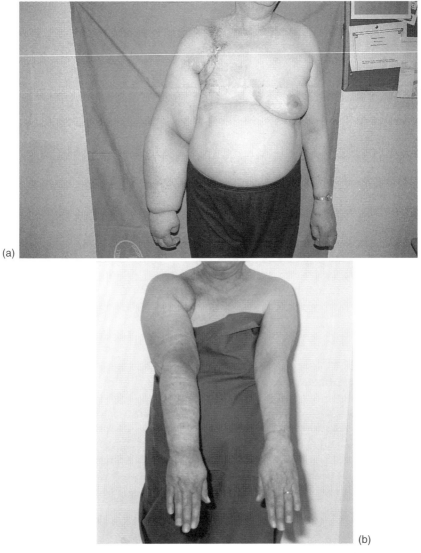

Figure 7.2 Breast cancer-related lymphoedema (a) before and (b) after intensive therapy.

Multilayer lymphoedema bandaging

MLLB works in conjuction with exercise to reduce the limb size and improve limb shape. Unlike elastic bandages, short-stretch bandages apply a semi-rigid casing when applied to a limb. These bandages exert a high working pressure with a low resting pressure (*see* p.165).

Exercise

The aim of exercise during intensive therapy is to enhance lymphatic and venous return, and to improve function and mobility. Exercise enhances the effect of bandages on the muscle pump (*see* p.140).

Ongoing evaluation

Evaluation should include changes in limb size, the presence or absence of truncal oedema, joint movement, changes in shape, and the condition of the skin and underlying tissues. Treatment is adapted daily and should take into account how the patient is coping with the treatment. After intensive therapy the patient should continue to be monitored closely until the condition has stabilised. As a guide, monitoring should be carried out at 1, 3, 6 and 12 months. The evaluation should also include psychosocial status.

Maintenance phase

The maintenance phase comprises a daily regimen of self-care for long-term control of the lymphoedema. Patients who have mild uncomplicated lymphoedema are best suited for this approach (BLS group 2). A maintenance programme encompasses similar elements to the intensive phase but in modified form (Table 7.2). For example, bandages are replaced with containment garments which are worn in the daytime (*see* p.165).

Adherence to self-care regimens

The efficacy of maintenance therapy depends to a great extent on whether the patient is able and willing to take on the responsibility for daily self-care. Good communication between the therapist and the patient is crucial in this process. Emphasis should be placed on educating patients and other significant people in their lives in order to increase their understanding of lymphoedema and its management.[37–42] Honesty, openness and compromise are all necessary. Identification of adverse psychological factors is important, so that potential problems can be dealt with expeditiously.[12–15] Education will:

- help the patient to adapt and integrate the illness experience into their lives[12]

- enhance behaviours conducive to health maintenance

- help the patient to feel in control.

The use of clear concise written information with diagrams facilitates this process. Non-adherence occurs as a result of:

- a conscious decision by the patient not to adhere and to seek other methods of treatment

- a lack of understanding about their condition

- an inability to take part because of their health status

- the quality of the patient–carer relationship

- the absence of a supportive social support network

- beliefs and attitudes about health.

Iteration generally enhances a person's willingness to adhere to a self-care regimen.[43]

Clothing and footwear

It is generally difficult to find clothes that are comfortable, cosmetically acceptable and focus attention away from the swollen limb. The use of flowing garments, such as bat wings sleeves or a choice of plain colours with a patterned neckline draws attention away from a swollen arm. Jewellery can also be used to dress up the neckline. For people with leg swelling there is a range of compression garments available with different styles and colours. Lace-top stockings may be more cosmetically acceptable than tights to young women and the cost is not much more than a plain garment.

Well-fitting shoes are vital for those with lower limb swelling and will help control the swelling, encourage mobility and prevent falls. Referral to an orthotist is appropriate if the foot swelling does not allow standard sized shoes to be worn. Shoes with low heels are preferable, with more fashionable designs limited to special occasions.

Sometimes there needs to be compromise, and this should be based on informed choice. For example, a patient may decide to wear a lower class compression garment because of the greater choice of colours.

Children and adolescence

There are no published data in the UK on the prevalence of lymphoedema in children. Lymphoedema therapists therefore have a responsibility to maintain statistics and to share information. Children with lymphatic disorders often have other medical problems (*see* p.293). As with adults, the aim of management is to reduce and control the swelling, and to prevent complications.

General approach

Ideally all children should be managed in a paediatric centre or clinic with specialists to offer care and support to both the child and the family. Although the evaluation of the child is similar to the adult, there is a further requirement to monitor growth and general development – physical, cognitive, emotional and social.[20,44]

Each child is an individual within a family context, and all members of the family should be educated about lymphoedema and encouraged to take part in the various aspects of care. Education enables the family and the child to gain a sense of control. Emotional development is enhanced by a positive body image and high self-esteem. Early experiences can influence future coping mechanisms in areas such as relationships, career choices and feelings of self-worth.[44] A parent who has difficulty in accepting the child's disability may unwittingly transfer negative influences to the child, often with life-long consequences.

It is important that the child is able to live as normal a life as possible. Children's problems can be immense and challenging and an emphasis on meeting these challenges positively is important. The therapeutic relationship is built up over time and is a vital resource for both the child and family. In addition to the immediate and extended family, classroom teachers and adults who play a key role in any part of the recreational activities of the child require information on lymphoedema and pertinent aspects of care.

In small children the lymphoedema can be managed by skin care and the prevention of infection, lymphatic massage and exercise. As the child grows, low compression garments can be worn during the day or bandages at night to control the swelling. Garments need to be changed every 3 months because of growth. As with adults, bandaging children is a specialist technique and should be carried out only under the direction and supervision of an experienced therapist.

Information on skin care and the prevention of infection is particularly important because children succumb very quickly to infection. Parents should be encouraged to check the skin daily, treat any breaks in the skin by washing the area and applying antiseptic creams or lotions. Daily moisturising is advisable to keep the skin well-hydrated (see pp 118 and 130).

Parents often find difficulty in obtaining suitable footwear for their children. This problem may be compounded by plantar swelling and congenital malformations of the feet. Shoes should be well-fitting, comfortable, non-constrictive and preferably, provide gentle uniform pressure from the distal to proximal end of each foot. Well-fitting footwear will limit the foot swelling and prevent shape distortion. Referral to an orthotist is recommended if standard shoes are unsuitable.

Adolescence brings its own difficulties and a different approach is often needed if the young person is to respond to the challenge of puberty and peer aggression. They require the same treatment as adults with regard to their lymphoedema but may require additional support from health professionals who are sensitive to their specific psychosocial needs. Listening, providing honest information, offering choices and adjusting the treatment accordingly is a great help. Ideally, monitoring should be in an adolescent unit because of the integral psychological support available. Meeting other adolescents with lymphoedema lessens the sense of isolation.

Patient-centred care

People now generally take more of an active role in the maintenance of their own health.[22–24,42] Self-management is not possible without understanding. The main challenge for the health professional is to:

- empower the patient to take control of their own health responsibilities
- identify those who do not comply and those who are unable to take responsibility because of other health problems.

Regular re-evaluation helps to identify problems such as anxiety and depression before they begin to have a major chronic impact on a patient's life. Working within a multiprofessional and holistic framework ensures that the needs of most patients are met.

Outcome measures

Evaluation of treatment and cost-effectiveness is fundamental.[45] The collection of demographic and statistical data will ensure that the service is tailored to meet the needs of the population it serves. It can also be used to provide information for the ongoing development of services and to justify existing funding. Incidence and prevalence data on all types of chronic oedema are required to provide accurate figures on the size of the population with lymphoedema.

Limb volume is the main objective measure because it is relatively straightforward. However, there is as yet no standardised way of measuring limb volume; this can make it difficult to compare results between centres. Water displacement provides an accurate estimate of limb volume but is generally impractical. A perometer or volumometer is used in some clinics; these measure limb volume electronically but are both cumbersome and expensive. The most commonly used method of measurement in the UK is calculation of limb volume using the formula:

$$\text{Volume per 4cm} = \frac{\text{circumference}^2}{\pi}$$

Outcomes measures, however, should include a patient's perception of the treatment, level of satisfaction, quality of life, changes in shape and size, skin condition and joint mobility. Psychological morbidity is more difficult to quantify. Some tools do exist, for example the Nottingham Health Profile and the Hospital Anxiety and Depression Scale.[46] However, these are not condition-specific and have not been validated in people with lymphoedema.

Light on the horizon?

Although lymphoedema is a chronic progressive condition for which there is no known cure, conservative management is effective. Rehabilitation involving the patient in all aspects of care is the key to success; a holistic approach is essential.

Recent government initiatives on the development of cancer services in the UK have led to increasing interest by health professionals about cancer-related lymphoedema and its management. This is linked with a shift towards more patient-centred care. In the past patients had to struggle to obtain effective treatment for lymphoedema – and still do if their condition is not cancer-related (*see* p.1). Over the last decade, however, considerable progress has been made in the UK in raising awareness about lymphoedema and how it can be managed effectively. The BLS has recently developed a core curriculum for training courses for health professionals. This is both unique and exciting.

References

1   Casley-Smith JR (1985) Discussion of the definition, diagnosis and treatment of lymphoedema (Lymphostatic disorders). In: JR Casley-Smith and NB Piller (eds) *Progress in Lymphology: Proceedings of the Xth International Congress of Lymphology.* University of Adelaide Press, SA, pp 1–16.

2   Földi M and Földi E (1991) Conservative treatment of lymphoedema. In: W Olszewski (ed) *Lymph stasis: Pathophysiology, Diagnosis and Treatment.* CRC Press, Inc., USA, pp 469–82.

3   British Lymphology Society (1997) *Definitions of Need Document.* BLS Publication, Caterham, UK.

4   British Lymphology Society (1995) *Strategy for Lymphoedema Care Document.* BLS Publication, Caterham, UK.

5   Casley-Smith JR and Casley-Smith JR (1997) *Modern Treatment for Lymphoedema,* 5th edn. The Lymphoedema Association of Australia, Adelaide.

6   Földi E *et al.* (1985) Conservative treatment of lymphoedema. *Angiology.* **36**: 171–80.

7   Mason M (1993) The treatment of lymphoedema by complex physical therapy. *Australian Physiotherapy.* **39**:41–5.

8   Brorson H (1998) *Liposuction and Controlled Compression Therapy in the Treatment of Arm Lymphoedema Following Breast Cancer.* Wallin and Dalholm Boktryckeri. PHD Thesis, Malamo University, Sweden.

9   Matthews K and Smith J (1996) The effectiveness of modified complex physical therapy for lymphoedema treatment. *Australian Physiotherapy.* **42**:323–7.

10 Daane S *et al.* (1998) Post mastectomy lymphoedema management: Evolution of the complex decongestive therapy technique. *Annals of Plastic Surgery.* **40**: 128–33.

11 Dicken S *et al.* (1998) Effective treatment of lymphoedema of the extremities. *Archives of Surgery.* **133**:452–7.

12 Chin P *et al.* (1998) *Rehabilitation Nursing Practice.* The McGraw-Hill Companies Inc., USA.

13 Loomis M and Conco D (1991) Patients' perceptions of health, chronic illness, and nursing diagnosis. *Nursing Diagnosis.* **2**:162–70.

14 Swanson B *et al.* (1989) The impact of psychosocial factors on adapting to physical disability: A review of the research literature. *Rehabilitation Nursing.* **14**:64–8.

15 Taylor S (1995) *Health Psychology.* McGraw-Hill Inc., USA.

16 Sandler G (1980) The importance of the history in the medical clinic and the cost of unnecessary tests. *American Heart Journal.* **100**:928–31.

17 Smitt B and Weiner S (1986) The diagnostic usefulness of the history of the patient with dyspnoea. *Journal of General Interim Medicine.* **1**:386–93.

18 Bordage G (1995) Where are the history and the physical? *Canadian Medical Association Journal.* **152**:1595–7.

19   Stewart M *et al.* (1995) *Patient Centred Medicine.* Sage Publications, USA.

20   Bates B (1995) *A Guide to Physical Examination and History Taking,* 6th edn. J B Lippincott Company, Philadelphia.

21   Cook D (1993) *Patients Choice.* Hodder and Stoughton, London.

22   Fitzpatrick R and Hopkins A (1997) *Measurement of Patient Satisfaction with Their Care.* Royal College of Physicians, London.

23   Royal College of Physicians (1997) *Improving Communication Between Doctors and Patients.* A working party report. Royal College of Physicians, London.

24   Brown S (1995) An interviewing style for nursing assessment. *Journal of Advanced Nursing.* **21**:340–3.

25   Sackett D and Rennie D (1992) The science of the art of the clinical examination. *Journal of the American Medical Association.* **297**:19.

26   Read S (1995) *Catching the Tide: New Voyages in Nursing?* Sheffield Centre for Health and Related Research, Sheffield University.

27   Manley K (1997) A conceptual framework for advanced practice. *Journal of Clinical Nursing.* **6**:179–90.

28   Ford P and Walsh M (1994) *Nursing Through the Looking Glass: New Rituals for Old.* Butterworth-Heinemann Ltd, Oxford.

29   Ranade W (1997) *A Future for the NHS?* Addison Wesley Longman Ltd.

30   Von Winiwarter (1892) Chirurgischen Krankheiten der Haut. In: *Deutsche Chirurgie.* Enke, Stuttgart, Chapter 17.

31   Twycross R (1997) *Symptom Management in Advanced Cancer.* Radcliffe Medical Press, Oxford.

32   Veitch J (1993) Skin problems in lymphoedema. *Wound Management.* **4**:42–5.

33   Mallon E and Ryan T (1994) Lymphoedema and Wound Healing. *Clinics in Dermatology.* **12**:89–93.

34   Leduc O *et al.* (1988) Manual lymphatic drainage: scintigraphic demonstration of its efficacy on colloidal protein reabsorption. In: H Partsch (ed) *Progress in Lymphology – IX.* Exerpta Medica, Elsevier, Amsterdam, pp 551–5.

35   Wittlinger G and Wittlinger H (1995) *Textbook of Dr Vodder's Manual Lymphatic Drainage. Volume 1: Basic Course.* Haug International, Brussels.

36   Kurz I (1995) *Textbook of Dr Vodder's Manual Lymphatic Drainage. Volume 3: Treatment Manual.* Haug International, Brussels.

37   Fietcher-Alywahby N (1989) Principles of teaching for individual learning of older adults. *Rehabilitation Nursing.* **14**:330–3.

38   Cameron C (1996) Patient compliance: recognition of factors involved and suggestions for promoting compliance with therapeutic regimes. *Journal of Advanced Nursing.* **24**:244–50.

39   Sauer R and Seitz T (1988) Psychological and social support of cancer patients. *Recent Results in Cancer Research.* **108**:311–5.

40   Curran C (1985) Shaping an image of competence and caring. *Nursing and Health Care.* **6**:371–3.

41   Wingate A and Lackey M (1989) A description of the needs of non-institutionalised cancer patients and their primary care givers. *Cancer Nursing.* **12**:216–25.

42   Speechley V (1992) Patients as partners. *European Journal of Cancer Care.* **1**:22–5.

43   Ley P (1982) Satisfaction, compliance and communication. *British Journal of Clinical Psychology.* **21**:241–54.

44   Ricci-Balich J (1996) Paediatric Rehabilitation Nursing. In: S Hoeman (ed) *Rehabilitation Nursing*. Mosby Year Book, New York.

45   National Health Service (1997) *The New NHS, Modern – Dependable*. HMSO.

46   Sitzia J and Sobrido L (1997) Measurement of health related quality of life of patients receiving conservative treatment for limb lymphoedema using the Nottingham Health Profile. *Quality of Life Research*. **6**:373–84.

8   Skin management in lymphoedema

Nina Linnitt

This chapter outlines the reasons why meticulous skin care is arguably the most important aspect in the management of lymphoedema. Skin care is important for everyone with – or at risk of – lymphoedema, and necessitates lifelong vigilance and attention.

The skin is the largest organ in the body and consists of two layers, the epidermis and the dermis (Figure 8.1). The dermis is composed of connective tissue including collagen and elastin fibres. These fibres provide the skin with its durability and elasticity. The subcutaneous adipose tissue allows the skin to move over the underlying tissues. It also contributes to the shape of the body.

The dermis contains minute initial lymphatic vessels which are connected by the pre-collectors through the subcutaneous adipose tissue to deeper collecting lymphatics.[1] The lymphatics play an important role in controlling the microcirculation in the skin. In lymphoedema, this is disrupted and results in the stasis of fluid, protein and other macromolecules in the tissues. The body's immunological responses are dependent on an efficient lymphatic system. Lymphatic failure results in an altered immune surveillance. This will have an adverse effect on wound healing which will, in turn, increase the likelihood of secondary infections/acute inflammatory episodes (AIE) (*see* p.130).[2]

Functions of the skin

The skin has several functions, including:

- organ of communication
- regulation of body temperature
- protection from infection
- excretion of waste
- prevention of tissue dehydration
- supporting and shaping the body.[3]

Substances which penetrate into the skin will, at least in part, be cleared from the skin by the superficial initial lymphatics. Such substances include the solvents of cosmetics, injected substances (e.g. vaccines and drugs), stain from tattoos and the products of inflammatory reactions.[4]

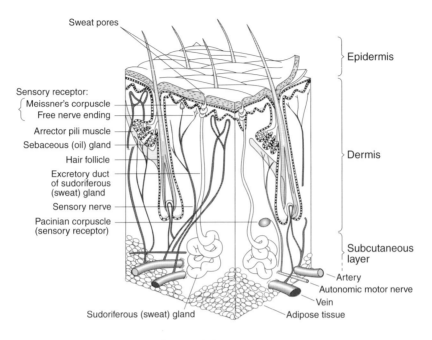

Figure 8.1   Cross-section of normal skin.

In lymphoedema, the superficial lymphatics are compromised. Whatever is placed on or in the skin may have an impact on the management of the swelling. AIE damage subcutaneous tissue by accelerating fibrosis, leading to increased oedema and an increased risk of further AIE.[5] The characteristic skin changes of lymphoedema are the result of the combined impact of poor skin condition, high-protein oedema, chronic inflammation and increased fibrosis. Skin changes are more common in lymphoedema of the lower limbs. They include:

- thickening – giving rise to Stemmer's sign (*see* p.45)[6]

- enhanced skin folds

- papillomatosis – a cobblestone appearance to the skin surface

- hyperkeratosis – a warty, scaly change in the skin

  } caused by cutaneous fibrosis

- lymphangiomas – dilated skin lymphatics which look like blisters on the skin surface; they sometimes leak and are a potential portal for infection.[5]

Skin evaluation

Details of any skin problems (e.g. allergic reactions, eczema, psoriasis) past and present, or within the immediate family, should be noted. Examination includes comparing the swollen limb with the unaffected limb. Much information can be gathered by *inspection*:

- colour (normal, erythema, cyanosis?)
- nails
- hair (folliculitis?)
- bites, scratches
- bullae, papules, plaques
- ulceration.

For measuring outcome, it is helpful to develop a straightforward grading system (Table 8.1).

Table 8.1   Grading for skin condition

Grade	Skin condition
0	Well-hydrated, no skin abnormalities
1	Slightly dry
2	Dry and flaky
3	Scaly/hyperkeratotic
4	Presence of skin problems
5	AIE ± other skin problems

Inspection with *palpation* reveals whether the skin is hot, cold, moist, dry or flaky. Heat may imply local infection or underlying chronic inflammation. The depth and extent of the oedema is determined by *visual examination* and *palpation*, noting particularly whether it extends into the adjacent trunk.

Following evaluation, the importance of continuing skin care at home must be explained to the patient, and the condition of the skin monitored regularly. If this does not improve, further explanation to the patient or a change of treatment may be needed. Patient education, motivation and adherence in skin care are essential if problems are to be detected and dealt with promptly.

New lesions should be recorded and investigated, with the possibility of lymphangiosarcoma kept in mind (*see* p.50).

Aims of skin care

The aims of skin care are:

- to maintain a healthy tissue condition
- to reduce the risk of infection.

Daily care of the affected limb should include:

- meticulous hygiene
- moisturisation of the limb and adjacent trunk with emollients
- inspection of the limb and adjacent trunk.

Particular attention must be paid to skin folds. The skin in the fold tends to be macerated and this may be exacerbated by the application of cream.

Even patients with hydrated skin must be encouraged to moisturise their skin regularly, and must be educated about the importance of skin care (Box 8.A).[7,8] Moisturising at bedtime is best because the limb is not sticky in the morning when the compression garment is put on again.[9]

Emollients

Several factors contribute to dry skin, for example dehydration, smoking, stress, medication, exposure to the sun and ageing.[10] The aim of moisturising is to re-establish the integrity of the stratum corneum (the most superficial layer of the skin), thereby enhancing hydration of the epidermis. The result will make dry, scaly skin much smoother. This can be achieved by using bland emollients which moisturise and soothe dry irritated skin, for example, aqueous cream and Diprobase.[11] Perfumed products should not be used because of the risk of skin sensitisation, leading to inflammation.

Emollients can be divided into three categories:

- bath oil
- soap substitutes
- moisturisers – lotions, creams, ointments.

Box 8.A   Additional written information for patients about skin care[7,8]

General information

If an arm is swollen, protect hands when washing up or gardening.

If a leg is swollen, wear protective footwear at all times. Do not walk in bare feet.

Wear a thimble when sewing.

Dry well in between digits after bathing to protect from fungal infections.

Treat any cuts or grazes promptly by washing and applying antiseptic.

Notify your general practitioner immediately if the limb becomes hot or more swollen.

Use an electric razor to reduce the risk of cutting the skin.

Other important points about the swollen limb:
• do not have blood taken from it
• do not have injections into it
• do not allow your blood pressure to be measured on it.

Summer advice

Avoid insect bites – use repellent sprays.

Treat bites with antiseptics and/or antihistamines.

Protect the limb from the sun:
• sit in the shade when possible
• use a high-factor sun block.

Equipment to take on holiday:
• usual emollients
• high-factor sun block
• insect repellents/sprays
• antihistamine tablets
• antiseptic solutions.

If you have had recurrent infections, you should also take antibiotics with you when you go on holidays in case of need.

Bath oil

When bathing, water is absorbed by the skin and hydrates it. However, the absorbed water is rapidly lost to the atmosphere and has minimal long-term benefit.[12] Bath oil (e.g. Balneum) should be used to help restore the integrity of the skin and thereby help prevent the skin from drying out; 15 ml added to the bath or foot-bowl is adequate. Bath oil should ideally be used together with other emollients such as a soap substitute and a moisturiser. Soaps and perfumed cosmetic bath oil additives should be avoided as they cause further drying of the skin. They are also potential sensitising agents for allergic dermatitis.[13] Bath oil makes the bath or foot-bowl slippery and care should be taken to prevent patients from slipping and falling, particularly those who are elderly or less mobile.

Soap substitutes

The untoward effects of soaps and other surfactants include drying of the skin, irritant contact reactions, contact allergy and enhanced skin penetration by other substances, for example bacteria. This increases the risk of infection. Patients should be advised, when washing, to use a soap substitute instead of a perfumed cosmetic soap.

Soap substitutes are emulsions of oil-in-water and contain more water than oil. This enables them to be mixed with water. Aqueous cream is an example of a soap substitute. With dry skin, soap substitutes should be used together with other emollients to help rehydrate the skin.

Creams

Creams are a mixture of ointment and water. To prevent the two elements separating, stabilisers and emulsifiers are mixed together. Creams also contain preservatives, for example hydroxybenzoates (parabens) and cetylstearyl alcohol. Both of these preservatives may become important sensitisers in leg ulcer patients.[14] Lanolin, extracted from wool, is present in some creams, emollients and bath additives.[15] It is inadvisable to use any product containing lanolin on leg ulcers because of the high incidence of contact dermatitis.[16] Lymphoedematous limbs are immunosuppressed and the regular use of creams with preservatives and/or lanolin can cause similar problems.

Creams can be divided into *cold creams* (emulsions of water-in-oil) and *vanishing creams* (emulsions of oil-in-water).

Cold creams:

- do not mix well with exudate
- are easy to apply
- are cosmetically acceptable.

Vanishing creams:

- have a high water content
- *may make a dry skin worse as the water in the cream evaporates*

- mix well with water and can therefore be used as a soap substitute
- rub easily into the skin.

Lotions:

- are liquid creams
- are less moisturising
- are cooling on hot skin
- may be more sensitising.

Generally, lotions are *not* used in the skin care of patients with lymphoedema.

Ointments

Ointments differ from creams in that they:

- contain little or no water
- are greasy but prevent evaporation of water by diminishing trans-epidermal water loss
- form an impermeable layer over the skin.

Ointments are therefore used in patients with more marked dryness of the skin, particularly in those whose skin does not improve adequately with the daily application of a bland cream (*see* p.126).

Skin sensitivity in lymphoedema

Sensitisation is unlikely to develop in healthy skin.[16] In contrast, inflamed or damaged skin has the potential to become a site of primary sensitisation. Lymphoedema patients can therefore suddenly become sensitive to products they have used for years without trouble. An allergic reaction (contact dermatitis) will have a knock-on effect; the integrity of the skin may be disrupted by the inflammatory response and associated pruritus. It results in further damage to the underlying tissues and an increase in oedema. If the skin condition fails to respond to treatment, it is vital to identify which topical agents are being used. The patient may require referral to a dermatologist for patch-testing to identify specific allergens.

If problems arise with an emollient which has been used for a long time, it may be that the contents of that emollient have changed. By law, the contents of cosmetics have to be listed; this does not apply however to pharmaceutical products, and companies can change the ingredients of their products without having to notify the public.[17] Hence, if a patient presents with a sudden change in the skin condition (e.g. a rash), it is important to check if there has been a change in the formulation of the products being used. These risks would be reduced if patients used only bland moisturisers, for example aqueous cream.

Potential skin complications and their management

Common skin problems include:

- hyperkeratosis
- fungal infections
- contact dermatitis
- lymphorrhoea
- folliculitis.

Hyperkeratosis

Patients with hyperkeratosis or other fibrotic skin changes may initially need to moisturise twice daily until the skin condition improves. A good choice of ointment is 50% white soft paraffin and 50% liquid paraffin (50/50 WSP/LP). It only rarely leads to skin sensitisation.[15] In severe cases of hyperkeratosis it may be necessary to apply small amounts of a keratolytic agent (e.g. 5% salicylic acid ointment) beneath a hydrocolloid dressing, for example Comfeel or Granuflex.[16,18] If left in position for a few days, it softens the hyperkeratosis and enables the scales to be lifted off easily without damage to the underlying skin. As long as the skin is well moisturised, massaging using small circular motions will lift off the hyperkeratosis.

Once the skin is hydrated the patient can use a bland emollient such as aqueous cream. This is inexpensive and generally well-tolerated despite containing preservatives. It is very important that the patient is told to switch back to an ointment (e.g. 50/50 WSP/LP) if the condition deteriorates (Figure 8.2).

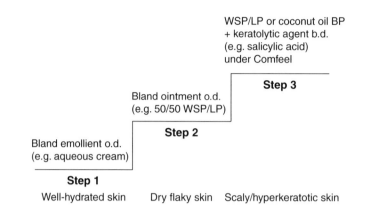

Figure 8.2   3-step ladder for skin care in lymphoedema; if the skin does not improve, refer to a dermatologist.
WSP = white soft paraffin; LP = liquid paraffin (mineral oil); BP = British Pharmacopoeia.

Fungal infections

Fungal infections are common in lymphoedema. Untreated fungal infections may lead to recurrent cellulitis and be a difficult problem to eradicate. Conventional antifungal creams can exacerbate the condition if they lead to increased maceration of the skin. Antifungal powders used in socks and shoes regularly are both beneficial and safe. Ointment containing 3% benzoic acid (half-strength Whitfield's ointment) used prophylactically helps prevent tinea interdigitale (athlete's foot), and can be used safely over long periods.[19]

Contact dermatitis

Dermatitis (synonym, eczema) is a common inflammatory skin condition characterised by weeping, irritated erythematous skin.[15,20] Contact dermatitis is caused by external factors which have either irritated the skin or caused an allergic reaction. Typically it occurs at the point of contact with the irritant.

Irritation of the affected area may lead to scratching which results in further breakdown of the tissues and secondary infection. This is common in dermatitis.[15] Patients presenting with this problem need to be educated appropriately and advised on necessary treatment. They require advice on how to monitor and maintain the health of the skin, and have raised awareness of how to deal with dermatitis if it arises in the future.

Treatment of dermatitis includes emollients and topical corticosteroids. It is more beneficial to apply the corticosteroid to moisturised skin, i.e. apply the emollient and, preferably, then wait 15–20 minutes before applying the corticosteroid. It may be necessary to refer to a dermatologist for patch-testing to identify the allergen if the dermatitis recurs or chronic dermatitis develops.

Topical corticosteroids are available only on prescription. Several different corticosteroids are available as ointments, creams and lotions. They are classified into potency groups of mild, moderate, potent and very potent.[20,21] When used correctly, topical corticosteroids are very helpful in controlling the dermatitis. Many people are fearful about using them and generally will under-use rather than over-use them.

Problems may arise when patients are not educated about the need to reduce the potency of the corticosteroid as their skin improves. A rebound phenomenon may occur if the patient's skin clears after a few days on a potent corticosteroid and the patient then stops using it and the skin condition deteriorates again. The patient restarts the potent corticosteroid and the cycle of events is repeated.

Adverse effects of topical corticosteroids are seen in adults when potent or very potent corticosteroids are used for long periods, and may occur in children with mild or moderate strength preparations. Adverse effects include bruising, skin atrophy and striae. The risk of adverse effects also depends on the extent of the area treated, the daily volume applied and the age of the patient.[20,22] Systemic adverse effects can also occur as a result of prolonged systemic absorption.

Lymphorrhoea

The term lymphorrhoea is a term used to describe the weeping of lymph through the skin surface. Lymphorrhoea can soak through dressings and clothes, and pool in shoes. To the patient, the skin feels cold and uncomfortable.[8] It often occurs in palliative patients where the skin is fragile and thin. It can also occur in acute oedema when the skin is rapidly stretched. In this case the skin literally springs a leak. Lymphorrhoea places the patient at risk of infection and appropriate treatment is essential. Treatment of lymphorrhoea comprises:

- emollients around the affected site
- elevation of the limb to reduce hydrostatic pressure
  raise an affected arm to shoulder level
  use a foot-rest for the leg

- support bandaging to prevent or minimise further leaking until the skin heals (see p.165).

Folliculitis

This is inflammation of hair follicles. When using a lot of greasy moisturisers, folliculitis can occur as the oil gets trapped in the hair follicle. Folliculitis causes tiny spots but can lead to cellulitis. If a patient appears to have folliculitis, they should be shown how to apply the emollient appropriately, i.e. after the emollient has been rubbed onto the skin, the last movement should be downward in the direction of the hair growth. This reduces the risk of oil getting trapped in the follicles and causing an AIE (see p.130).

Conclusion

Skin care is a crucial part of the treatment of lymphoedema. Health professionals should educate patients about the importance of skin care. Specific advice needs to be given, for example, about the use of non-perfumed emollients. Patients at risk of developing lymphoedema must be advised about ways of reducing the risk. If patients understand the importance of skin care, they are able to make informed choices and respond to problems should they arise.

References

1   Ryan TJ (1998) The skin and its response to movement. *Lymphology.* **31**:128–9.
2   Burri H *et al.* (1996) Skin changes in chronic lymphatic filariasis. *Transactions of the Royal Society of Tropical Medicine and Hygiene.* **90**:671–4.
3   Clancy J and McVicar AJ (1995) The Skin. In: *Physiology and Anatomy – A Homeostatic Approach.* Edward Arnold, London, pp 505–21.
4   Ikomi F and Schmid-Schonbein GW (1995) Lymph transport in the skin. *Clinics in Dermatology.* **13**:419–27.
5   Mortimer PS (1990) Investigation and management of lymphoedema. *Vascular Medicine Review.* **1**:1–20.
6   Stemmer R (1976) Ein klinisches zeichen zur Früh-und differential-diagnose des lymphödemse. *VASA – Journal for Vascular Diseases.* **5**:261–2.
7   Regnard C *et al.* (1991) *Lymphoedema, Advice on Treatment,* 2nd edn. Beaconsfield Publishers Ltd, Beaconsfield.
8   Summer advice and skin care in lymphoedema (1998) *Lymphoedema information leaflet.* Oxford Lymphoedema Clinic.
9   Veitch J (1993) Skin problems in lymphoedema. *Wound Management.* **4(2)**: 42–5.
10   Anderson HM (1996) What can you do about your patient's dry skin? *Journal of Gerontological Nursing.* **5**:10–16.

11 Hill M (1994) *Skin Disorders*. CV Mosby, St Louis.
12 Watts J (1998) Out on a Limb. *Nursing Times*. **94(50)**:63–6.
13 Ryan TJ and Mallon EC (1995) Lymphatics and the processing of antigen. *Clinics in Dermatology*. **13**:485–92.
14 Hannuksela A and Hannuksela M (1996) Soaps and detergents in skin diseases. *Clinics in Dermatology*. **14**:77.
15 Cameron J (1995) The importance of contact dermatitis in the management of leg ulcers. *Journal of Tissue Viability*. **5(2)**:52–5.
16 Mallon EC and Ryan TJ (1994) Lymphoedema and wound healing. *Clinics in Dermatology*. **12**:89–93.
17 Cameron J (1998) Red card for allergies. *Nursing Standard*. **13**:3.
18 Venables J and Williams A (1996) Managing skin problems in uncomplicated lymphoedema. *Journal of Wound Care*. **5(5)**:223–6.
19 Mortimer PS (1995) The dermatologists contribution to lymphoedema management. *Scope – on Phlebology and Lymphology*. **2(3)**:17–19.
20 Venables J (1995) The management and treatment of eczema. *Nursing Standard*. **9(44)**:25–8.
21 British National Formulary (1999) Topical corticosteroids. In: *British National Formulary*. British Medical Association and the Royal Pharmaceutical Society of Great Britain, No: 32 (March), pp 493–500.
22 McHenry PM (1995) Management of atopic eczema. *British Medical Journal*. **310**:843–7.

9 Acute inflammatory episodes

Peter Mortimer

Acute inflammatory episodes (AIE) is a term used to describe the attacks of apparent infection, simulating cellulitis, which afflict lymphoedema patients. Various names have been used for such attacks:

- cellulitis

- lymphangitis

- episodic dermatolymphangio-adenitis

- erysipelas

- pseudo-erysipelas.

The variety reflects certain differences from classical cellulitis. The term *secondary acute inflammation* has been proposed by the International Society of Lymphology as a more accurate description of acute inflammation within an area of lymphoedema.[1] *Acute* distinguishes the episode from the ever-present chronic inflammation of lymphoedema and *inflammation* allows for the absence of infection.

Apart from lymphangiosarcoma (Stewart-Treves syndrome) and other skin cancers, AIE is probably the most serious complication of lymphoedema. It causes severe constitutional upset and often emergency admission to hospital.

Clinical characteristics

Typical AIE start rapidly, often without warning. Patients feel unwell as if influenza is starting. Severe attacks can produce fever, rigors, headache, vomiting and even delirium. A feeling of heat together with redness and increased swelling occur within 24 hours in the lymphoedematous area. Pain may precede any rash and sometimes antedates the constitutional upset. Some patients recall that an accidental skin puncture, for example a gardening injury or an insect bite, preceded the attack but the majority have no warning and can, within 30 minutes, change from apparent normal health to malaise, vomiting and rigors. Many learn to carry antibiotics with them at all times and self-medicate when necessary. Nonetheless, attacks can be sudden and frightening.

Atypical AIE

Episodes vary considerably in presentation so that, unless the condition is considered, the diagnosis may be missed. Pain may occur without any obvious inflammation and, occasionally, constitutional upset may be minimal. Sometimes the condition may 'grumble' in a chronic manner for days or weeks and only with complete recovery after prolonged antibiotic treatment can a firm diagnosis be made.

Recurrent AIE

A characteristic of lymphoedema is for AIE to recur. Intervals between episodes may be more than 12 months or as short as 3 weeks so that there is barely any time for recovery between attacks, resulting in severe debility. With each attack, a stepwise deterioration in the lymphoedema occurs, presumably from further damage to lymphatics, so setting up a vicious circle.

Classical cellulitis

Cellulitis is the term used for inflammation of subcutaneous tissue in which an infective cause, generally bacterial, is proven or assumed.[2] Erysipelas is a bacterial infection of the dermis with involvement mainly of the upper subcutaneous tissue. The two conditions often overlap and makes distinction impossible and therapeutically unnecessary. Cellulitis and erysipelas are both caused by bacteria, and the presence of Streptococcal antigens in the dermis and subcutis in both conditions supports this view. Nonetheless, bacteria can be difficult to isolate. Culture of biopsy specimens yielded a positive result in only 26% in one series.[3] Because the cause of the cellulitis cannot be determined even by exhaustive culture techniques in most patients with classical cellulitis, it is possible that the inflammation is not always microbiological in origin.

In the immunocompetent patient, cellulitis is generally caused by Streptococcus. *Staphylococcus aureus* is occasionally isolated but, because of positive serology for Streptococcus, it is possible that both organisms are jointly responsible in these patients.[4] Lymphangitis and lymphadenitis often co-exist with AIE and may even be the predominant feature, thereby emphasising the importance of the lymphatic route as a defence against infection.[5]

Differences from classical cellulitis

In lymphoedema, AIE often do not produce an area of clearly demarcated erythema with a migrating border as is seen in classical cellulitis and erysipelas. This may be because the inflammatory process spreads rapidly throughout the oedematous tissues. An AIE may manifest as confluent erythema but often it is blotchy or just focal inflammatory spots (Plate 9.1). Rarely can an offending micro-organism be isolated from skin swabs so prompting the term *pseudo-erysipelas*.[5] Sometimes AIE fail to resolve despite standard treatment with antibiotics. Recurrent AIE can be a characteristic feature and in some patients even prophylactic antibiotics fail to prevent attacks, thus questioning infection as the sole explanation.

Lymphoedema and regional immunodeficiency

Lymphatics convey antigens together with lymphocytes, macrophages and Langerhans cells to lymph nodes. Without intact lymphatics a primary immune response cannot develop. T lymphocytes constantly recirculate between central organs, blood and tissues for the purpose of immunosurveillance.[6] In lymphoedema, disturbances in lymphocyte trafficking may interfere with host defence mechanisms within the lymphatic drainage area, thereby predisposing to AIE.

Evidence supporting the role of the lymphatics in immunosurveillance was provided during the early days of experimental organ transplantation. Interruption of lymph drainage obstructs the afferent arm of the immunological cycle and delays rejection.[7] Total afferent lymphatic interruption in inbred guinea-pigs allowed temporary tumour allograft growth from a tumour cell inoculum which was readily rejected when injected into an area with normal lymphatic drainage.[8]

The small risk of malignant disease arising in longstanding lymphoedema, the most serious of which is lymphangiosarcoma, has led to suggestions that lymphoedema presents a site of 'acquired immunodeficiency' or 'immuno-privilege'.[9] Cutaneous immune responses in breast cancer-related lymphoedema are significantly impaired in the oedematous arms.[10]

Prevalence

In one series 24% of 131 primary lymphoedema patients developed AIE, whereas only 5% of 37 patients with lymphoedema after cancer treatment did.[11] A higher incidence of AIE in primary lymphoedema was also found in another series attending two different lymphoedema clinics in the UK.[12] Of

402 patients attending the London clinic, 23% had experienced at least one AIE; of 99 Newcastle patients the figure was 32%. In both clinics primary lymphoedema patients were more likely to suffer cellulitis than patients with secondary lymphoedema. The chronicity of the swelling affected prevalence; the longer the duration of oedema the more likely were AIE to occur.

AIE of the arm after curative treatment for breast cancer was reported in 15/273 patients (6%) over 42 months.[13] All patients with AIE had lymphoedema. The mean interval between cancer surgery and the AIE was 38 months. In another series 41% of patients with postmastectomy lymphoedema developed an AIE. Interestingly, AIE occurred in 63% of patients who developed lymph-oedema > 1 year after cancer treatment compared with 35% who developed lymphoedema < 1 year after mastectomy.[14] There are also reports of breast AIE after breast radiation for cancer. It is likely that impaired lymph drainage from the breast predisposes to AIE because breast oedema often co-exists.[15] Distinction from an erythematous radiation reaction (i.e. skin burn) may be difficult.

Of more than 300 women who had had a hysterectomy with pelvic lymph-adenectomy, only 9 patients developed leg AIE, all of whom had received radiation therapy.[16]

Causes

The naïve view of AIE is that stagnant lymph fluid provides an ideal medium for bacterial growth. The reality is almost certainly more complex. The low yield of bacteria in microbiological specimens does not necessarily exclude infection and the good response of AIE to penicillin in most initial episodes, and as prophylaxis for recurrent episodes, supports the view that bacteria are a causal agent.

The substantial number of non-group A Streptococci isolated from AIE asociated with lymphoedema suggests that opportunistic infection as a result of the 'regional immunodeficiency' may be a factor. In classical cellulitis of a limb, organisms other than group A Streptococci and *Staphylococcus aureus* are rarely found.[3] Pathogenic mechanisms responsible for cellulitis by non-group A Streptococci in lymphoedema are not understood.

Streptococcal pyogenic exotoxins are capable of causing inflammation which may be partly direct toxicity and partly hypersensitivity. In experimental animals such exotoxins have been shown to enhance hypersensitivity reactions against unrelated proteins such as purified protein derivatives of *Mycobacterium tuberculosis* and enhance the development of passive Arthus reactions to antigen–antibody complexes. The extent to which Streptococcal pyogenic exotoxins are involved in any form of cellulitis remains speculative.[17]

It is assumed that the portal of entry for the infection in AIE is through the skin, hence the recommendation for good skin care and hygiene in all patients with lymphoedema. Only a minority of patients, however, notice a direct relationship between an accidental penetrating injury and subsequent AIE. The majority of patients receive no warning of an impending attack. There is certainly a widely held belief that breaches in skin integrity from dermatitis, fungal infection (tinea pedis), and at points of lymphorrhoea (lymph leakage) increase the likelihood of AIE.[18] Some patients notice a relationship between foci of infection elsewhere, such as pharyngitis or dental infection, and the onset of an AIE.

It has been suggested that, once infection has gained entry to lymph-oedematous tissue, it is never fully eradicated but remains quiescent with varying episodes of re-activation – somewhat akin to herpes simplex. It is my experience that a relapse often occurs on discontinuation of phenoxy-methylpenicillin even after successful prophylaxis for 1–2 years. In some patients, circumstances such as long car journeys, excessive exercise and even treatment with multilayer lymphoedema bandaging (MLLB) can precipitate AIE, despite good skin care.

Predisposing factors

Predisposing factors for recurrent AIE include:

- penetrating skin injury
- weeping skin lymphangiomas (lymphorrhoea)
- fungal skin infection (tinea pedis)
- skin disease in general
- elephantiasis.

Tinea pedis is an almost constant association of leg lymphoedema (Plate 9.2). Although the close apposition of swollen toes leading to skin maceration may be the main causal factor, underlying immunodeficiency is also likely to contribute. In one report, all 25 cases of recurrent 'lymphangitis' had co-existent fungal infection of their feet. Of the 15 patients in whom fungal infection was eradicated none had further AIE. The remainder, in whom the fungus persisted, continued to have AIE.[18]

Acute fungal infection is best treated either with topical or oral terbinafine. Long-term, half-strength Whitfield's ointment is recommended at night as prophylaxis. For deep cracks and crevices where bacteria readily colonise, regular hygiene is necessary followed by an antiseptic drying agent, for example, eosin, brilliant green or magenta paint.

It is commonsense not only to treat skin fungal infection but any dermatitis which results in a breach of skin integrity so permitting entry of micro-organisms. Persistent or relapsing dermatitis, particularly of the blistering type on palms or soles will frequently result in lymphangitis. If lymphoedema exists, a vicious circle of recurrent AIE and deteriorating oedema will be established. Dermatological advice with regard to the control of dermatitis is essential.

Weeping lymphangiomas can be difficult to control. Compression should be first-line treatment but if this fails or they exist at sites where compression is not possible, for example genitalia, then gentle cautery or LASER therapy under anaesthetic may be necessary.

The fact that AIE are sometimes induced by multilayer lymphoedema bandaging (MLLB), excessive walking or a long car journey suggests that continuing infection may exist in a quiescent form ready to erupt at any time in the right circumstances. Such a scenario would parallel recurrent attacks of herpes simplex, for example cold sores, but there is no evidence that AIE are viral in origin.

Tropical elephantiasis

Fever is the earliest symptom of filariasis. Severe rigors and fever precede tender lymph nodes, generally accompanied by lymphangitis. Such attacks respond well to diethylcarbamazepine indicating that microfilaraemia is the cause. Secondary bacterial infections frequently complicate filarial lymphoedema and are the result of lymphatic obstruction, not specifically the filariasis. Nonetheless, distinction may not be easy and the term *episodic dermatolymphangio-adenitis* (DLA) has been coined to describe the clinical features ranging from skin changes to inflamed lymph vessels and nodes. Bacteria can be cultured from tissue fluid, lymph and lymph nodes. The term DLA should be reserved for the chonic inflammatory, episodically-exacerbated changes in lymph-oedema presenting as erythema of the skin in the swollen limb with red streaks along the superficial lymphatics and enlarged painful regional nodes.[19]

Non-filarial or endemic elephantiasis arises from the uptake of microparticles of silica and aluminosilicates through the soles of the feet (*podoconiosis*).[20] Acute episodes characteristically occur when one leg begins to swell and feels hot, and the groin nodes are swollen. Fever, rigors, headache and malaise accompany the local symptoms. Although attacks resemble AIE, antibiotics do not seem to influence the course of the episode. Interestingly, the condition may be associated with excessive use of the leg or after an excess of alcohol. The frequency of episodes varies from one a month to occasional attacks, depending on the activity of the patient. Each attack results in worsening of the lymphoedema.

Diagnosis

AIE are easily diagnosed when accompanied by constitutional upset, fever and rigors. If constitutional upset is minimal, distinction from other forms of inflammation such as thrombophlebitis or dermatitis is not easy. Occasionally erythema may not be evident and the suspicion of cellulitis is based solely on pain and increased swelling.

As in classical cellulitis, identification of an infectious agent is unlikely and the decision to treat is based on clinical judgement. Exclusion of alternative diagnoses such as deep vein thrombosis (DVT) using compression ultrasonography may be necessary. In one study the differentiation between AIE and DVT was investigated by measuring the protein concentration of oedema fluid. Values were significantly higher in AIE with no overlap between high tissue fluid protein concentrations in AIE and the much lower ones in DVT.[21] In the leg, skin changes associated with varicose dermatitis or lipodermatosclerosis may cause confusion because they can predispose to AIE (Plate 9.3).

Management

The acute episode

Treatment of a single AIE does not differ from treatment for classical acute cellulitis, i.e. rest and antibiotics. In severe cases, when there is marked systemic upset and concern for the patient's welfare, admission to hospital and IV benzylpenicillin is advisable. The addition of flucloxacillin may be sensible as cover for *Staphyloccocus aureus* (Figure 9.1).

Penicillin, however, may fail to control severe Streptococcal infection. This is probably due to a reduction of penicillin-binding proteins and/or too low a dose. The greater efficacy of clindamycin in experimental models of Streptococcal infection is probably related to its mechanism of action – the inhibition of protein synthesis including that of bacterial toxins. It is recommended in addition to penicillin in severe cases.[22]

Although exercise as a stimulant to lymph flow is always recommended as treatment for lymphoedema, rest is essential (and should be enforced) during an AIE. Anecdotal evidence for this was provided by a doctor with lower limb lymphoedema and an AIE. In an attempt to continue working, and after two courses of oral antibiotics, he self-administered IV benzylpenicillin and flucloxacillin but after 2 weeks was no better. At this point he came to see me. He had a swollen, red leg which was hot and tender up to the knee. He had a low-grade pyrexia and was exhausted. A Doppler examination excluded thrombosis. Bed rest with leg elevation for 48 hours produced a

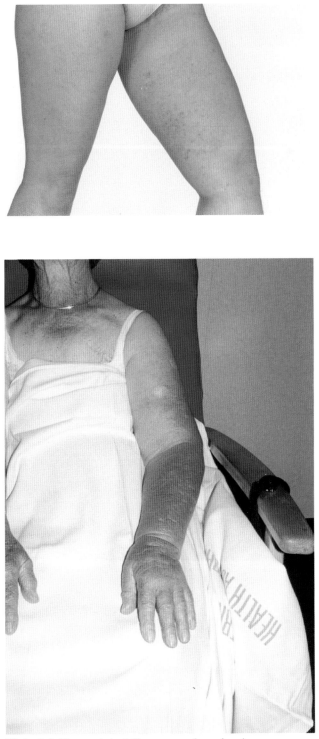

Plate 9.1 The rash in AIE can vary from focal inflammatory spots (above) to confluent erythema (below).

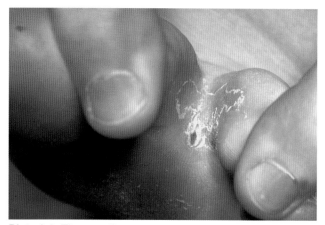

Plate 9.2 Tinea pedis.

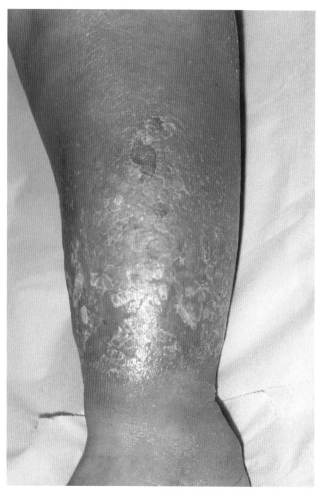

Plate 9.3 Lipodermatosclerosis.

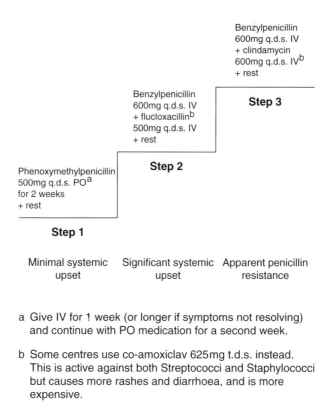

a Give IV for 1 week (or longer if symptoms not resolving)
   and continue with PO medication for a second week.

b Some centres use co-amoxiclav 625mg t.d.s. instead.
   This is active against both Streptococci and Staphylococci
   but causes more rashes and diarrhoea, and is more
   expensive.

Figure 9.1   3-step treatment ladder for AIE.

dramatic recovery and confirmed the importance of traditional rest for settling inflammation. At what point should exercise to stimulate lymph drainage be re-introduced is a question of judgement as is the re-application of compression garments.

Recurrent AIE

Although there is general agreement that AIE should be prevented, no randomised controlled trials of prophylaxis exist. Accepted practice is to give long-term penicillin. In one open prospective study of long-acting, benzathine penicillin 1 200 000 units IM was given every 3 weeks for 1 year.[23] AIE were abolished in 41/45 patients. Interestingly, some patients continue to suffer 'breakthrough' attacks of inflammation despite penicillin, and it is not unusual for AIE to recur as soon as prophylaxis ceases. In the UK, common practice is to use oral phenoxymethylpenicillin 500–1000mg/day. Experience suggests that stronger broad-spectrum antibiotics convey no additional benefit but trial data are lacking.

There is a general belief that a reduction in oedema through physical therapy reduces the incidence of AIE. In one prospective open study of 229 consecutive patients treated with manual lymphatic drainage (MLD) massage and MLLB, remedial exercise and skin care, with a maintenance regimen of compression garment, exercise and nocturnal bandaging, the incidence of 'infection' decreased from 1.1 attacks per patient per year to 0.65.[24] Other groups have also reported similar reductions in the incidence of AIE after physical therapy.[25]

Conclusion

There are clearly deficiencies in our knowledge of the cause(s) of AIE, and therefore of their management. Even so, education of patients and families (and of health professionals generally) about the importance of prompt antibiotic treatment and rest will help considerably to reduce the severity of these episodes and their sequelae in terms of increased fibrosis and more treatment-resistant swelling.

References

1   Casley-Smith JR et al. (1985) Summary of the 10th International Congress of Lymphology Working Group Discussions and Recommendations, Adelaide, Australia, August 10–17. Lymphology. 18:175–80.
2   Highet AS et al. (1992) Bacterial infections. In: RH Champion, JL Burton, FJG Ebling (eds) Textbook of Dermatology, 5th edn. Blackwell Scientific Publications, Oxford, pp 968–73.
3   Hook EW et al. (1986) Microbiologic evaluation of cutaneous cellulitis in adults. Archives of Internal Medicine. 146:295–7.
4   Bernard P et al. (1989) Streptococcal cause of erysipelas and cellulitis in adults. Archives of Dermatology. 125:779–82.
5   Edwards EA (1963) Recurrent febrile episodes in lymphoedema. Journal of the American Medical Association. 184:858–62.
6   Streilen JW et al. (1980) Langerhans cells: functional aspects revealed by in-vivo grafting studies. Journal of Investigative Dermatology. 75:17–21.
7   Barker CF and Billingham RE (1968) The role of afferent lymphatics in the rejection of skin homografts. Journal of Experimental Medicine. 128:197–221.
8   Futtrell JW and Myers GH (1972) Role of the regional lymphatics in tumour allograft rejection. Transplantation. 13:551–7.
9   Futtrell JW and Myers GH (1972) The burn scar as an immunologically privileged site. Surgical Forum. 23:129–31.

10 Mallon E *et al.* (1997) Evidence for altered cell mediated immunity in post-mastectomy lymphoedema. *British Journal of Dermatology.* **137**:928–33.

11 Schriger A *et al.* (1965) Acute lymphangitis and cellulitis – diagnosis and therapy. *Minnesota Medicine.* **48**:191–4.

12 Badger C (1997) A study of the efficacy of multi-layer bandaging and elastic hosiery in the treatment of lymphoedema and their effects on the swollen limb. PhD Thesis, University of London.

13 Simon MS and Cody RL (1992) Cellulitis after axillary lymph node dissection for carcinoma of the breast. *American Journal of Medicine.* **93**:543–8.

14 Mozes M *et al.* (1982) The role of infections in postmastectomy lymphedema. *Surgery Annual.* **14**:73–83.

15 Hughes LL *et al.* (1997) Cellulitis of the breast as a complication of breast conserving surgery and irradiation. *American Journal of Clinical Oncology.* **20**:338–41.

16 Dankert J and Bouma J (1987) Recurrent acute leg cellulitis after hysterectomy with pelvic lymphadenectomy. *British Journal of Obstetrics and Gynaecology.* **94**:788–90.

17 Baddour LM and Bisno AL (1985) Non-group A beta-hemolytic streptococcal cellulitis. *American Journal of Medicine.* **79**:155–9.

18 Young JR and de Wolfe VG (1960) Recurrent lymphangitis of the leg associated with dermatophytosis: report of 25 consecutive cases. *Cleveland Clinic Quarterly.* **27**:19–24.

19 Olszewski WL *et al.* (1994) Bacteriological studies of skin tissue fluid and lymph in filarial lymphoedema. *Lymphology.* **27**:345–8.

20 Price EW (1990) *Podoconiosis: Non-Filarial Elephantiasis.* Oxford University Press, Oxford.

21 Berlyne GM *et al.* (1989) Oedema protein concentrations for differentiation of cellulitis and deep vein thrombosis. *Lancet.* **2**:728–9.

22 Bisno AL and Stevens DL (1996) Streptococcal infections of skin and soft tissues. *New England Journal of Medicine.* **334**:240–5.

23 Olszewski WL (1996) Episodic dermatolymphangioadenitis (DLA) in patients with lymphoedema of the lower extremities and benzathine penicillin administration. *Scope – on Phlebology and Lymphology.* **3(4)**:20–24.

24 Ko DSC *et al.* (1998) Effective treatment of lymphedema of the extremities. *Archives of Surgery.* **133**:452–8.

25 Földi E (1996) Prevention of dermatolymphangioadenitis by combined physiotherapy of the swollen arm after treatment for breast cancer. *Lymphology.* **29**:48–9.

10   Exercise and lymphoedema

Karen Hughes

Exercise is universally considered to be an important component of the conservative management of lymphoedema. There is, however, a dearth of published data about it or evidence of efficacy. In approaching the subject of exercise in lymphoedema, it is essential to understand the complexity of movement and its probable effects on oedema if patients are to be given correct and relevant advice. This chapter provides background information about the effect of different types of muscle activity on both the vascular and the lymphatic circulations.

Effect of exercise on the circulation to the limbs

Arterial supply

Arteries supply nutrients and oxygen to all parts of the body. The walls of arteries are thick and muscular and maintain their patency during muscle contraction. Pressure exerted by contraction of the left ventricle drives the blood around the body rhythmically. Skeletal muscle has an excellent arterial supply. The more work a muscle does the greater the need for nutrients and oxygen. To meet this demand the body diverts more arterial blood to the muscles and the heart beats faster. Lymph formation is directly proportional to arterial flow (*see* Chapter 4); hence the more vigorous the activity the more lymph is formed.

In an average day, 40% of the body's lymph is formed within skeletal muscle.[1,2] Muscles can work anaerobically for short periods but then demand a very high arterial supply to restore the metabolic equilibrium. Patients should be advised not to exercise too vigorously or for too long or their swelling will increase as a result of extra lymph formation. Further, overexertion of the muscles leads to a build-up of lactic acid. This causes arterial vasodilation and increased arterial flow but, if pain is limiting movement, there is no compensatory increase in venous return.

Venous return

It is essential for patients with lymphoedema to maximise venous return, even though this can never fully compensate for poor lymphatic drainage. On average at rest, 60% or more of the blood is in the venous system.[3] The veins act as a reservoir for storing blood, particularly in the legs. The blood is stored in superficial capacitance veins which are small but numerous. These play an important part in regulating venous return to the right atrium; they lie outside the deep connective tissue fascia which surrounds the muscle compartment and their capacity to expand is therefore not restricted.

The deep transport veins lie within the muscle compartment, mostly between individual muscles. The muscle itself is drained by small veins which empty directly into the large transport veins. The position of the transport veins means that they inevitably respond to muscular movement.

Perforating veins connect the two systems. These pass obliquely through the connective tissue and are occluded when a muscle contraction tenses the fascia (Figure 10.1). The walls of veins have weak muscles and are unable to pump blood upwards by their own action. The muscles in the vein wall will maintain the integrity of the vein if the applied external pressure is low, and so allow the veins to redistribute blood to compensate for postural changes. Valves determine the direction of flow and allow blood to flow only in the direction of the heart. Blood from the head and neck is drained by gravity and the veins in this region contain few valves. Venous return from all other areas of the body generally takes place against gravity, and relies on external pressure being applied to the veins.[4,5] For blood to be returned to the heart

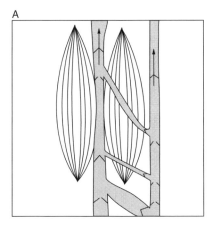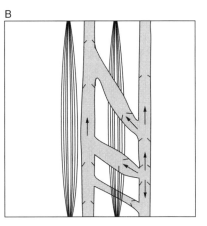

Figure 10.1 The venous leg pump.
A Every time the leg muscles contract the veins are compressed, pushing the blood upwards.
B Every time the leg muscles relax blood is sucked in from the periphery.

against gravity, the external hydrodynamic pressure needed to force fluid from an area of high pressure to an area of low pressure must exceed the hydrostatic (gravitational) pressure. In the average human, the hydrostatic pressure from the heel to the diaphragm is about 120cm H_2O.[6] The necessary hydrodynamic pressure is less than this because of the residual arterial pressure transmitted to the venous capillaries and the negative pressure applied by the diaphragm on inspiration. As the diaphragm moves down and the chest wall out, a negative pressure (potential vacuum) is formed in the thorax which results in inspiration. At the same time, the negative pressure pulls the blood in the veins up towards the heart. This has most effect on the thoracic venous drainage.

The hydrodynamic pressure achieved by the body is far in excess of the body's needs under normal circumstances. Elongated bodies have maximum volume when they are cylindrical. At rest, veins are circular in cross-section and deformity of the veins as a result of pressure from contracting muscles or movement will cause an increase in pressure within the veins. Provided there are properly functioning venous valves, fluid will move to an area of lower pressure, i.e. towards the heart. When the pressure is removed the veins return to their normal state and refill by drawing fluid from the veins below, again moving fluid from an area of high pressure to an area of low pressure. The greater the movement or the stronger the muscle contraction the greater the hydrodynamic force. Further, each time the foot strikes the ground, the veins in the foot contract and propel blood into the lower leg.[7] This is important because the muscles of the foot are small and there is relatively little movement in the foot compared with the leg.

Venous return is increased by a combination of movement and muscle activity. It is therefore important to maintain a good range of movement and normal muscle tone. Movement is optimum when it is slow and rhythmical. This enhances the emptying and refilling of the deep veins (which drives blood out of the limb) and allows the superficial veins to empty into the deep veins via the perforating veins. During prolonged isometric activity (*see* p.145), the perforating veins are occluded as they pass through the deep fascia; this prevents drainage and increases the pressure in the superficial veins. This will cause difficulty with the uptake of fluid into the venous capillaries in the skin and lead to an increased load on the lymphatic system.

In addition, by resting the limb in elevation with the foot above the level of the heart, hydrostatic pressure will act in the required direction of blood flow and so reduce the need for the muscle pump. Resting in this position will also reduce capillary filtration because of a decrease in the arterial capillary pressure now that arterial flow is having to work against hydrostatic pressure.

Lymphatic return

The lymphatic system is fundamentally different from the venous system in that the larger vessels and collectors have a well-developed smooth muscle wall. Lymphatic return is influenced by three main forces:

- *vis a tergo* (literally, compulsion from behind)
- *extrinsic pump*
- *intrinsic pump.*

Vis a tergo is a classical term used to describe lymph flow from an area of high lymphatic pressure in the initial lymphatics to an area of low pressure in the ascending thoracic duct, particularly on inspiration.[8] However, this alone would not account for the flow because pressures required to shift fluid would exceed any decrease in pressure between the initial lymphatics and the thoracic duct. Further, direct measurements have shown that the pressure in the initial lymphatics is lower than in the thoracic duct for most of the respiratory cycle.[9]

Inspiration has a major effect on thoracic lymphatic drainage because of the proximity of the vessels to the heart and where the hydrostatic pressure requirements are low. Sudden increases in intra-abdominal pressure such as occur with coughing and laughing will greatly increase abdominal drainage and empty the cisterna chyli.

There is controversy about whether the extrinsic or intrinsic pump has the most effect on lymphatic return from the limbs. In practice, this is not a problem because both are helped by slow rhythmical movement. In relation to the extrinsic pump, the pressure applied to veins by muscle contractions, movement, arterial pulsation and respiration push fluid from the limb in the direction of the heart.[10,11] This mechanism is important when lymphatics travel adjacent to contracting muscles. For the extrinsic pump to function effectively, the initial lymphatics must open when the pressure in the tissues is low during periods of rest and close when the pressure is high during exercise. Alternating pressures cause the initial lymphatics to act as tiny pumps and propel the lymph towards the collecting vessels. It is well-recognised that paralysed limbs swell, supporting the concept of a functional extrinsic pump. Indeed, it has been recognised for more than a century that there is little lymph flow in the resting limb.[12] Studies have shown that movement and muscle contraction are important for both the uptake of lymph into the initial lymphatics and the propulsion of lymph through collecting and transport vessels in a similar manner to veins.[10,11] *Advise on exercise given for improving venous return is applicable to lymphatic return.*

Lymphatics also have an intrinsic pump.[13-15] The lymphatics contract spontaneously to propel lymph from the periphery. When lymphatics contract and move fluid towards the heart they produce a negative pressure in the initial lymphatics which 'pulls' lymph in from the surrounding tissues. It has been shown that in the initial lymphatics the pressure is lower than that in the surrounding tissues over a substantial portion of the contraction cycle. This has led to the conclusion that the intrinsic muscle pump is more important than the extrinsic pump. During muscle contraction the frequency of pulsation can increase 6–10 times.[16,17] Increases in intraluminal pressure of the lymphatics have been shown to increase both the frequency and amplitude of contractions of this pump. There is an increase in protein uptake when exercising in rigid bandages (see p.173). There is also an increase in lymphatic flow without any movement from an area with a local increase in temperature.

It has been shown, in patients suffering from lymphoedema, that these spontaneous contractions can be absent and, because of changes in pressures, the extrinsic pump may play a more important role.[13] It is believed that passive movements of the limb will also increase the contractions of the intrinsic pump.

Movement between the skin and the underlying tissues is essential for the filling of the initial lymphatics. This has been shown in studies on massage and the uptake of lymph (see p.204).[18] The skin is a very mobile organ and slides over the underlying tissues as the body moves but becomes less mobile during inactivity or during sustained muscle contractions. It is therefore essential that any muscle activity produces skin movement.

If the body does not move normally there tends to be minor trauma on movement. If trauma occurs more lymph is produced. Trauma will also occur in limbs which are not adequately supported at rest.

The circulation is under the control of the sympathetic nervous system. Patients who have had radiotherapy may have some damage to this system and responses to change in activity or the environment may be absent or take longer to initiate.[19,20]

Muscles and movement

The body moves in a very complex way and exercise programmes must be planned to encourage a good pattern of movement.

Definitions of muscle activity[21]

Muscle contractions are of two main types:

- *isotonic contraction* which constitutes an increase in intramuscular tension accompanied by a change in the length of a muscle to either lengthen or shorten a muscle
- *isometric contraction* which involves the development of a force by an increase in intramuscular tension without any change in muscle length.

There are three main forms of muscle work:

- *static muscle work*, when muscles contract isometrically to counter-balance opposing forces and maintain stability. The contraction needed will increase with increasing load, e.g. when using heavy weights
- *concentric muscle work*, when a muscle contracts isotonically and *shortens* to produce movement. The origin and insertion of the muscle are drawn together in the direction of muscle pull
- *eccentric muscle work*, when a muscle contracts isotonically and *lengthens*. The origin and insertion are drawn apart as the muscle works to oppose a force which is greater than its own contraction. Movement is in the direction of the opposing force and in the opposite direction to the muscle pull.

Muscles generally act in groups. Muscles will act in one of four ways to produce efficient, controlled and functional movement. Movement will take place in different groups in different ways at the same time:

- *agonists* (prime movers) are the muscles which contract concentrically to provide the force required to produce the required movement
- *antagonists* are the muscles which act eccentrically to inhibit and control the prime mover or oppose an outside force, e.g. gravity
- *synergists* work with the agonists to provide a suitable background of activity and to facilitate movement; they act so as to modify the direction of pull of the agonist and to stabilise a joint when a muscle acts over more than one joint
- *fixators* work to stabilise the bones of origin of the other muscle groups and to increase the efficiency of movement and the stability of the body as a whole. They can be used to fixate the body in such a way that the agonist can effectively reverse the function of its origin and insertion. This type of work is always static. For controlled movement, the fixators should be initiated fractionally before the other groups (Boxes 10.A and 10.B).

Box 10.A   Flexing the elbow with no rotation with the arm held in the anatomically neutral position

Biceps and brachialis act as the *agonist* group; these muscles also act as forearm pronators and shoulder flexors.

Triceps act as an *antagonist* controlling the rate of flexion.

The *synergists* are the shoulder extensors and the forearm supinators, in this case acting concentrically and statically.

The *fixators* are the rotator cuff muscles and the scapula stabilisers, providing a stable origin for the prime movers.

If the arm is moved out to the side for this activity, the deltoid becomes first a *prime mover* but then works extremely hard as a *fixator* for the activity to take place. If the arm is carrying a weight, the activity increases in the agonist, synergist and fixator groups but decreases in the antagonist group.

When activity is in the same direction as gravity, such as the elbow extension in the same starting position, there is no prime mover because gravity takes on this function and the original agonists will act eccentrically for control.

Box 10.B   Flexing the knee while lying prone on a plinth

The *agonists* are the hamstrings; these muscles also act as hip extensors.

The *antagonists* are the quadriceps to help control the rate of flexion.

The *synergists* are the hip flexors, which include the quadriceps which now acts in two capacities.

The *fixators* are the large muscles of the trunk, which fix the pelvis and the muscles of the hip and so fix the position of the femur.

If the same action is performed sitting on the edge of a chair, gravity becomes the *prime mover* until the knee reaches 90° of flexion after which the hamstrings again become the *prime mover.*

Imagine the same exercise when standing. The side flexors on the opposing side of the body at first become *prime movers* to shift weight and then become very powerful *fixators* to balance the body.

Unless people are very co-ordinated, they find it difficult to stand on one leg for more than 30–60 seconds and the muscles of the shoulder girdle and arms are brought into play as fixators.

In general the fixators are the deeper muscles and the prime movers are the large superficial muscles. When looking at exercise and lifestyle it is important to look at the activity as a whole and not just at the prime movers, particularly if certain tasks are noted to be causing an increase in swelling.

Evaluation

Patients should be evaluated on the first visit and subsequently monitored to ascertain any changes in movement ability. Changes reflect either deterioration (as a result of radiation fibrosis, recurrent disease, increasing oedema etc.) or improvement (less oedema and a decrease in fibrosis).

Evaluation must include the following in comparison with the unaffected limb taking normal ranges into consideration:

- posture, particularly the position of the pelvis/shoulder girdle
- joint range[22]
- muscle power[11]
- function
- ease of movement[23]
- changes in sensation.

Ideally the evaluation should test myofascial length, adverse neural tension and normal movement patterns.[24,25]

It is necessary to check that the patient is not using extra movements of the trunk to compensate for decreased range, for example side flexion to increase shoulder abduction and back extension to compensate for poor hip extension.

Swollen limbs should move in the same pattern and plane as the unaffected limb. Generally, a dominant limb is stronger than the non-dominant limb. In longstanding oedema the body may compensate for the extra weight by increasing muscle bulk, or there may be muscle wastage as a feature of the lymphoedema.[11]

Management

People with lymphoedema should be advised to rest with their affected limb in elevation, ideally with the hand/foot above the level of the heart. This will maximise both lymphatic and venous return as well as reducing capillary bed pressure in the arteries.

Positioning

Positioning of the leg

It is impossible to raise the foot above the level of the heart when sitting. Even so, when sitting the leg should be supported on a stool or equivalent. Ideally the leg should be supported along its entire length with the knee in slight flexion. If the knee is straight, the patient will slump to release the stretch on the sciatic nerve and the hamstring muscles causing discomfort in the lumbar spine. Practical strategies need to be worked out with patients. These could include a foot-stool under the desk at work and repositioning furniture, together with a general review of daily routine.

At night, limb elevation can be achieved by standing the end of the bed on 7–10cm blocks or placing a pillow under the mattress at the foot-end of the bed. It is important not to raise the bed too high or venous return from the head and neck will be reduced. The ideal position is lying with the trunk horizontal, the head on a pillow and the legs elevated up to 60° of hip flexion. This position is easily achieved, for example when watching television, by lying on a couch with the leg supported by pillows on the arm of the couch. It is best to avoid standing still for long periods. This is not always possible, so patients should be advised to stand on tiptoe every few minutes to activate the muscle pump.

Positioning of the arm

The arm should be supported along its length (including the hand) with the shoulder at approximately 90°. *The arm must not be raised above this position otherwise the first rib moves up towards the clavicle and obstructs the venous return from the arm.* It can also be extremely uncomfortable and may lead to neural symptoms. Appropriate elevation can easily be achieved by placing a pillow on the arm of a chair, when sitting at home etc. At work, the arm can be rested on the arm of a chair.

It is important not to let the arm hang down for long periods. This can be achieved by tucking the hand in a pocket or the front of a coat, or by supporting the arm with the other limb. If the arm has to hang at the side of the body for any period, making a fist and then stretching out the fingers every few minutes helps to reduce fluid collection. A hanging position must be avoided at all costs in the flaccid limb because of the risk of subluxation of the shoulder. When active, a sling should be used to prevent this.

Exercise programmes

The following points should be noted (*see* Appendix 1–3):

- patients should always exercise wearing external support (*see* pp 173 and 193)

- patients should be given an exercise programme to be followed each day at a time which is convenient to their routine

- patients with specific problems of decreased movement or pain should be referred for specialised physiotherapy

- previous musculoskeletal conditions such as rheumatoid arthritis, neck pain and back pain must be considered

- exercise programmes should always be tailored to the individual patient's need taking their age, fitness and general health into account

- avoid static exercise as much as possible. This can be quite difficult if doing strengthening exercises, e.g. straight leg raising. If isometric activity is necessary, intersperse with isotonic activity and periods of rest

- lower quadrant exercises should to a large extent be aimed at strength while upper quadrant exercises should be aimed at mobility

- starting positions for exercise should always be such that the fixators need to do minimal work. In general this is achieved by supporting the limb proximal to the area being exercised, e.g. placing an arm on a pillow or cushion while the hand is exercised

- exercises should be slow and rhythmical with rest periods. For instance, in bending and straightening the elbow, it is important to relax after straightening because only one group of muscles (the elbow flexors) has been used

- all joints in the affected quadrant should be moved through the pain-free range

- pushing into the painful range can cause trauma and increase oedema

- all muscle groups in the affected quadrant should be used through the pain-free range, e.g. straightening the arm above the head or against gentle resistance to exercise the triceps

- programmes should be easy to follow and not too time-consuming

- it is important that the patient moves normally and 'trick' movements are avoided, e.g. side flexion to give the appearance of increased shoulder flexion

- it is important that patients maintain a good posture during their exercise programme because this will carry forward into other activities. Good posture promotes good quality movement and this is important for preventing soft tissue injury
- exercise programmes should include deep breathing exercises to promote good thoracic venous and lymphatic return.

Passive exercise

Patients with a significant degree of paralysis as a result of nerve injury should have the affected limb(s) moved passively. The movements should be slow and rhythmical with the limb well-supported. The joints should be moved through the pain-free range and with surrounding joints in several different positions to prevent muscle shortening. There is no evidence to indicate what number of repetitions is ideal.

Advice to patients

The following advice should be given to patients:

- patients should be warned against the dangers of overvigorous activity and static activity, e.g. carrying heavy bags. Coping strategies could be to load shopping into lots of relatively small bags at the supermarket for easy transfer into the car
- patients need to understand the importance of maintaining normal muscle tone so that muscles can support the veins and lymphatics
- patients need to be educated about the importance of posture and maintaining a good range of movement. Practical strategies might include a correctly positioned keyboard, cues to correct posture and set times to move the limb during the day
- it is impossible to avoid all static activity and patients should be advised to grip and relax the hand or move the foot slowly up and down during these times and have a period of rest with the limb elevated once the task is completed
- discussion on lifestyle and work is essential so that activities can be managed with the minimal detrimental effect on swelling. Practical strategies could be to change the position of a filing cabinet, so that heavy repetitive work is done by the normal arm, and for manual workers to plan tasks so that heavy activities are interspersed with gentler activities. Gardening

can be broken into areas of the garden so digging is alternated with pruning and weeding, and similar strategies can be devised for housework

- sport can be a difficult area for some people. A sport should be taken up gently, gradually building up until it has a detrimental effect on the oedema. As fitness improves, patients may be able to increase their activity. The level achieved varies and much support is needed through this period. The patient may benefit from higher compression garments during sporting activities. Contact sports such as football can lead to an increased risk of infection. All sports carry a risk of trauma which is likely to have an adverse effect on the swelling

- swimming is ideal exercise; as the body is supported by water, the need for the global fixators to work hard is considerably reduced. The water acts as gentle resistance and helps build up muscle tone. There is little risk of injury and the water gives some degree of external compression

- walking and cycling are good for patients with lower limb oedema because they are rhythmical and use the calf and foot muscle pumps; on the other hand, prolonged walking on hard surfaces such as pavements may lead to more swelling. This could be helped with advice on footwear, i.e. well-supporting cushioned heels

- exercise helps to prevent or reduce obesity. Obesity tends to exacerbate lymphoedema. Weight stability and loss can be helped by physical activity as well as a controlled diet.

Conclusion

It is important that discussion about changes in lifestyle stem from a clear theoretical knowledge about lymphoedema. For many patients work is essential both financially and psychologically. Co-operation with occupational health departments may enable many people to continue with their present employment. Hobbies and other interests can often be continued with some modification. Contact sports are best avoided because of the risk of injury. Maintenance of good function is essential for quality of life. For patients who lack muscle strength and range of movement, adaptations recommended by occupational therapists often improve function. An acceptable level of function varies with each individual and advice should be given accordingly. The most important aspect of lymphoedema is patient education because people have to cope most of the time without immediate professional help. Patients need a good understanding of exercise and its effect on their swelling to be able to adapt their lifestyle with minimum detriment to quality of life.

References

1 Reed RK (1981) Interstitial fluid volume, colloid osmotic and hydrostatic pressures in rat skeletal muscle. Effects of the venous stasis and muscle activity. *Acta Physiologica Scandinavica.* **112**:7–17.

2 Aukland K (1989) *Textbook of Nephrology,* 2nd edn (Vol 1). Williams and Wilkins, Baltimore, p 214.

3 Hincliff S and Montague S (1988) *Physiology for Nursing Practice.* Ballière Tindall, London, pp 358–60.

4 Stuckmann J *et al.* (1986) Venous muscle pump function in patients with lymphoedema. *British Journal of Surgery.* **73**:886–7.

5 Qvarfordt P *et al.* (1983) Intramuscular pressure, venous function and muscle blood flow with lymphoedema of the leg. *Lymphology.* **Sept 16(13)**:139–42.

6 Holbaun G (1986) *Compression Stockings.* Schattner, New York, p 7.

7 Binns M and Pho R (1988) Anatomy of the venous foot pump. *Injury.* **19**:443–5.

8 Kampmeier OE (1969) *Evolution and Comparative Morphology of the Lymphatic System.* Thomas Springfield, Illinois.

9 Zweifach BW and Panther JW (1975) Micromanipulation of pressure in terminal lymphatics on mesentery. *American Journal of Physiology.* **228**:1326.

10 Kinmonth JB (1982) *The lymphatics – Surgery, Lymphography and Diseases of the Chyle and Lymph Systems,* 2nd edn. Edward Arnold, London, pp 80–1.

11 Casley-Smith JR and Casley-Smith JR (1997) *Modern Treatment for Lymphoedema.* Terrace Printing, Adelaide, pp 188–90.

12 Generish H (1879) Die Aufranhre der lymph dürsch die sehnew und Fascian der Skelettmuskein *Arb Physiol Anst.* **5**:53.

13 Olszewski WL (1991) *Lymphostasis, Pathophysiology, Diagnosis and Treatment.* CRC Press, Boca Raton, Florida, p 121.

14 Ferguson M (1992) Modulation of lymphatic smooth muscle contractile responses by the epithelium. *Journal of Surgery and Research.* **52**:359–63.

15 Szuba A and Rockson G (1997) Lymphoedema: anatomy and physiology and pathogenesis. *Vascular Medicine.* **2**:321–6.

16 Mason M (1993) *Exercise for Lymphoedema of the Arm.* Pirie Press, Adelaide, p 26.

17 Eisenhoff J *et al.* (1995) Importance of valves and lymphangion contractions in determining pressure gradients in isolated lymphatics exposed to elevations in outflow pressure. *Microvascular Research.* **49**:97–110.

18 Keeley V (1997) The pathophysiology of lymphoedema associated with treatment for breast cancer – recent developments. *Progress in Palliative Care.* **5(3)**:107–10.

19 Svensson W *et al.* (1994) Colour Doppler demonstrates venous flow abnormalities in breast cancer patients with chronic arm swelling. *European Journal of Cancer.* **30A(5)**:664–70.

20 Svensson W *et al.* (1994) Increase arterial inflow demonstrated by Doppler ultrasound in arm swelling following breast cancer treatment. *European Journal of Cancer.* **30A(5)**:661–4.

21 Gardiner MD (1971) *Principles of Exercise Therapy.* Bell and Sons, London pp 22–4.

22 Sugden EM *et al.* (1998) Shoulder movement after early treatment of breast cancer. *Clinical Oncology.* **10**:173–81.

23 Todd J (1999) A study of lymphoedema patients over their first six months of treatment. *Physiotherapy.* **85**:65–76.
24 Wall D and Melzach R (1992) *Textbook of Pain.* Churchill Livingstone, Edinburgh.
25 Bergmark A (1989) Stability of the lumbar spine. A study in mechanical engineering. *Acta Orthopaedica Scandinavica* (suppl). **230**:1–54.

Appendix I

Suggested exercises for patients with oedema

Exercise for the arm

It is important that any exercises performed should not cause pain.

Preparation

1 Plan to take 20 minutes.

2 Patients sit on armless chairs with their feet placed flat on the floor. If a chair is too high, place a pillow under the feet.

3 Encourage patients to maintain correct spinal curves throughout the exercise programme, e.g. sitting up straight and not slouching.

4 Accessory/extra movements such as side flexion, thoracic and lumbar extension, shoulder elevation, to give the appearance of extra range, should be avoided.

5 Support the affected limbs proximal to the joint being exercised.

6 Encourage patients to breathe normally throughout.

7 Advise patients to stop when the movement becomes painful.

8 The exercises should be slow and rhythmical.

I General

a Abdominal breathing – 3 sets of 5 breaths – avoid dizziness.

b   Flex alternative legs at the hips and knees and pull into abdomen using the arms (some patients find this very difficult).

c   Gentle posture correction – pelvis, lumbar spine, thoracic spine and neck. Correct curves should be maintained throughout the programme and a slumped posture should be avoided.

2 Neck

Only for patients with no history of rheumatoid arthritis or severe neck problems. Patients must stop if they become dizzy or lightheaded.

a   Flex the neck and lower the chin onto the chest wall and then extend the neck and look at the ceiling. Repeat 5 times.

b   Side flex the neck to the right and to the left. Avoid rotation. Repeat 5 times.

c   Rotate the head to the right then to the left. Repeat 5 times.

d   Circle the head to the right 5 times. Circle the head to the left 5 times.

3 Girdle

a   Elevate the shoulders then depress the shoulders. Repeat 10 times.

b   Protract the shoulders then retract the shoulders. Avoid elevation. Repeat 10 times.

c   Circle shoulders forwards. Repeat 10 times. Circle shoulders backwards. Repeat 10 times.

4 Shoulder and girdle

a   Elevate the arms through flexion – encouraging the patient to laterally rotate as they elevate then lower and extend the arm at the same time encouraging the arm to medially rotate. Keep the elbow relaxed. Repeat 10 times.

b   Elevate the arms through abduction again laterally rotating during elevation. Touch hands above the head if possible. Then lower and adduct the arms at the same time as medially rotating. Repeat 10 times.

c   Place hands behind the neck and then behind the back. Repeat 10 times.

d   For patients who are reasonably fit and who have good movement. With a straight arm – circle forwards 5 times. Circle backwards 5 times.

e   Breast stroke with shoulders at approximately 90°. Repeat 10 times.

5 Elbow

a   Start with the elbow bent and the forearm supinated ('palm-up'), then extend the elbow and pronate the forearm ('palm-down'). Repeat 20 times. Patients may find supination difficult when bandaged.

b   With the elbow supported with the opposite hand and flexed to 90° – pronate and supinate the forearm. Repeat 10 times right arm, then 10 times left arm.

6 Wrist

Supporting the forearm at the wrist with the opposite hand:

a   Flex and extend at the wrist keeping the fingers relaxed. Repeat 10 times right arm, then 10 times left arm.

b   Abduct (lateral side flexion) and adduct (medial side flexion) the wrist keeping the fingers relaxed. Repeat 10 times right arm, then 10 times left arm.

c   Circle the right wrist in one direction 10 times, then in the other direction 10 times. Repeat with the left wrist.

7 Hand and fingers

With the arm resting on a pillow on the knee:

a   Make a tight fist, then extend the fingers. Repeat 20 times.

b   Abduct (separate) and adduct (bring together) the fingers and thumb. Repeat 10 times.

c   Oppose the pad of the thumb to the pad of the little finger. Repeat 10 times.

d   With the wrist and the metacarpophalangeal (MCP) joints extended, flex the interphalangeal joints. Repeat 10 times.

e   With the interphalangeal joints extended, flex the MCP joints and extend the wrist. Repeat 10 times.

8 Stretches

a   Abduct the shoulder to 90° if possible, then extend and laterally rotate the arm at the shoulder, supinate the forearm, extend the elbow, wrist and fingers. Hold for a count of 10 and repeat 3 times. Repeat with opposite arm.

b   Flex the shoulders to 90° if possible and adduct the shoulders. Extend the elbows and hold the wrist in neutral. Then protract the shoulder girdle and hold for a count of 10. Repeat 3 times.

c   Make a fist and flex the wrist, then with an extended elbow extend and medially rotate at the shoulder. Hold for a count of 10 and repeat 3 times.

9 Relaxation

a   Sitting in a relaxed position with the hands on the abdomen, slowly breathe in and out using the diaphragm.

b   Imagine somewhere pleasant and sit quietly for a few minutes to allow heart rate and muscle tone to return to normal.

Exercise for the leg

These exercises should not be undertaken by patients with a history of severe back problems.

Preparation

1   Plan to take 20 minutes.

2   Good posture should be maintained at all times.

3   Avoid trick movements to compensate for normal movements, i.e. back extension, side flexion, rotation.

4   In lying – anterior iliac crests level with each other and approximately level with posterior iliac crest. In sitting – both feet placed evenly on the floor, hips and knees at approximately 90° – a pillow or foot-support may be needed for small patients. Good spinal curves and pelvic position. In standing – near a wall or plinth for support. Good pelvic position and correct spinal curves. It is often necessary to correct posture after each set of movements.

5 Support patient's limb proximal to the joint being exercised when practical.

6 Encourage patients to breathe normally.

7 Advise patients to stop when the movement becomes painful.

8 The exercises should be slow and rhythmical.

1 Supine lying

a Three sets of 5 deep abdominal breaths.

b Flex alternate hips and knees and gently draw into the abdomen applying pressure with the arms. Repeat 5 times. This is difficult for some patients and impossible in bandages.

2 Crook lying

a Posteriorly tilt the pelvis by flattening the back into the plinth then anteriorly tilt the pelvis by arching then flattening the back. Repeat 10 times.

b Flatten the back into the bed then slide hands forwards on the thighs. Repeat 10 times.

c Tighten the gluteal muscles and lift the pelvis off the bed to form a bridge. Hold for a count of 3 and lower. Repeat 10 times.

d Extend one leg, hold for a count of 3 then flex the knee to the starting position. Repeat with the opposite leg. Repeat 10 times.

3 Supine

a Hip hitch alternate legs. Repeat 10 times.

b Dorsiflex the feet and extend and lock the knees to clear the heel from the plinth with no hip movement. Hold for a count of 3 then relax. Repeat with alternate legs 10 times.

c As above then flex at the hip and lift heel 4 inches from the bed. Hold for a count of 3 then lower the leg slowly and relax. The calf should touch the bed before the heel. Repeat with alternate legs 10 times.

d As above but instead of hold then abduct, adduct the leg and return the hip to neutral before lowering. Repeat with alternate legs 10 times.

e Dorsiflex ('toes up') then plantar flex ('toes down') both feet. Repeat 10 times.

f Invert then evert both feet. Repeat 10 times.

g Circle feet 10 times in one direction then 10 times in the opposite direction.

4 Side lying with lower leg bent for support

a Abduct upper leg approximately 20°, hold for a count of 3 and slowly lower then relax for a count of 3. Repeat 10 times.

b As above but instead of hold, flex and extend hip before lowering the leg. Repeat 10 times. Lie on opposite side and repeat.

5 Prone lying with head turned to the side

a With knee flexed to 90°, extend the hip, hold for a count of 3, slowly lower then relax for a count of 3. Repeat with opposite leg. Repeat 10 times.

b As above but with knee extended. Repeat 10 times.

c Extend and flex alternate knees. Repeat 10 times.

6 4-point kneeling, i.e. crawling position (if able)

a Anteriorly and posteriorly tilt the pelvis by humping and hollowing the back. Repeat 10 times.

b Extend alternate hips and knees keeping pelvis even. Repeat 10 times.

7 Sitting

a While sitting in a chair, 'walk' legs backwards and forwards to encourage hip hitching. Repeat 10 times.

b With knees flexed to 90°, lift alternate legs by bending the hip. Repeat 10 times.

c Straighten the knee and lock, hold for a count of 3, then slowly bend the knee. Repeat with the opposite leg. Repeat 10 times.

d   Dorsiflex then plantar flex at the ankles. Repeat 10 times.

e   Invert then evert both feet. Repeat 10 times.

f   Circle feet 10 times in one direction then 10 times in the opposite direction.

g   With feet flat on the floor and the toes extended, flex at the tarsal/metatarsal joint and the metatarsal joints to raise the longitudinal arches of the feet. Repeat 10 times.

8 Standing

a   Hip hitch while keeping the shoulders level. Repeat 10 times on alternate legs.

b   Stand on alternate legs without pelvic drop on side of the raised leg. Repeat 10 times.

c   Stand on toes, hold for a count of 3, slowly lower and relax for a count of 3. Repeat 10 times.

d   Stand on the inside borders of both feet, hold for a count of 3, slowly lower and relax for a count of 3. Repeat 10 times.

e   With feet flat on the floor and the toes extended, flex at the tarsal/metatarsal joint and the metatarsal joints to raise the longitudinal arches of the feet. Repeat 10 times.

9 Relaxation

a   Gentle abdominal breathing.

b   Imagine somewhere pleasant and lie still for a few minutes to allow heart rate and muscle tone to return to normal.

Appendix 2

Suggested home exercise programme for patients with arm oedema

The sleeve or bandaging must be worn during exercising.

Exercise 1

Sit or lie in a relaxed position and gently rest the hands on the abdomen. Take gentle breaths so the abdomen rises on breathing in and falls on breathing out. Breathing in this way uses the deep areas of the lungs. Take 5 breaths.

Exercise 2

Sitting or lying, gently bend the hip and knee so that the thigh comes into contact with the abdomen. Gently increase the pressure on the abdomen by squeezing the knee gently against the abdomen with your hands. Repeat 3 times with each leg.

Exercise 3

Sitting in a relaxed position:

a   Gently raise the shoulders to the ears and then push the shoulders down as far as they will go. Repeat 5 times.

b   Gently brace the shoulders back as far as possible and then bring the shoulders forwards as far as possible. Repeat 5 times.

c   Gently circle the shoulders forwards. Repeat 5 times.

d   Gently circle the shoulders backwards. Repeat 5 times.

Exercise 4

Either standing or sitting forward in a dining chair. Take care to keep a good posture and do not lean back:

a   Lift both arms forward and then as high as possible above the head and then take both arms as far back as you can. The elbows should be kept straight but relaxed. Repeat 5 times.

b   Lift both arms out to the side and then touch the hands above the head. Bring both arms down and as far across the front of the body as possible. Repeat 5 times.

c   Reach as far behind the neck as possible and then as far up the back as possible. Repeat 5 times.

d   With the arm held straight circle the arm forwards. Repeat 5 times.

e   With the arm held straight circle the arm backwards. Repeat 5 times.

Only do exercises (d) and (e) if your shoulder moves freely and take care you have plenty of space.

Exercise 5

Sitting comfortably with the arm supported on the arm of a chair or a table:

a   Gently bend and straighten the elbow. Repeat 10 times.

b   Turn the palm of the hand to face up to the ceiling and then down to the floor. Repeat 10 times.

This exercise is difficult if the arm is in bandages.

Exercise 6

Sitting in a chair with the forearm supported on the arm of a chair or on a table with the hand free and the palm facing towards the floor:

a   Lift the hand as far back as it will go so that your fingers point up to the ceiling and then bend the hand as far as it will go so that your fingers point to the floor. Repeat 5 times.

b   Move the hand at the wrist from side to side. Take care not to move at the elbow. Repeat 5 times.

c   Circle the wrist 5 times in one direction and then 5 times in the opposite direction.

d   Make a tight fist and then straighten the fingers as far as possible. Repeat 5 times.

e   Make a fist and straighten the fingers individually. Repeat 3 times.

f   Touch the tip of the thumb to the tip of the little finger and then spread the fingers out. Repeat 5 times.

Exercise 7

Sitting in a chair or lying down shake the arms so they feel relaxed, take gentle breaths as in Exercise 1 and relax for a few minutes to let the heart rate return to normal.

Appendix 3

Suggested home exercise programme for patients with leg oedema

The exercise programme always begins with abdominal breathing. Either sitting in a chair or lying on a bed with the knees slightly bent place the hands gently on the abdomen. As you breathe in slowly let the abdomen rise and as you breathe out the abdomen will fall. Breathing in this way draws air to deep areas of the lungs. This can take a little practice. Take 5 breaths.

Again either sitting or lying, bend one leg at the hip and knee and gently squeeze the thigh into the abdomen using your arms. Repeat 3 times with each leg.

Exercise 1

Lying on your back with the knees bent and the feet on the bed:

a   Place one hand in the small of the back and tilt the pelvis so the small of the back presses into the hand and relax. Repeat 5 times.

b   Tilt the pelvis as above then slowly raise the bottom off the bed to make a bridge then lower and relax. Repeat 5 times.

c   Tilt the pelvis as before then gradually slide the hands up the thigh towards the knees and try to sit up. This will strengthen the abdominal muscles without putting strain on the lower back. You will not get a lot of movement. Repeat up to 10 times.

d   Straighten one leg, hold for a count of 3 and then bend the knee. Repeat 5 times with each leg.

Exercise 2

Lying flat on your back with your legs straight:

a Pull the foot towards you from the ankle, brace the knee back, hold for a count of 3 and relax. Repeat 5 times.

b Tighten the knee as above, then lift the heel about 4 inches off the ground, hold for a count of 5 and relax. Repeat 5 times.

c Tighten and lift as before, then take the leg out to the side, then across the body, back to the centre, lower and relax. Repeat 5 times.

d Move the foot slowly up and down at the ankle. Repeat 5 times.

e Turn the foot in and out at the ankle. Repeat 5 times.

f Circle the foot at the ankle 5 times in one direction and 5 times in the opposite direction.

g Curl up the toes and stretch them out. Repeat 5 times.

Exercise 3

First lying on one side and then on the other with the lower leg slightly bent:

a With the knee straight lift the top leg up about 4 inches, hold for a count of 3, lower and relax. Repeat 5 times.

b Lift the leg as above then bend and straighten the knee before lowering. Repeat 5 times.

Exercise 4

Lying on your front if able:

a Lift one leg back from the hip, hold for a count of 3, lower and relax. Repeat 3 times with each leg.

b Bend at the knee to raise the foot about 4 inches off the ground, hold for a count of 3, lower and relax. Repeat 5 times with each leg.

Exercise 5

Sitting in a straight chair with the hips and knees at right angles:

a   Straighten one knee and pull the foot up at the ankle, hold for a count of 3, lower and relax. Repeat 5 times with each leg.

b   Slowly raise the heels off the ground and push the toes into the ground, hold for a count of 3, lower the heels and relax. Repeat 5 times.

c   With the heels remaining on the floor, bend at the ankle so the front of the foot rises off the floor, hold for a count of 3, lower and relax. Repeat 5 times.

d   Straighten the affected leg so the heel is on the ground. Circle the foot at the ankle 5 times in one direction and 5 times in the opposite direction.

Exercise 6

Do not do these exercises if you are not fully mobile or have poor balance.

Exercises in standing. Stand straight with the legs slightly apart and weight evenly distributed:

a   Slowly raise up onto the toes, hold for a count of 3 and lower. Repeat 5 times.

b   Slowly bend at the knees and straighten to the starting position. Repeat 5 times.

c   Slowly lift the affected leg out to the side, count to 3 and lower.

d   Repeat with the unaffected leg.

11 Containment in the management of lymphoedema

Jacquelyne Todd

Introduction

Containment is the action of enclosing, restricting and keeping under control.[1] In the management of lymphoedema, this refers to the application of a wrapping to enclose a part of the body. This is achieved through the use of *multilayer lymphoedema bandaging* (MLLB) or *compression garments*:

- *support* is used to provide retention and control without the use of compression.[2] The bandages used in the management of lymphoedema produce a firm encasement to swollen tissues. Voluntary muscle contraction and relaxation within inelastic bandages cause variations in tissue pressure and stimulate lymph flow

- *compression* implies the direct application of pressure.[3] In the management of lymphoedema, elastic garments are frequently used to compress the tissues of a swollen limb.

Although containment is not curative, it is used to reduce swelling and thereafter to maintain the reduction. External support in combination with muscular activity stimulates both lymphatic and venous drainage.

Containment has been described as one of the foundations of good lymphoedema management.[4-8] It is particularly useful in treating limb lymphoedema because bandages or garments can be applied with relative ease. It can also be used as part of the management in other sites of swelling, such as the external genitalia.

MLLB is used in the first intensive phase of management (also known as complex physical therapy – CPT and complex decongestive therapy – CDT). They need to be re-applied daily for a limited period of time. Bandages contribute to:

- the speedy reduction of swelling

- improvement in skin condition

- the softening of fibrotic tissue.

Compression garments are fitted in the second (maintenance) phase of management, when the individual is shown how to combine their use in a programme of self-care. Garments enable the individual to control their swelling and to maintain the management outcomes achieved during the intensive phase.[9] In a number of cases, MLLB is not necessary and the individual can move directly into a programme of maintenance therapy using compression garments. Management in the UK has been largely modelled on methods pioneered in Europe, in which external support is integrated in a two-phase programme of care (*see* p.103).[10,11] In palliative care, the same principles of management are adopted. In this situation, it is often necessary to adapt methods to accommodate individual needs.

The use of binding for swollen limbs can be traced back over many centuries to descriptions in Greek and Egyptian history. In the Middle Ages, combinations of bandages and plaster dressings were used as well as laced stockings made of dog leather. Bandages were initially made of woven cotton and were inextensible. Later, to provide elasticity, rubber was incorporated within the fabric and, more recently, elastomer products.[12]

Descriptions of bandaging in lymphoedema management is confusing as several contradictory terms and concepts abound in the literature. Bandaging is often referred to as compression bandaging. This raises some questions, such as how does bandaging in lymphoedema management differ from other methods of compression bandaging – and why? What are the special features and techniques that distinguish bandaging in the management of lymphoedema?

Multilayer lymphoedema bandaging

The first part of this chapter will cover:

- the use of bandages in the management of lymphoedema

- indications for MLLB

- an outline of techniques of application.

Although the following discussion will contribute to a theoretical framework for future practice, it must be emphasised that bandaging is a specialist technique. The skill can be mastered only by practice under the supervision and guidance of an experienced therapist.

Rationale of application

The types of bandage used in lymphoedema management produce a distinct effect. They do not contain elastomer and therefore do not perform in the same way as elastic bandages. When applied within a multilayer system, these bandages provide a semi-rigid encasement of the tissues. Skeletal muscle activity brings about circumferential changes in limb size and results in an increase in pressure within the bandage encasement. To describe this type of bandaging as compression bandaging is misleading because the increase and variations in pressure under the bandages is largely dependent on skeletal muscle activity (i.e. forces generated within but not by the bandages). The main function of bandages in lymphoedema management is to provide support for underlying tissues and to act as a counterforce to voluntary muscle activity. MLLB is a recognised part of conservative lymphoedema management[10,13] and is particularly important in complicated lymphoedema. Complicated lymphoedema is identified by several clinical features, any one of which may indicate the need for MLLB.[14]

Pathophysiology

Inadequacy or obstruction of lymph drainage results in low output lymphatic failure.[13] Initially this causes pitting oedema. In time there is deposition of fibrin and fat, and the swelling becomes irreversible and non-pitting ('brawny oedema'). There is progressive fibrosis of the skin and subcutis, resulting in characteristic changes such as hyperkeratosis and deepened skin folds. There is progressive distortion of limb shape, with increasing loss of mobility and an increased risk of acute inflammatory episodes (AIE).

Chronic venous insufficiency also leads to chronic oedema.[15] This is associated with a 'dynamic insufficiency' of lymphatics.[16] MLLB plays an important role in the management of chronic venous insufficiency by:

• reducing the blood pressure in the superficial venous system

• improving deep venous return

• reducing the oedema.[17]

In the case of elderly and immobile individuals, swelling may be the result of a combination of chronic venous hypertension and reduced lymph drainage, leading to dependency oedema.[9] In this situation, MLLB can play a part in the reduction of swelling especially if mobility or exercise is possible. MLLB is an effective method of management in all these forms of chronic oedema, subject to medical and psychosocial evaluation, and screening of the patient's physical and functional abilities.

Bandaging may also play a role in the management of *lipoedema*. This condition is frequently misdiagnosed as obesity or lymphoedema. Lipoedema affects females and is often distinguishable by its characteristic distribution (*see* p.56). The non-pitting swelling is often tender on palpation and may bruise easily.[18] MLLB may be more comfortable than elastic compression, although the volume reductions are often disappointing. Further, long-term success is often compromised by a poor tolerance to compression garments.

MLLB in the management of lymphoedema:

- enhances lymph formation (i.e. the movement of interstitial fluid into the initial lymphatics)

- improves lymph drainage (i.e. the passage of lymph through the lymph vessels)

- reverses fibrotic changes in the skin and subcutis
    softens fibrosis
    restores shape

- minimises chronic inflammatory changes in the skin

- eliminates lymphorrhoea

- provides support for overstretched inelastic tissues

- enhances muscle pump action by providing a semi-rigid encasement for working muscles.

Why multilayer bandaging?

The bandages used in lymphoedema management have a high cotton or synthetic fibre content and do not contain elastomer. They have some stretch and extensibility produced by the weave of the fabric,[19] and are described as short-stretch bandages. The relatively low pressures under the bandages exerted at rest increase considerably during exercise (Figures 11.1 and 11.2). This contrasts with elastic compression bandages which stretch as the muscle expands but maintain a high resting pressure. Bandaging in lymphoedema management causes an alteration in total tissue pressures and stimulates lymph drainage.[13]

The use of extensible bandages has been shown to stimulate lymph drainage[20,21] and to reduce oedema.[22] General principles relating to graduated external compression are implemented in lymphoedema bandaging. In graduated compression, greater pressure is applied at the distal end of the limb to compensate for the relatively high hydrostatic pressures exerted on the blood capillaries.[23]

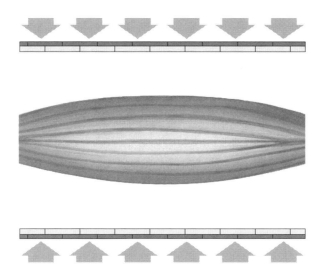

Figure 11.1   Resting pressure = Pressure provided by the applied bandages at rest.

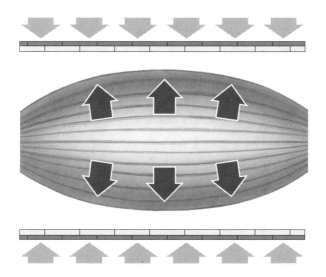

Figure 11.2   Working pressure = Pressure exerted by the contraction of the muscles within the bandaged limb during activity.

Although the bandaging used in lymphoedema will have the predominant effect of supporting the underlying tissues, a graduated pressure can be achieved during limb movement by altering the firmness and rigidity of the bandage system.

The law of Laplace

There are a number of physical principles that relate to the application of MLLB. These are summarised in Laplace's law:[4]

$$p \propto \frac{n \times t \times constant}{c \times w}$$

p = sub-bandage pressure
n = number of layers
t = bandage tension
c = limb circumference
w = width of bandage
constant = 4630.

The function of a bandage is determined by:

- relevant physical principles

- the fabric components of the bandage

- the method of application.

Sub-bandage pressure

Sub-bandage pressure refers to the pressure exerted by applying a bandage under tension to a curved surface[24] and is determined by a number of factors.

Bandage tension

Bandage tension is the force achieved when the bandage is stretched. It is determined by the force used on application and subsequently by the properties of the fabric. Sub-bandage pressure is directly proportional to the tension of the applied bandage.

Elastic bandages will stretch considerably before they reach the stage of lock-out (the point when the textile nature of the bandages resists further extension) and are capable of exerting very high pressures on the underlying tissues. Conversely, short-stretch bandages reach a lock-out point relatively quickly and will exert a lower sub-bandage pressure. There are major variations between the pressures achieved by different individuals on applying a bandage.[25] The tension at which an extensible bandage is applied should remain constant. Any graduation in rigidity should be achieved by increasing layers. Written guidance about the optimum tension with extensible bandages in lymphoedema is difficult to find. However, there appears to be agreement that the bandages should not be stretched to their maximum length.[19] Other determinants of appropriate tension will be the textile composition of the bandage and the patient's estimation of comfort and their ability to move the limb freely when bandaged.

The elasticity of the bandage is instrumental in influencing its tension. The fabric's elastic properties will determine its ability to resist any change in its length and to return to its original dimensions once the stretching force has been removed.[26] Elastic bandages have a high resting pressure and a low exercise pressure. This type of bandage will stretch to accommodate to the changing limb dimensions produced by skeletal muscle activity with a minimal increase in sub-bandage pressure. Elastic bandages can exert high pressures on underlying tissues which will be maintained for relatively long periods (up to 1 week). For this reason, they form an attractive management option in the management of venous ulcers and are used in the four-layer bandaging technique.[27]

There is some evidence to show that elastic bandages will maintain their pressure[28] and accommodate large or awkwardly shaped limbs.[29] However, the high degree of compression means that there is an increased risk of tissue damage and necrosis if poorly applied or used in cases of arterial insufficiency.[30,31] Short-stretch bandages will exert a low resting sub-bandage pressure which will be maintained for around 24 hours. These bandages are particularly valuable in stimulating lymph drainage because of the variations of sub-bandage pressure that can be achieved between resting and exercise. Other factors which will influence the performance of a bandage include:

* the age of the bandage (irrespective of its use)
* the number of times it has been used
* the length of time it has been in place.

Number of layers

The sub-bandage pressure is directly proportional to the number of layers used in the bandage application. In lymphoedema, several bandages are applied with an even pressure to achieve a graduated pressure, with more bandages being used to wrap the distal part of the limb. More layers will probably sustain pressure for longer periods.[17]

Width of the bandage

The sub-bandage pressure is indirectly proportional to the width of the bandage. A narrower bandage will exert more pressure than a wide bandage.

More turns are required to cover an area with a narrower bandage, contributing to the higher sub-bandage pressure.

Circumference of the limb

The sub-bandage pressure is indirectly proportional to the circumference of the limb. This principle is in accordance with Laplace's law which, in this context, states that pressure is directly proportional to bandage tension and inversely proportional to limb radius.[32] The pressure which will be applied over a limb will be greatest at the point of smallest circumference. In a normally shaped limb, this means that the same number of layers applied with the same degree of tension will automatically result in a graduated compression. The relatively small circumference of the upper limb requires a reduced number of layers than is required in the management of lower limb swelling. Because lymphoedema can result in enhanced skin folds and distorted limb shape, it is important to ensure that any distortions or skin folds are padded out before bandaging.

The sub-bandage pressure can be measured on the surface of the skin, under the bandages, using a device known as an Oxford pressure monitor (Tally Medical UK). Although this device is a useful indicator and useful as a teaching tool, it has several limitations:

- the pressure is only measured at certain points on the skin
- the subcutaneous tissues absorb the majority of the pressure.[33]

Therefore the pressure available to stimulate deep lymphatic and venous drainage remains unknown.

Evidence of efficacy

MLLB has an acknowledged role within decongestive lymphoedema therapy (DLT) in the UK.[14,34] However, evidence of its efficacy is limited and is largely dependent on a number of small scale studies. In fact, most of the evidence on the use of bandages is related to the management of vascular insufficiency. Several papers compare the respective healing rates of leg ulcers using different compression bandaging systems, sometimes with the addition of garments.[27,28,35] Some authors acknowledge the vital role of external compression in promoting the healing process through oedema control and an improvement of venous and lymph drainage.[36,37] Compression has been described as 'the most important component in venous ulcer management'.[38]

In lymphoedema management, MLLB is part of an integrated programme of physical therapies and it is difficult to isolate the evidence relating to bandaging alone. Currently available evidence is generally drawn from small studies. Although many of the results are not statistically significant, they provide some insight into the role of external support and compression in the management of lymphoedema.

Several studies have shown a reduction in limb volume when containment is part of the management programme.[39–41] Walking while wearing an elastic stocking increases tissue fluid and lymph pressures, and enhances the propulsion of tissue fluid and lymph.[42]

Some small studies provide insight into the role of bandaging in management. A controlled study of the movement of colloids in wrist flexors of patients with postmastectomy lymphoedema showed that the application of bandages increased protein transport through the lymphatics and that this was further increased by exercise while bandaged.[19] Interestingly, the increased transport of protein by the lymphatics continued after the cessation of exercise. Non-elastic bandages have been shown to produce a significant improvement in deep venous flow and in the reduction of ambulatory venous hypertension. There is evidence to indicate the presence of increased intramuscular pressure, accompanied by a decreased muscle blood flow and venous emptying.[43] By providing a semi-rigid encasement for working muscles, it is likely that extensible bandages will stimulate more effective blood flow and venous drainage.

An 11-day management programme of daily multilayer bandaging and self-massage showed that most of the reduction in limb volume occurred during the first 4 days.[44] In a study of 7 patients over an average of 12 weeks, the use of inelastic bandages (Unna's boot) combined with remedial exercises produced limb volume reductions in individuals with advanced lower limb lymphoedema.[45]

Although volume reduction is a useful and measurable management outcome, this does not encompass other important factors, such as:

* improvement in the condition of the skin

* a reduction in the protein content of the oedema

* softening of the skin and subcutis as a result of disruption of fibrosis.

There is a clear need for collaborative multicentre studies, in which a more comprehensive set of outcome measures are incorporated. Such a proposition is dependent on the development of condition-specific validated measurement tools.

Indications for MLLB

Indications for MLLB include:

- fragile or damaged skin, including ulceration
- fibrotic skin changes, including hyperkeratosis and papillomatosis
- lymphangioma
- lymphorrhoea
- fibrotic changes in the subcutis resulting in solid, non-pitting areas of tissue where the swelling is constant and does not reduce in elevation
- pronounced skin folds
- irregularity of limb shape caused by the swelling
- an excess limb volume of $\geqslant 20\%$ (compared with the normal unaffected limb).

Bandaging is sometimes indicated in the case of advanced malignant disease when it is applied for symptom relief (e.g. to reduce heaviness and discomfort, and to control lymphorrhoea). In these situations, individual needs will influence the choice of bandages and methods of application.

There are situations in which physical problems prevent patients from applying garments themselves, for example immobility, frailty. Arrangements for appropriate long-term management must be established so that a compression garment can be worn subsequent to MLLB.

It may be necessary to continue with bandaging for some time following a course of intensive management. For example, a patient may be directed to apply a short-stretch bandage over the top of their garment during exercise or as a more comfortable method of maintaining external support overnight.

Contra-indications to the use of MLLB

Contra-indications to the use of MLLB include:

- AIE: an increase in lymph drainage spreads infection but, in any case, MLLB is not tolerated because of pain and discomfort
- arterial insufficiency: MLLB will lead to further ischaemia and possibly tissue necrosis. It is important to check the arterial circulation as part of the initial evaluation; a calculation of the resting pressure index (RPI) can be made using Doppler ultrasound[17]

- deep vein thrombosis (DVT): the clinical features of DVT are pain, swelling, erythema, heat and tenderness.[46] An urgent medical referral is required

- severe cardiac failure: an increase in pressure over a limb can result in the rapid removal of fluid from the swollen part. This will result in an increase in central venous pressure which could cause cardiac overload.

As a general indicator, MLLB should not cause pain, discolouration of the fingers or toes, or altered sensation such as 'pins and needles' (paraesthesiae) or numbness. In these situations, the bandages should be removed and re-applied with less tension.

Situations requiring caution

The patient's medical history may indicate the need for caution if there is a possibility of sensory or vascular deficit or of mild cardiac failure (e.g. diabetes, paralysis, hypertension, bronchial asthma). In these situations, management should be undertaken with caution and the patient's medical status should be re-evaluated at frequent intervals.

Management programme

MLLB is part of a management programme which is likely also to include skin care, exercise and a manual drainage technique. The programme is decided after a comprehensive evaluation and in full consultation with the patient and relevant members of the multiprofessional team. MLLB is generally applied in the first intensive phase of management, progressing to the use of compression garments once the condition of the swollen limb permits.

Preparation

Before commencing the programme of management, the patient will require information regarding suitable clothing to wear during the course of bandaging. Footwear can be a problem and it is useful to have a stock of oversized shoes and plaster boots in the treatment centre. In order to allay any anxieties or concerns, a full explanation of the plan of care and a demonstration of the bandages to be used should be provided. This verbal explanation should be accompanied by written information, including contact names and guidelines on what to do if problems occur – as in the case of signs of ischaemia. Recommendations should be given regarding suitable activities and regular exercise to be undertaken during management. Arrangements for the provision of laundry facilities and any requirements for transport should be included in the planning process. The timing of appointments may need to accommodate family or work commitments.

MLLB is likely to continue for 2–3 weeks, during which time the bandages are changed daily. The suspension of management over a weekend may have an impact on the volume reduction achieved through the course of bandaging.[47] However, the service implications of daily care need to be considered, especially if there is only one therapist. Strategies such as teaching the patient or carer to re-apply the outer layer of bandages may help to overcome these difficulties.

Two sets of bandages are required over the course of management, with additional finger/toe bandages. The bandages will require laundering according to the manufacturer's instructions. They are dried flat so that the fabric can rest and restore its shape before re-use. There are several ways in which a bandage can be applied. In all cases, the following principles should be observed:

- bandages are applied within a multilayer system over appropriate stockinette and padding. It is important to ensure that there are no creases or wrinkles in the stockinette as this will cause discomfort and chafing. The stockinette should be changed daily to avoid problems such as folliculitis (see p.128)

- all areas of the limb should be bandaged with an overlap of each wrap of the bandage. Bandaging should include fingers or toes. If the digits are not covered during MLLB, there is a probability that they will swell during the course of the management.

Padding

Padding is used:

- to protect sensitive areas, such as ankle/foot; wrist/hand; antecubital or popliteal fossa

- to 'iron out' shape distortions and skin folds; a loosely applied retention bandage is generally necessary to hold pieces of padding in place on the limb

- to produce a regular cylinder shape of the limb prior to the application of pressure. Special attention is paid to areas such as the hand and foot, where the shape of the limb could result in more pressure being exerted on lateral borders

- to soften and reshape areas of fibrosis.

Materials

A number of materials may be used as padding:

- undercast padding bandages and low density foam; to prevent chafing and provide bulk to the area to produce the required shape prior to applying bandages

- foam chippings (approximately 1cm square), lightly packed and secured into pouches of stockinette. These chipping bags are useful for increasing bulk in the palm of the hand and for padding out skin folds

- high density foam to soften fibrotic areas. This is added into the bandage system following the stockinette. If the skin is fragile, a layer of undercast padding is applied first to prevent chafing. Shaped pieces are commercially available; alternatively, pieces can be individually prepared by the therapist. All edges should be trimmed and bevelled before use to minimise any possibility of skin abrasion

- high density foam cut into small cubes and/or longitudinal strips and then placed within two layers of 10cm wide adhesive strapping (e.g. Mefix). The small cubes of foam are placed over the fibrotic area where they can exert a massaging effect on the skin and tissues. Longitudinal strips are positioned in such a way as to redirect superficial lymph drainage towards functioning collateral pathways.[13]

Bandaging

There are several ways of applying bandages, for example spiral bandaging and a reverse spiral ('figure of eight') technique. The effectiveness of any technique is dependent on the skill of the health professional applying the bandage. Applying bandages takes time and can be uncomfortable for both the patient and the therapist because of the prolonged need to remain in one position or because of stretching and twisting the limb. Such problems can be reduced by ensuring that all materials are at hand and by the use of equipment such as an adjustable couch.

Bandages are applied in order to achieve a graduated sub-bandage pressure; this is *not* produced by altering the tension of the bandage on application. Graded pressure is achieved by the appropriate selection of bandage width, bandage overlap and the use of layers of bandage. The individual bandage should not be stretched to its maximum length.[25] While bandaging, guide the bandage close to the limb using the other hand to smooth out the bandage during application. All bandages are held in place with tape and not the metal fasteners which are supplied with some bandages. These fasteners, although useful for holding the unused roll intact, could injure the skin if used to secure bandages.

The appropriate positioning of joints in the affected limb during bandaging is important so as to ensure that comfort and mobility are maintained. For example:

- the fingers or toes should be relaxed and not extended

- when applying the hand bandage, the patient is asked to spread their fingers apart

- the foot should be in 90° flexion at the ankle

- the elbow and knee should be slightly flexed

- in order to achieve the tension required for a comfortable degree of exercise pressure, the patient is asked to make a fist during arm bandaging, and to bend their ankle and pull their toes up during leg bandaging.

Each bandage is started distally and taken proximally, with more layers of bandage being used at the distal end of the limb. It is important to scrutinise progress at every stage, both by observation and by using hands to judge the quality of application.

A method for applying MLLB to the upper limb

Materials required:

- tubular bandage (cut to approximately twice the length of the limb to accommodate the sideways stretch)

- elastic gauze bandages, 4cm width (2)

- undercast padding (4 or 5) or low density foam, depending on the limb size and shape

- short-stretch bandages in the following sizes; 6cm (1); 8cm (1); 10cm (2 or 3)

- high density foam pieces – if necessary.

Bandaging the upper limb

1 Applying stockinette
A hole is made for the thumb and the stockinette is applied to the arm, from the base of the fingers to the axilla.

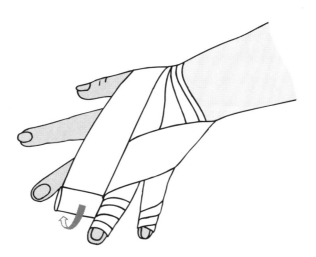

Figure 11.3   Finger bandaging.

2 Applying finger bandage (Figure 11.3)

The elastic gauze bandage is secured by a turn with minimal tension at the base of the hand and then taken across the dorsum of the hand to wrap each finger in turn. Always coming from the dorsum of the hand, the first turn is taken at the base of each finger nail, followed by circular turns around each finger, moving proximally. Padding may be incorporated into the bandage if required. In most cases, the thumb and finger tips are left free of bandage as this greatly improves dexterity and function and in most circumstances, does not adversely affect the reduction in finger swelling.

3 Applying undercast padding (Figure 11.4)

Padding bandage is applied to the hand, wrist and arm to achieve a cylindrical shape of the limb and to protect areas which are vulnerable to pressure.

Padding can be double- or triple-folded to achieve extra protection. Any foam pads are held in place by a retaining bandage.

4 Applying hand bandage

A 6cm bandage is secured by a turn with minimal tension at the wrist and then taken across the dorsum of the hand to wrap twice around the hand adjacent to the base of the fingers. The fingers should be held apart while the hand is bandaged. All the hand is covered in successive wraps, ensuring that the circles overlap and that there are no gaps in the bandage.

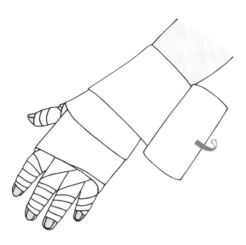

Figure 11.4 Applying undercast padding to the hand and arm.

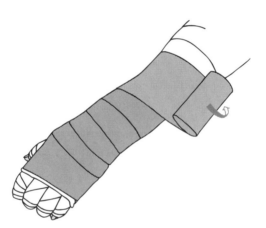

Figure 11.5 Applying arm bandage.

5 Applying arm bandage (Figure 11.5)

When the hand bandage is completed, the remaining bandage is wrapped around the forearm as a spiral bandage. The next bandage (8cm width) is started at the wrist and taken up to cover the forearm. Each bandage turn should overlap the previous one by two thirds. The next bandage is wider (10cm) and starts at the distal end of the forearm, applied in the reverse direction to the previous bandage. This bandage extends up to the top of the arm (Figure 11.6).

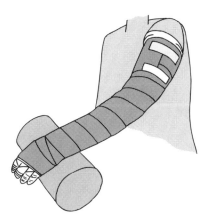

Figure 11.6   Completion of arm bandage.

A method for applying MLLB to the lower limb

Materials required:

- tubular bandage (cut to approximately twice the length of the limb to accommodate the sideways stretch)

- one elastic gauze bandage, 4cm width (unrolled, folded in half lengthways and re-rolled)

- undercast padding, depending on the size and shape of the limb (approximately 6–8)

- short-stretch bandages, in the following sizes; 6cm (1); 8cm (1 or 2); 10cm (3 or 4); 12cm (4–6).

Bandaging the lower limb

1 Applying stockinette to cover the leg from the toes to the groin.

2 Applying toe bandage (Figure 11.7)
The elastic gauze bandage is secured by a turn with minimal tension at the distal end of the foot. The bandage is taken across the dorsum of the foot and wrapped around each toe in turn, coming from the top of the foot. The first turn is taken at the base of the toe nail, followed by circular turns around each toe, moving distally. Padding may be incorporated into the bandage if necessary.

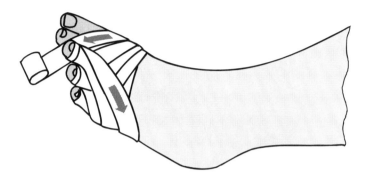

Figure 11.7   Toe bandaging.

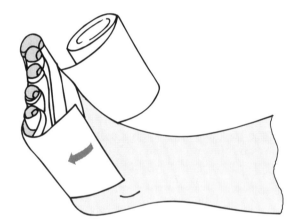

Figure 11.8   Applying undercast padding to the foot.

3 Applying undercast padding (Figure 11.8)

Padding bandage is applied to the foot, ankle and leg to achieve a cylindrical shape of the limb and to protect areas which are vulnerable to pressure. To achieve extra protection, the padding can be double- or triple-folded or low density foam can be cut and shaped to incorporate with padding bandage. High density foam pads are incorporated as required, for example in the concavities of the malleolar region. Any foam pads are held in place by a retaining bandage.

4 Applying first foot bandage (Figure 11.9)

The first bandage (6 or 8cm) commences with a complete turn around the base of the toes. With the foot at 90°, the bandage is taken across the dorsum

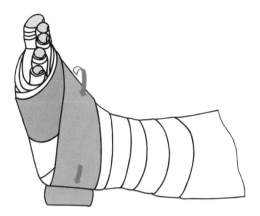

Figure 11.9   Applying first foot bandage.

of the foot and around the ankle. This is repeated a number of times to form a figure of eight to give the required degree of firmness at the base of the foot. Any surplus bandage is taken up the leg with minimal tension.

5 Applying second foot bandage (Figure 11.10)

The second bandage (8cm) commences with a turn with minimal tension just above the ankle. The bandage is taken obliquely down to cover the heel. The next circle overlaps the preceding one, but this time covers the ankle. The bandage is then taken obliquely down to cover the sole of the foot and to overlap the circle which covered the heel. The remainder of the bandage is taken up in circles around the calf.

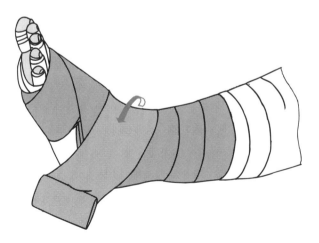

Figure 11.10 Applying second foot bandage.

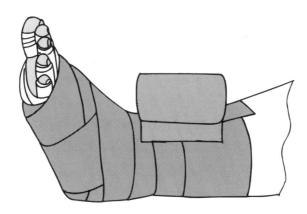

Figure 11.11 Applying bandage to the lower leg.

6 Applying bandage (lower leg) (Figure 11.11)

The next bandage (10cm) is applied in the reverse direction, commencing on the foot or above the ankle, depending on the degree of tension required on the foot. Each overlap covers two thirds of each previous circle. The bandage is taken to below the knee (Figure 11.12) In some cases, a fourth bandage is added to the lower leg.

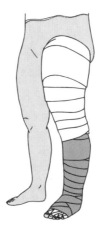

Figure 11.12 Completion of bandage to knee level.

7 Applying bandage (upper leg)

The next bandage (10cm) commences below the knee and is taken in circles up the leg, with an overlap of two thirds at each turn. After this, a 12cm bandage is applied to complete the circular turns up to the groin. On

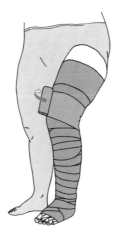

Figure 11.13 Completion of bandage to top of the leg.

completion, another 12cm bandage is applied in a reverse direction, commencing below the knee and up to the top of the leg (Figure 11.13).

A figure of eight style of application can be used on the outer layer of bandage to help keep the bandage layers in place. It produces greater pressure than the simple spiral method.[22] The use of a figure of eight style of bandage in the cubital and popliteal fossa offers further protection and support to the soft tissues in these areas.

Cost and availability

Bandages and materials used in MLLB have, to date, been unavailable on prescription. Bandaging in lymphoedema management has been largely confined to specialist centres, where trained therapists have had the necessary resources to carry out this procedure. Since early 1999, several short-stretch bandages have been available on prescription in the UK. Undercast padding of varying widths has also been available on Drug Tariff since mid-1999. It remains to be seen how improved availability will influence the use of MLLB in the UK.

The personal impact of MLLB

There is limited information on the personal impact of bandaging. It generally forms part of an intensive management programme in which rapid improvements can be achieved. A rapid reduction in limb volume is a visible outcome and a positive experience. Physical improvements are likely to form an incentive to persevere with long-term self-management.

As has already been discussed, MLLB is time-consuming and can be quite tiring for the patient, particularly when combined with other treatments. It forms part of the 2-phase management programme where the patient is dependent on the therapist. Even during this part of their care, it is important to allow the individual to maintain as much independence and self-control as possible. An explanation should always be given of the techniques used, the likely outcome and the underlying rationale. Whenever possible, the patient should be encouraged to participate actively in the bandaging at whatever level they feel comfortable with. Ultimately, the therapist may wish the patient to continue with a bandaging technique in the next phase of management. This will be more easily achieved if the patient has developed confidence in applying the bandages themselves.

Conclusion

This section has provided an introduction to the principles, materials and methods used in multilayer lymphoedema bandaging. MLLB is recognised as an important part of lymphoedema management. There is evidence to show its efficacy within a programme of therapy. Knowledge of the principles underlying bandaging is crucial to an understanding of the technique and its application. An appropriate selection of methods and materials is vital to the safe and successful application of MLLB. It forms the first part of the application of external support in the management of a person with lymphoedema.

It is possible that the bandaging techniques may be continued by the patient following the first phase of management and used to supplement the effect of compression garments. For this reason, it is important to promote their active participation and to monitor their progress carefully.

Knowledge of the role of MLLB in lymphoedema management is informed by physiological and physical principles. Current evidence supporting the specific role of bandaging in lymphoedema is drawn from related fields and several small scale studies. More information is needed regarding the effects of bandaging and the use of different materials and methods. Collaborative multicentre studies may be the best way of obtaining such data. Current research has largely focused on limb volume reduction as the single management outcome measurement. Future research will depend on the development of validated and condition-specific outcome measurements. A wider set of quantitative and qualitative measures would provide clearer insight into the effect of MLLB in lymphoedema management.

Compression garments in the management of lymphoedema

The use of elastic sleeves or stockings is one of the cornerstones of lymphoedema management.[34] Garments used in lymphoedema management are of a higher compression class than those used to treat venous disorders. Sleeves or stockings form part of a daily self-management programme. It is essential that the health professional can make a selection that is appropriate to the physical and psychosocial needs of the patient. The safe and effective use of compression garments is dependent on knowledge of their use and the health professional's ability to apply this knowledge in the clinical setting. This section will provide an introduction to the rationale of treatment and the issues relating to evaluation and implementation of care. To complement this knowledge, health professionals should acquaint themselves with the stocks that are available in their clinical setting. A comprehensive clinical evaluation should take place. Lymphoedema is a chronic condition and it is probable that garments will become a constant feature of daily life. For this reason, educational and psychosocial issues are of primary concern to the health professional.

The use of stockings became possible in the late 19th century due to advances in fabric technology. The elastic nature of earlier garments was due to the use of strengthened rubber. Recent technological advances have provided lighter synthetic fibres that are used in the production of sleeves and stockings (Figures 11.14–11.17). Garments are available in a number of different compression classes, sizes and styles. There are two main methods of manufacture; circular and flat bed knit. A flat bed garment is made as a flat piece to specific measurements and then joined with a seam. These garments are generally custom-made to a specific order. Custom-made garments are necessary when individual need determines a specific requirement of style, level of compression and size. They are more expensive and accurate measurements are vital, in line with the manufacturers' instructions. The circular knit garments are produced in one piece with no seam and are available as off-the-shelf garments. These have the advantage of being relatively cheap and easily accessible.

Aesthetic issues play an important part in garment provision. The shade and colour of the sleeve or stocking is often an important consideration for the patient. Although there are several choices for stockings of the lower compression classes, this is not the case with arm sleeves or high compression stockings. A number of textile fabrics are used to provide different thicknesses of materials and a variety of compression classes. Smooth yarns produce light and sleeker garments, which may be an option in lower compression classes. Although some of the lower compression stockings have a closed toe, the higher compression class stockings are toe-less. It is common to leave the

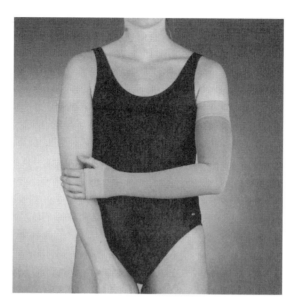

Figure 11.14 Arm sleeve (combined).

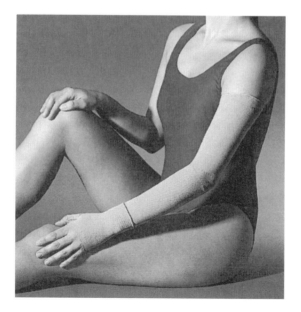

Figure 11.15 Arm sleeve and separate hand piece.

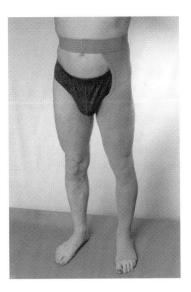

Figure 11.16 Thigh stocking with waistband.

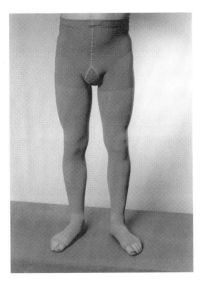

Figure 11.17 Panty tights.

fingertips free of compression when using handpieces or some gloves. This method aids comfort and functional ability as well as providing a means of ensuring vascular competence at the limb extremities.

In the UK, compression is an established and recognised treatment for venous disorders. These stockings are available on prescription in the community, according to the British Standard Specification for Graduated Compression Hosiery 1985 (Figure 11.18).[48] They are useful for treating venous disorders, but are of a lower compression than is generally required for the treatment of lymphoedema. The compression gradient reduces from 100% at the ankle to a maximum of 40% at the top of the thigh (Figure 11.19). This compression gradient is not sufficient to control lymphoedema where swelling extends to the root of the limb and causes distortion in limb shape. In general, the garments used to treat lymphoedema are made to the International Standard, which provides stronger compression than the British Standard (Figure 11.18).

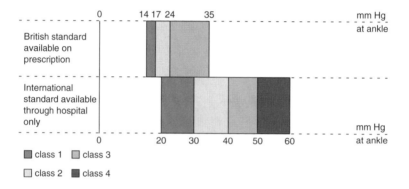

Figure 11.18 Comparison of British and International compression class.

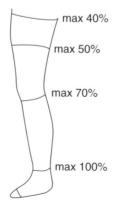

Figure 11.19 Compression profile of a stocking.

Garments used for lymphoedema are not available on British standard prescriptions (FP10, GP10). The stronger compression class stockings, tights and sleeves are only available through prescription from a hospital consultant or from a lymphoedema therapist.

Rationale of application

The principles discussed in the section on MLLB also apply to the use of compression garments. Stockings and sleeves contain elastomer, which gives elastic properties to the garment. The fabric's elasticity will determine its ability to resist any change in its length and to return to its original dimensions once the stretching force has been removed.[3] The degree of elasticity is dependent on the textiles used and the weave of the material and will produce a compressive force on the underlying skin and tissues. Compression can be defined as the direct application of pressure.[3] As from 1988, elastic stockings are measured according to their performance, rather than their material composition. The degree of pressure they exert on the skin can be measured in the laboratory and then used to calculate the compression class of the garment. In general, lymphoedema management requires sleeves in compression classes 1 and 2 (< 40mmHg) and stockings in compression classes 3 and 4 (> 40mmHg).

All garments provide a gradient of compression, with the strongest pressures being exerted at the distal part of the limb (Figure 11.19). In this way, the compression garment can effectively limit increased intravascular hydrostatic pressure and promote venous and lymphatic drainage. In making the appropriate selection of garments, the principles of Laplace's law should be applied.[17] The sub-bandage pressure will be directly proportional to the tension in the stocking or sleeve. This will be determined by the elastic properties of the garment and will also be influenced by how the garment has been applied. The pressure – if constant throughout the length of the garment – will be inversely proportional to the circumference of the limb. The pressure exerted by the same compression class garment will be greatest over a limb of smaller circumference. For this reason, a lower compression class garment is indicated on limbs of smaller proportions.

It is important to pay particular attention to the fit of the garment at the wrist or ankle. At this point, the pressures are relatively strong in relation to the circumference of the limb. Off-the-shelf garments are designed for regularly shaped limbs. The compression gradient and respective pressures may be adversely affected if fitted on an irregular limb shape. In these cases, reshaping using MLLB and the use of custom-made garments can play a role in management.

The actions of compression garments

Compression garments:

- prevent re-accumulation of fluid following the first intensive phase of management
- limit capillary filtration
- raise interstitial pressure
- enhance lymph formation (i.e. the movement of interstitial fluid into the initial lymphatics)
- improve lymph drainage (i.e. the passage of lymph through the lymph vessels)
- minimise chronic inflammatory changes in the skin
- provide support for inelastic tissues
- enhance muscle pump action by providing external counterforce for working muscles.

The description of elastic sleeves and stockings as containment garments is useful as it depicts the two main functions of compression garments in lymphoedema management:

- the limitation of capillary filtration by opposing capillary hydrostatic pressure
- the enhancement of the effect of voluntary muscle action in promoting venous and lymphatic drainage.

Compression garments play an important role in maintaining the improvements in size and shape achieved through intensive treatment.[10,49] Elastic garments do not provide the same rigid counterforce to skeletal muscle activity as MLLB.[50,51] However, some reduction in limb volume is possible, particularly if there is a small degree of pitting oedema.[2,3] In the absence of other complicating factors, an excess limb volume of $<20\%$ can be controlled immediately with garments and without the use of MLLB.[14] Elastic garments, unlike short-stretch bandages, have the advantage of providing sustained pressure over long periods of time. Sleeves or stockings can be applied independently by the patient and can be worn throughout the day with minimal re-adjustment. Garments will provide adequate control of the swelling over a period of months, provided that they are used and cared for as recommended by the manufacturers.

Evidence of efficacy

Most data about compression garments relate to their use in the management of leg ulcers.[52–54] Although their use is discussed in most lymphoedema literature, there is a limited number of studies regarding their value in a programme of lymphoedema management.

Two studies have shown the benefits of compression sleeves in the management of postmastectomy lymphoedema.[7,55] A significant reduction in limb measurements was shown over 6 months.[7] The use of a sleeve alone resulted in a moderate improvement, which could be further improved by the addition of other physical methods. *Interestingly, weight gain was the sole negative factor in relation to reduction in limb volume.* An increase in adipose tissue may limit the effectiveness of the garment. Other studies also report a loss in limb volume after the provision of elastic garments, although management was not always limited to the use of garments alone.[39,56,57]

Calf muscle pump exercises in stockings have been shown to raise both tissue fluid and lymph pressure.[58] This suggests that exercise within garments produces a similar effect on lymph drainage as exercise within bandages.[19] There is some evidence to show that garments reduce venous pooling.[49,51] Exercise within a class 2 compression stocking (30–40mmHg) was shown to stimulate venous return.[59] The use of garments subsequent to drainage prevented refilling of the tissues.[49] By minimising capillary filtration and stimulating venous drainage, garments minimise the formation of oedema. By improving venous return, garments may play a role in improving muscle pump efficiency in oedematous limbs.[43] Further work is required to identify the level of compression required to stimulate this effect.

Evaluation for the use of compression garments

Compression garments are selected following a full evaluation of the patient's physical and psychosocial status. Sleeves or stockings are an important part of the management programme. High levels of compression are often required and adequate measures must be taken to ensure that management is safe and effective.

An evaluation of vascular status, including arterial competence should be undertaken. In lower limb oedema this evaluation should include the measurement of ankle-brachial pressure index (ABPI) by Doppler ultrasound. Garments are not applied when a DVT is suspected. However, a number of authors have argued for the provision of stockings at an early stage following anticoagulation.[60,61] Compression garments are also not used during an AIE as they can aid the spread of the infection and increase reactive fibrosis.

Indications for the use of compression garments

Indications for the use of compression garments include:

- swelling ≤ 20% excess volume
- the limb shape is regular and not distorted
- the skin is intact and resilient
- the patient is able to apply and remove the garments independently or with the help of a spouse, partner or carer who can be available when required.

Contra-indications to the use of compression garments

Contra-indications to the use of compression garments include:

- AIE
- arterial insufficiency
- severe cardiac failure
- fragile or damaged skin, including ulceration
- lymphorrhoea
- pronounced skin folds
- irregularity of limb shape caused by the swelling
- limbs where the swelling is > 20% excess volume.

Psychosocial issues

Several studies have investigated the psychological and physical problems associated with breast cancer-related arm swelling (see p.89).[62-64] Findings indicate increased psychosocial maladjustment and increased morbidity, together with functional impairment. Women with arm swelling reported feelings of resentment, embarrassment and of being overwhelmed by the condition. Problems with clothes were frequently identified, with the subjects often losing interest in their appearance.[62] A significant impairment in the patients' adjustment to work and the home environment has been shown, together with a greater disruption to sexual relationships.[63] The effect of a swollen limb on body image is a major issue for some people with lymphoedema.[44,65,66]

Although available evidence relates to arm swelling, the issues are pertinent to people with lymphoedema in other parts of the body. In each case, lymphoedema is a chronic condition requiring life-long adaptation and adjustment. The evaluation of a patient for compression garments requires careful consideration of these psychosocial issues. The constant use of a sleeve or stocking may be seen as an additional stigma that increases feelings of embarrassment and reduces self-esteem. The person may perceive the garment as drawing attention to the swollen limb and as an obstacle in relationships with partner, family or friends.

On the first few occasions, the patient may feel uncomfortable about discussing these personal issues, particularly in the presence of another family member. Individual needs and expectations should be discussed sensitively and in an environment that provides plenty of opportunity for the person to express their feelings. It may be apparent that the patient requires more emotional support and help prior to garment fitting. Psychosocial issues may influence the style and compression class of garment and the time when it is provided.

The success of compression garments will be largely dependent on the motivation of the patient to persevere with their use. Garments are more likely to be accepted and valued when measures are taken to promote an understanding of their role within a management programme.[67] In a recent study including patient expectations, over 70% of patients expressed a desire for information on lymphoedema and self-help measures.[41] Patient education should include the establishment of clear and agreed goals and the use of written information to supplement verbal advice. Although there is limited information relating psychosocial status with the specific use of garments, there is evidence to show the psychosocial benefits of lymphoedema therapy.[62,68,69] A reduction in swelling and increasing confidence and competence in self-management skills are powerful tools of motivation. After a period of successful management, the patient is more likely to persevere with a programme of self-care, including the use of compression garments.

Getting started

If garment fitting is to take place after a course of intensive management, the sleeve or stocking should be available for fitting on completion of this phase of management. This means that preparations for garment selection take place before MLLB is completed. This is possible and successful if measurements are taken at the point where volume reduction is reaching a plateau. Measurements for compression garments should be made in accordance with the manufacturer's instructions.

Sometimes, patients cannot tolerate compression garments. When this is the case, different forms of lightweight support may be acceptable to the patient.

Although this will not provide the same control as higher compression classes, it may be a more acceptable way of introducing the concept of wearing a compression garment. For example, low compression graduated support stockings are now available from commercial outlets. The patient may be happy to wear these as a single or double layer. Likewise, some of the lycra materials used in clothes manufacture may provide some support, particularly in the case of truncal oedema. Conversely, any tight fitting clothing or narrow straps of material that produce ridging or lines on the skin is likely to impede lymph flow and can counteract the benefits gained by wearing compression garments.

Patient instruction and information

The patient will require a full explanation and instruction on the use of garments (Box 11.A).

Box 11.A Application of compression garments

Garments are applied by folding them back on themselves to wrist or ankle level. After the hand or foot is positioned, the garment is gradually pulled on in segments. This method ensures accurate positioning and avoids overstretching of the material.

Rubber gloves should be worn during application to prevent damage to the fabric and to ensure the even distribution of material.

There are several commercially available application aids that may assist the patient in applying their garment.

Some garments are designed with certain features to keep them in place on the body, e.g. straps that attach around the trunk or stockings which include a grip top.

A water-based glue is available which can be applied in vertical strips to the skin and which will then hold the garment in place.

When in place, there should be no folds, wrinkles or tight bands of fabric in the garment. It should never be folded back on itself during use, nor cut or reshaped.

The length of time for which the garment is worn will be agreed on an individual basis. In general, it is worn during the day and removed at night. It should be worn every day and is most valuable during warm weather or during exercise (contrary to what the patient may prefer). There are occasions when the patient is required to wear a garment all the time.[13,70] This is particularly the case after a course of MLLB when the tissues are likely to refill. However, the compressive nature of garments can make them uncomfortable at night and a lower compression class or the alternative use of night banda-ging may be more appropriate. *Skin care should be done after the garment is taken off at the end of the day because emollient cream can damage the fabric and make garment application difficult.*

As comfort is a primary consideration in management, accurate measurement and fitting is essential. The choice of compression garment is made after a comprehensive evaluation. The appropriate style and compression class will be selected after consideration of both physical and psychological factors. In addition to the initial vascular screening, it is important to re-evaluate arterial competence at follow-up appointments to ensure continuing vascular integrity. Clear verbal and written instructions should be given on how to recognise any ischaemic changes and of necessary actions to take in this event.

In certain situations, a double layer of garments are used. Examples of when this method is indicated include:

* when firmer compression is required at the distal part of the limb in order to maintain control of the oedema

* patients who cannot apply one stocking of sufficient compression strength due to limited mobility and dexterity, but who can apply two sets of garments of a lower compression class

* when the massaging effect produced by the simultaneous wearing of two garments is beneficial, as in the case of some patients with lipoedema.

Although there are some descriptions of the use of double layer garments,[9] there is limited evidence regarding the rationale or effect of this approach. The degree of pressure achieved by doubling garments remains questionable, although it is unlikely to be the sum of the two separate garment pressures. All the limb should be contained and the garments should provide a comfortable gradient of pressure. It is important to evaluate the possible effect of any extra compression in an area of overlap. If distal swelling is a potential problem, an alternative selection of garments should be made. Sleeves and stockings should be washed and cared for in accordance with the manufacturer's instructions. In order to preserve the quality of elasticity within the garment, two sets should be provided and worn alternately. Sleeves will need renewal after approxi-mately 6 months and stockings will need changing every 4 months.

Cost and availability

The stockings available on prescription in the community are a lower com-pression class (< 40mmHg) and more useful for the management of venous disease. Each stocking counts as a separate item for prescription charges. The garments used in the management of lymphoedema can be obtained through a surgical appliance form which is completed by a hospital consultant or specialist nurse. In many cases, compression garments are provided through the lymphoedema clinic or therapist.

If the clinic is situated in the independent sector (such as a palliative care unit), it is necessary to negotiate the cost of providing garments with the purchasers of the service. A system for monitoring the throughput of garments is essential to ensure that appropriate stocks are available and that an accurate calculation of cost can be made. Garments are a relatively expensive part of management which will increase progressively as the patient list and number of return visits grows.

Conclusion

Compression garments play an important role in the long-term management of lymphoedema. In order to select effective and safe garments, the health professional will require a sound knowledge of their role in management. Sleeves or stockings are selected after a comprehensive evaluation of the patient's physical and psychosocial needs. The continuing use of compression garments is dependent on the acceptance of their value and the patient's willingness to continue with their use. A fundamental role of the lymph-oedema therapist is to educate the patient regarding the use of compression garments. Knowledge about their role and value will encourage the patient to wear them regularly and apply them effectively. There may be situations when the feelings and emotional needs of the patient influence the sort of garments that are provided in the first instance. It is important to ensure that the use of compression garments does not increase psychological morbidity. They will be most valued and effective when they are perceived as a means of improving quality of life and promoting independence. Garments should be comfortable to wear and as aesthetically pleasing as possible. As a long-term method of containing the swelling, compression garments are an important part of lymphoedema management.

Acknowledgements

The author thanks Medi UK and Vernon-Carus Limited for providing information for this chapter.

References

1   Oxford University Press (1983) *The Shorter Oxford English Dictionary*, 3rd edn. Book Club Associates, London.

2 Thomas S (1990) Bandages and Bandaging. *Nursing Standard.* **4(39)**:4–6.
3 Badger C and Jeffs E (1997) Macmillan *lymphoedema education and practice. Cancer Relief.* Macmillan Publishers, London, 1.8–1.9.
4 Mortimer PS (1990) Lymphatics. In: RH Champion and R Pye (eds) *Recent Advances in Dermatology.* Churchill Livingstone, London.
5 Jeffs E (1992) Management of lymphoedema: putting treatment into context. *Journal of Tissue Viability.* **2(4)**:127–31.
6 Alliott F *et al.* (1996) Compression in lymphatic pathology and quality of life. *European Journal of Lymphology.* **6**:17.
7 Bertelli G *et al.* (1992) An analysis of prognostic factors in response to conservative treatment of postmastectomy lymphoedema. *Surgery, Gynecology and Obstetrics.* **175**:455–60.
8 Ohkuma M (1998) The less elastic bandage: comparison of two commercial products. *Lymphology.* **31(Suppl 16)**:503–5.
9 Mortimer PS (1995) Managing Lymphoedema. *Clinical and Experimental Dermatology*, **20**:98–106.
10 Földi E *et al.* (1985) Conservative treatment of lymphoedema of the limbs. *Angiology.* **35**:171–80.
11 Kurz I (1990) *Textbook of Dr Vodder's Manual Lymph Drainage. Volume 3, Treatment Manual*, 2nd edn. Haug Publishers, Heidelberg.
12 Browse NL *et al.* (1988) *Diseases of the Veins, Pathophysiology, Diagnosis and Treatment.* Edward Arnold, London.
13 Casley-Smith JR and Casley-Smith JR (1997) *Modern Treatment for Lymphoedema*, 5th edn. Terrace Printing, Adelaide.
14 British Lymphology Society (1997) *Definitions Relating to the Population and Needs of People With or At Risk of Developing Chronic Oedema.* BLS Publication, Caterham, Surrey.
15 Mortimer PS (1996) Lymphoedema. *Vascular Surgery.* 73–7.
16 Földi E *et al.* (1989) The lymphoedema chaos: a lancet. *Annals of Plastic Surgery.* **22**:505–15.
17 Morison MJ and Moffatt CJ (1995) *A Colour Guide to the Assessment and Management of Leg Ulcers*, 2nd edn. Mosby, Aylesbury.
18 Beninson J and Edelglass JW (1984) Lipedema – The non-lymphatic masquerader. *Angiology.* **35**:506–10.
19 Klose G (1994) *Lymphedema bandaging.* Lohmann, Neuwied.
20 Leduc O *et al.* (1990) Bandages: scintigraphic demonstration of its efficacy on colloidal protein reabsorption during muscle activity. *Progress in Lymphology XII.* Elsevier Science Publishers, BV.
21 Olszewski WL and Engeset A (1988) Vasometric function of lymphatics and lymph transport in limbs during massage and with elastic support. *Progress in Lymphology XI.* Elsevier, Excerpta Medica International Congress Series.
22 Leduc A *et al.* (1991) *Le Traitement Physique de l'Œdème du Bras. Monographies de Bois-Larris*, 2nd edn. Masson, Paris.
23 Thomas S (1996) High-compression bandages. *Journal of Wound Care.* **5**:40–3.
24 Nelson EA (1996) Compression bandaging in the treatment of venous leg ulcers. *Journal of Wound Care.* **5(9)**:415–8.
25 Logan RA *et al.* (1992) A comparison of sub-bandage pressures produced by experienced and unexperienced bandagers. *Journal of Wound Care.* **1(3)**:23–6.

26   Thomas S (1990) Bandages and bandaging: the science behind the art. *Care Science and Practice.* **8(2)**:56–60.

27   Blair SD *et al.* (1988) Sustained compression and healing of chronic venous ulcers. *British Medical Journal.* **297**:1159–61.

28   Duby T *et al.* (1993) A randomized trial in the treatment of venous leg ulcers comparing short-stretch bandages, four layer bandage system, and a long stretch-paste bandage system. *Wounds: A Compendium of Clinical Research and Practice.* **5(6)**:276–9.

29   Thomas S *et al.* (1992) Compression therapy in an obese patient. *Journal of Wound Care.* **1(1)**:19–20.

30   Callam MJ *et al.* (1987) Hazards of compression treatment of the leg: an estimate from Scottish surgeons. *British Medical Journal.* **195**:1382.

31   Moffatt CJ and Dickson D (1993) The Charing Cross high compression four layer bandage system. *Journal of Wound Care.* **2(2)**:91–4.

32   Stillwell GK (1973) The law of Laplace: some clinical applications. *Mayo Clinic Proceedings.* **48**:863–9.

33   Stemmer R *et al.* (1980) Compression treatment of the lower extremities particularly with compression stockings. *The Dermatologist.* **31**:355–65.

34   British Lymphology Society (1997) *Strategy for Lymphoedema Care.* BLS Publication, Caterham, Surrey.

35   Pierson S *et al.* (1983) Efficacy of graded elastic compression in the lower leg. *Journal of the American Medical Association.* **249(2)**:242–3.

36   Hofman D (1998) Oedema and the management of venous ulcers. *Journal of Wound Care.* **7(7)**:345–8.

37   Prasad A *et al.* (1990) Leg ulcers and oedema: a study exploring the prevalence, aetiology, and possible significance of oedema in venous ulcers. *Phlebology.* **5**:181–7.

38   Moffatt C (1997) Prevention of venous ulcer recurrence. *Scope on Phlebology and Lymphology.* **(December)4**:10–15.

39   Tomson D *et al.* (1992) The treatment of lymphoedema of the upper limb according to the Földi method: results. *European Journal of Lymphology.* **3(11)**:88–96.

40   Hutzschenreuter PO *et al.* (1991) Post-mastectomy arm lymphedema: treated by manual lymph drainage and compression bandage therapy. *Physical Medicine and Rehabilitation.* **1(6)**:166–70.

41   Todd JE (1999) A study of two lymphoedema clinics. *Physiotherapy.* **85(2)**:65–75.

42   Olszewski WL and Bryla P (1994) Lymph and tissue pressures in patients with lymphedema during massage and walking with elastic support. *Lymphology.* **27 (Suppl)**:1–893.

43   Qvarfordt PO *et al.* (1983) Intramuscular pressure, venous function and muscle blood flow in patients with lymphedema of the leg. *Lymphology.* **16**:139–42.

44   Rose K *et al.* (1993) Volume reduction of arm lymphoedema. *Nursing Standard.* **7(35)**:29–32.

45   Andrade MFC *et al.* (1996) Effectiveness of inelastic compression by Unna's boot in reducing advanced primary lower limb lymphedema. *Lymphology.* **29 (Suppl)**:430–3.

46   Collier M (1999) Brevet tx: anti-embolism stockings for prevention and treatment of DVT. *British Journal of Nursing.* **8(1)**:44–9.

47   Piller NB *et al.* (1994) Short-term manual lymph drainage and maintenance therapy for post-mastectomy lymphoedema. *Lymphology.* **27(Suppl)**:1–893.

48   British Standards Institution (1985) *British Standard Specification for Graduated Compression Hosiery (BS6612).* BSI, London.

49   Partsch H (1991) Compression therapy of the legs. *Journal of Dermatology, Surgery and Oncology.* **17**:799–805.

50   Partsch H (1990) *Contributions Towards Compression Therapy.* Lohmann, Neuwied.

51   Cornwall J *et al.* (1987) Graduated compression and its relation to venous refilling time. *British Medical Journal.* **295**:1087–90.

52   Fletcher A *et al.* (1997) A systematic review of compression treatment for venous leg ulcers. *British Medical Journal.* **315**:576–80.

53   Nelson EA (1996) Compression therapy for leg disorders. *Journal of Wound Care.* **5(4)**:162–4.

54   Jones JE and Nelson EA (1998) Compression hosiery in the management of venous leg ulcers. *Journal of Wound Care.* **7(6)**:293–6.

55   Zeissler RH *et al.* (1972) Postmastectomy lymphoedema: late results of treatment in 385 patients. *Archives of Physical Medicine and Rehabilitation.* **53**: 159–66.

56   Hutzschenreuter PO *et al.* (1991) Post-mastectomy arm lymphedema. *Physical Therapy and Rehabilitation.* **1(6)**:166–70.

57   Ferla F *et al.* (1992) Retrospective study on manual lymphatic drainage with or without combined use of elastic sleeve. *Progress in Lymphology, XIII.* Excerpta Medica, Elsevier Science Publications, The Netherlands.

58   Olszewski WL and Bryla P (1994) Lymph and tissue pressures in patients with lymphedema during massage and walking with elastic support. *Lymphology.* **27 (Suppl)**:1–893.

59   Partsch H (1984) Improvement of venous pumping in chronic venous insufficiency by compression dependant on pressure and material. *VASA – Journal for Vascular Diseases.* **13**:58–64.

60   McCollum C (1998) Avoiding the consequences of deep vein thrombosis. *British Medical Journal.* **317**:696.

61   Kmietowicz Z (1997) Complications of deep vein thrombosis are halved with compression stockings. *British Medical Journal.* **314**:849.

62   Woods M (1993) Patients' perceptions of breast cancer-related lymphoedema. *European Journal of Cancer Care.* **2**:125–8.

63   Tobin MB *et al.* (1993) The psychological morbidity of breast cancer-related arm swelling. *Cancer.* **72(11)**:3248–52.

64   Sitzia J and Sobrido L (1997) Measurement of health-related quality of life of patients receiving conservative treatment for limb lymphoedema using the Nottingham Health Profile. *Quality of Life Research.* **6**:373–84.

65   Carol D and Rose K (1992) Treatment leads to significant improvement. *Professional Nurse.* **8**:32–6.

66   Woods M (1995) Sociological factors and psychosocial implications of lymphoedema. *International Journal of Palliative Nursing.* **1(1)**:17–20.

67   Ley P (1977) Psychological studies of doctor–patient communication. In: S Rachman (ed) *Contributions to Medical Psychology*, 1. Pergamon Press, Oxford.

68   Mirolo BR *et al*. (1995) Psychosocial benefits of postmastectomy lymphedema therapy. *Cancer Nursing*. **18(3)**:1997–2005.

69   Hardy D and Taylor J (1999) An audit of non-cancer-related lymphoedema in a hospice setting. *International Journal of Palliative Nursing*. **5(1)**:18–27.

70   Leduc A and Leduc O (1992) *Le Drainage de la Grosse Jambe*, A Leduc (ed). Wilmart and Gilles, Belgium.

12   Manual lymphatic drainage

Albert Leduc and Olivier Leduc

In this chapter we discuss manual lymphatic drainage (MLD) as practised by ourselves. The historical context of MLD is referred to elsewhere (*see* p.97). Physical treatment is generally the best approach for managing lymphoedema. Although an accurate diagnosis is always necessary, treatment can be started after the completion of a comprehensive evaluation and on the basis of the clinical features. The physical treatment we use comprises:

- manual lymphatic drainage (MLD)

- pneumatic compression therapy (PCT) (low intensity)

- multilayer lymphoedema bandaging (MLLB) (foam and short-stretch bandages).

These methods go beyond symptomatic relief in that they modify the underlying disease process.[1,2]

Generally, the three techniques are combined. Indeed, we emphasise the necessity of using them together.[3,4] This view is based on many experiments in animals, volunteers without lymphoedema and patients.[4,5] MLD provided by a trained professional therapist should not be confused with 'manual lymphatic drainage' provided by many beauty specialists who have not undertaken the extensive training required for medical MLD. Although both are called MLD, the two methods are quite distinct.

MLD evacuates extracellular fluid from the interstitial space. At the same time many waste products of the cellular metabolism are removed. Two different phenomena make the evacuation of excess fluid from the swollen area possible:

- the fluid is 'captured' by the initial lymphatics

- the lymph is evacuated via the collector lymphatics.

First, the interstitial fluid is resorbed by the network of initial lymphatics. This resorption is the result of a local increase in tissue pressure. Then, the lymph is shifted from the pre-collectors to the collector lymphatics. Both these aspects of lymph drainage are facilitated by MLD.[6,7]

The place of MLD in the treatment of oedema

MLD alone may be sufficient to remove oedema initially. MLD has to be adjusted to the needs of the individual patient; the therapy depends on the particular response in each individual. The absolute rule is that the manipulations used in this technique must always be superficial and gentle.

Generally, MLD will be only a part of management. Our experiments show that MLD stimulates the resorption of proteins.[6] MLD thus aims to limit the swelling by reducing the protein content. It is the failure of this first step which necessitates the combination of MLD with other physical methods.

What does failure mean? Generally, we speak of failure if, after 10 sessions of MLD and exercises at a frequency of 3–5 sessions per week, there is no improvement at all, i.e. no softening of the skin, no reduction in pain and no functional improvement. At this moment it is recommended to start the second step. This is divided into two phases:

- phase A: MLD, exercises, PCT[8–11] and MLLB 5 times per week[12–15]
- phase B: MLD, exercises, PCT and compression garment, reducing from 5 times per week to 3 times and then once per week until the end of treatment.

MLD techniques

Manual contact

No emollients are used on either the hand of the therapist or the skin of the patient. The patient's skin is moved by the moving hand of the therapist. This stimulates the resorption of interstitial fluid by both lymphatics and veins.[6,7] The main difference between the lymphatic and venous systems is that the heightened lymphatic activity continues for some time after the cessation of the stimulation.[8,9]

Resorption ('re-absorption') technique

The hands are placed on the patient with the fingers slightly stretched (Figure 12.1). The wrist makes a rolling movement in a proximal direction (like a 'hand blotter') so allowing the fingers consecutively to exert a light pressure on the skin. The palm of the hand does likewise, increasing the tissue pressure and stretching the skin, thereby facilitating resorption into the initial lymphatics.

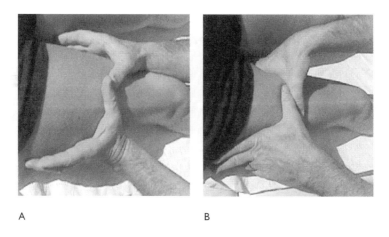

A   B

Figure 12.1   Resorption technique. A = start; B = end.

The pressure must be exerted in the direction of the lymphatic collectors, i.e. proximally. During the movement of the wrist, the shoulders of the therapist alternately abduct and adduct. Lymphoscintigraphy has confirmed the efficacy of this manipulation.[12]

Inciting ('call-up') technique

The hand placed on the patient's skin starts the movement proximally (Figure 12.2). The interdigital space between the thumb and fingers is held wide apart during this manoeuvre. This enables the span of the hand to stimulate all the lymphatic collectors. Although the collectors are generally near the veins,

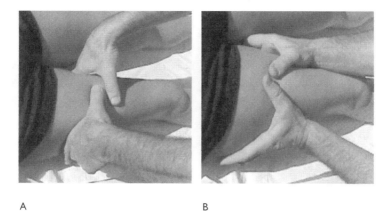

A   B

Figure 12.2   Inciting technique. A = start; B = end.

some are not. This is the reason why the fingers need to be spread out during this inciting ('call-up') technique. The pressure starts when the hand stretches the skin during the movement. This causes an attraction effect and a propulsion of the lymph in the collectors. These effects have also been confirmed by lymphoscintigraphy in humans.[12]

Although the position of the hands is important, most of the movement takes place at the shoulders and elbows. The wrist is bent to prevent the pressure becoming too great. The displacement of the fingers is almost non-existent. All movements are carried out gently and smoothly, and the pressure exerted is little more than a touch.

Specific movements of the resorption and inciting techniques

Circular movements of the fingers

The circular movements of the fingers (without the thumb) are carried out in a concentric way and with little pressure, moving the skin over the underlying tissues (Figure 12.3). The skin moves the underlying soft tissues causing a stretch. The movements are rhythmic and facilitate the resorption of interstitial fluid into the lymphatics. The pressure exerted is light and progressive. The pressure used should not collapse the superficial vessels. The circular movements must be repeated several times on the same place.

The hand of the therapist is removed without rubbing the patient's skin. The part is treated successively section by section and the pressure exerted is in the direction of the physiological drainage. The whole movement pattern is supported by repeated abduction and adduction of the therapist's shoulder; the elbow is bent and the forearm is successively rotated from palm-down to palm-up.

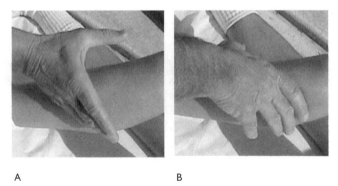

A   B

Figure 12.3   Example of resorption technique: circular movement of the fingers. A = start; B = end.

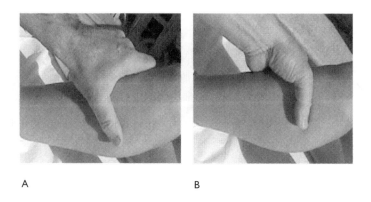

A   B

Figure 12.4   Example of resorption technique: circular movement of thumb. A = start; B = end.

Circular movements of the thumb

Just like the fingers, the thumb can carry out specific draining manipulations. The thumb is able to perform very fine movements and can adapt to the contours of the skin (Figure 12.4). As usual the pressure is in the direction of the local physiological drainage. The circular movement around the wrist is associated with an axial rotation of the thumb. Manipulation with either fingers or thumbs increases both the resorption and the inciting effects.

The fingers and/or the thumb placed on the patient's skin *start* the movement on the hand when the goal is to increase the inciting effect. The manipulation is repeated 4–5 times in the same place before moving the hand progressively in a proximal direction. The fingers and/or the thumb placed on the patient's skin *end* the movement of the hand when the goal is to increase the resorption effect. Numerous movements are undertaken in the same place until there is an apparent decrease in tissue turgor.

Combination of fingers and thumb movements

In this manipulation movements of the thumb and fingers are synchronised (Figure 12.5). The fingers and thumb move as described above. Care is taken not to pinch the skin. Recent experiments have shown that lymphatics can be damaged by deep massage.[16] Hence, all vigorous massage is contra-indicated in this technique. The different manipulations are done in a slow rhythm, once every 2–3 seconds. Intermittent pressure is better than constant pressure for moving interstitial fluid into the initial lymphatics.[13] The hand encloses the area being drained and exerts intermittent pressure in such a way that pressure is followed by relaxation.

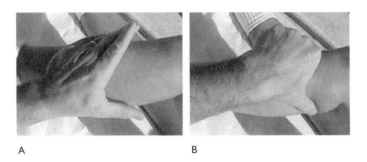

A   B

Figure 12.5   Example of resorption technique: combination of fingers and thumb movements. A = start; B = end.

Combination of both hands

Generally, both hands are used simultaneously during the drainage of the limb so as to encircle the lymphoedema (Figures 12.1 and 12.2). Encircling pressure is exerted if the area being treated is enclosed by both hands. This technique is used from the proximal part of the swollen limb gradually to the distal part in order to facilitate resorption into initial lymphatics and blood capillaries. During the inciting manipulation, both hands are wide open to cover the typical locations of the lymphatic collectors responsible for the removal of lymph.

Drainage of the lymph nodes

The drainage of the lymph nodes is carried out with the same care as the drainage of the lymphatic vessels. Both hands are placed on the skin. The distal hand starts the movement with the outer (radial) border of the forefinger. The proximal hand simultaneously starts with the inner (ulnar) border (Figure 12.6). The skin is smoothly and proximally stretched, and slightly pressed by a rolling movement of the hand. The position of the stretched fingers is perpendicular to the evacuation direction of the lymph nodes or, more precisely, the evacuation direction of the efferent lymphatics. It is also possible to perform this manipulation with both hands without exerting much pressure. Using both hands makes it possible to treat a greater area simultaneously. Some therapists habitually use the uppermost hand to give pressure and the underlying hand to balance and to regulate the pressure. This manipulation is repeated 8–10 times on the lymph nodes.

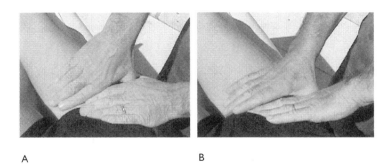

A   B

Figure 12.6   Drainage of the lymph nodes. A = start; B = end.

Examples of MLD

Primary lymphoedema of the lower limb

The patient lies supine with the head supported on a pillow and the lower limb(s) raised. Sitting with both legs horizontal is avoided, particularly if the patient is obese, because the abdomen compresses the superficial lymphatics of the groin and obstructs venous return. Some support can be used to lift the head and shoulders if there is difficulty in lying flat, for example if the patient is breathless. Venous flow is stimulated by raising the legs.

The sequence of events is shown in Figure 12.7:

1   drainage of the inguinal nodes (10 times)

2   inciting manipulation on the thigh (a,b,c)

3   drainage of popliteal nodes (10 times)

4   resorption of the lymphoedema; many manipulations until decreased tissue turgor is palpable

5   inciting technique from the distal part of the lymphoedema up to the root of the limb (once)

6   drainage of the inguinal nodes (twice).

These manipulations are repeated for about half an hour. In the same supine position, the patient should move the ankle up and down for a few minutes to stimulate venous return.

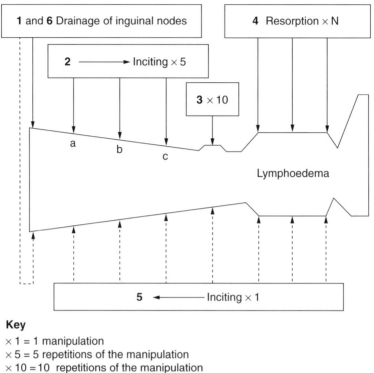

Key
$\times$ 1 = 1 manipulation
$\times$ 5 = 5 repetitions of the manipulation
$\times$ 10 = 10 repetitions of the manipulation
$\times$ N = many manipulations on the oedema

Figure 12.7 Primary lower leg lymphoedema; *see* p.209 for explanation.

Secondary lymphoedema of the lower limb

With oedema of the lower limb after inguinal or abdominal node removal, it is necessary to utilise alternative drainage pathways. Such pathways have been demonstrated in animals[17] and in humans.[18] These lympholymphatic anastomotic pathways still function when the normal pathway is destroyed by node removal:[19]

- the inguino-axillary pathway
- the inguino-inguinal or suprapubic pathway.

The therapist has to stimulate both pathways before draining the limb itself. The sequence of events is shown in Figure 12.8:

1   both axillary regions (10 times)

2   inciting manipulation from the axillary region down to the groin (5 times)

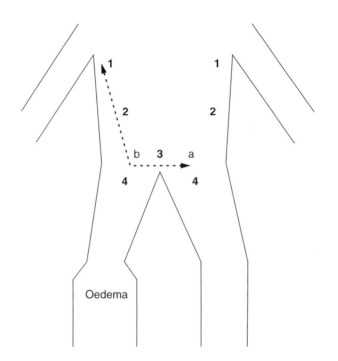

Figure 12.8 Oedema of the lower leg after oncological surgery; see p.210 for explanation.

3   suprapubic pathway (5 times)

4   both inguinal regions simultaneously (10 times).

After draining these alternative pathways, the therapist begins with the classical programme described earlier (Figure 12.7). It should be noted that, if there is a risk of bilateral leg swelling, working across the suprapubic pathway may lead to swelling in a previously unswollen leg.

Post-traumatic oedema of the arm

The patient lies supine with the head supported on a pillow and the upper limb about 30° in abduction and 15° in elevation. This positions the axillary vein in the optimal situation for drainage.[20] The sequence of events is shown in Figure 12.9:

1   both hands encircle the upper arm → inciting technique (5 times)

2   drain the trochlear nodes (5 times)

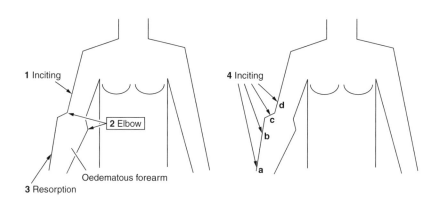

Figure 12.9   Post-traumatic oedema of the forearm; see p.211 for explanation.

3   resorption of the forearm oedema

4   inciting technique from the wrist up to the upper arm (once).

Postmastectomy lymphoedema

The following text should be read in conjunction with Figure 12.10. With the patient supine:

1   drain both subclavian regions (10 times)

2   drain both axillary regions (10 times).

With the patient lying on the unoperated side and the affected arm resting on the therapist's shoulder:

3   drain via alternative pathways along the back (3a, 3b, 3c) using the inciting technique.

Then with the patient supine:

4   drain the Mascagni pathway (a superficial secondary lymphatic pathway which crosses over the clavicle *en route* from the forearm to a chain of cervical lymph nodes)

5   inciting on the upper arm, beginning distally and working proximally to the axillary region

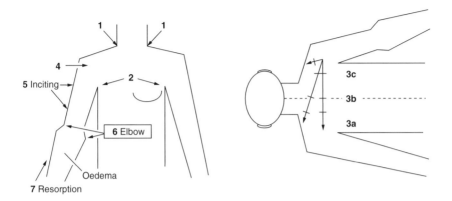

Figure 12.10 Forearm oedema after breast cancer surgery; see p.212 for explanation.

6   drain the trochlear nodes (5 times)

7   resorption of the oedema.

Results

The photographs were taken of the patients during outpatient treatment in a private treatment centre (Figures 12.11 and 12.12). Daily treatment lasts for 2 hours for a period of 2–3 weeks. The treatments were carried out by therapists trained in our techniques (Leduc method). For long-term follow-up, we aim to see the patient again 1–2 years after finishing the treatment.

Conclusion

MLD is part of our standard decongestive lymphoedema therapy. We have developed a non-aggressive form of MLD which generally reduces the volume of the limb considerably. With our physical treatment there is no risk to the patient. Equally important, treatment is on an outpatient basis and patients are able to continue their normal activities.

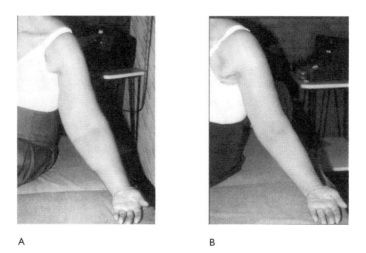

A   B

Figure 12.11 Postmastectomy oedema. A = before; B = after 2 weeks (10 treatments).

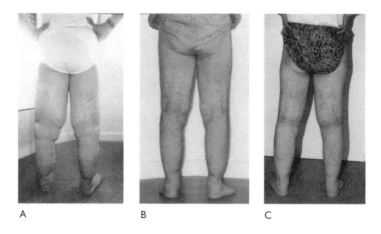

A   B   C

Figure 12.12 A = patient aged 51 after bilateral adenectomy; B = after 2 weeks of treatment; C = 1 year after treatment; the patient wears a compression stocking to maintain the improvement achieved with MLD.

References

1 Leduc A et al. (1991) Le Traitement Physique de l'Œdème du bras. Monographies de Bois-Larris, 2nd edn. Masson, Paris.
2 Leduc A and Leduc O (1992) Le Drainage de la Grosse Jambe, A Leduc (ed). Wilmart and Gilles, Belgium.

3 International Society of Lymphology, Executive Committee (1995) The diagnosis and treatment of peripheral lymphedema (consensus document). *Lymphology.* **28**:113–7.

4 Leduc A and Leduc O (1997) Kombination Verschiedener Therapie Masznahmen in der Behandlung des Lymphödem. *Zeitschrift für Lymph.* **1**:10–11.

5 Leduc O *et al.* (1998) The physical treatment of upper limb edema. *Cancer.* **83**:2835–9.

6 Leduc O *et al.* (1998) Manual lymphatic drainage: scintigraphic demonstration of its efficacy on colloidal protein reabsorption. In: H Partsch (ed) *Progress in Lymphology – IX.* Excerpta Medica, Elsevier, Amsterdam, pp 551–5.

7 Mortimer PS *et al.* (1990) The measurement of skin lymph flow by isotope clearance. Reliability, reproductibility, injections dynamics and the effect of massage. *Journal of Investigative Dermatology.* **95**:677–82.

8 Leduc A *et al.* (1985) Lymphatic resorption of proteins and pressotherapies. 6th Congress of the European Lymphology Group. Porto, Portugal, May 31.

9 Leduc O *et al.* (1990) Hemodynamic effects of pressotherapy. In: M Nishi, S Uchino, S Yabuki (eds) *Progress in Lymphology.* Elsevier Science, Amsterdam, pp 431–4.

10 Leduc O *et al.* (1998) Intermittent sequential pneumatic compression (ISPC). From the device to the patient. Progress in Lymphology. XVI. *Lymphology.* **31(suppl)**: 1–621.

11 Partsch H *et al.* (1980) Experimental investigations on the effect of a pressure wave massage apparatus (Lympha Press®). *Lymphedema, Phlebologie und Proktologie.* **2**:80.

12 Leduc O *et al.* (1990) Bandages: scintigraphic demonstration of its efficacy on colloidal protein reabsorption during muscle activity. In: M Nishi, S Uchino, S Yabuki (eds) *Progress in Lymphology.* Elsevier Science, Amsterdam, pp 421–3.

13 Leduc O *et al.* (1993) Dynamic pressure under bandages with different stiffness. In: H Boccalon (ed) *Vascular Medicine.* Elsevier Science, Amsterdam, pp 466–8.

14 Demeyer D *et al.* (1988) Etude comparative du comportement de bandages élastiques et non-élastiques utilisées dans le traitement de l'œdème lymphatique. *Annales de Kinésithérapie.* **15(10)**:461–7.

15 Mislin H (1961) Experimenteller Nachtweiss der Autochtonen Automatic der Lymphgefasse. *Experientia.* **17**:29–32.

16 Eliska O and Eliskova M (1995) Are peripheral lymphatics damaged by high pressure manual massage? *Lymphology.* **2**:21–30.

17 Leduc A and Lievens P (1976) Les anastomoses lympho-lymphatiques: incidences thérapeutiques. *Travaux de la Société Scientifique Belge de Kinésithérapie.* **4**:7–11.

18 Leduc A *et al.* (1993) Lymphatic drainage of the upper limb. Substitution lymphatic pathways. *European Journal of Lymphology and Related Problems.* **14**:11–18.

19 Piller NB *et al.* (1997) Lymphoscintigraphic evidence supports the existence of axilloinguinal anastomotic pathways in a patient with chronic secondary leg lymphedema subsequent to inguinal node clearance and radiotherapy. *European Journal of Lymphology and Related Problems.* **6**:97–9.

20   Belgrado J-P *et al.* (1998) Positioning of the axillary vein after breast surgery. 4th Meeting of the Latin-Mediterranean Chapter of the International Society of Lymphology and 24th Meeting of the European Group of Lymphology. June 18–20, 1998, San Marco di Castellabate (SA) Italie.

Further reading

Leduc A and Leduc O (1995) Le Drainage Lymphatique Théorie et Pratique 1980–1998. Masson, Paris.

13 Simple lymphatic drainage

Sarah Bellhouse

It is common practice in lymphoedema clinics to teach patients, and sometimes their relatives, simple lymphatic drainage (SLD) as part of the treatment
for lymphoedema. SLD is based on the principles of manual lymphatic drainage (MLD) but the hand movements have been simplified so that patients can
learn and apply the technique for themselves. SLD can be undertaken by
most patients (self-massage) and can help them feel more in control of their
condition. For patients who require SLD but cannot manage it themselves, a
relative or friend can be taught instead.

Patients and professionals have anecdotally reported good results and
benefits with SLD. Factors which influence the success of the treatment
include:

- the evaluation of the patient

- the type of training the therapist has received

- how the patient is taught

- whether the patient has experience of MLD or SLD before undertaking
  self-massage.[1]

It is not sufficient to hand out a leaflet on SLD and expect patients or their
relatives to teach themselves.

Indications for use of SLD

A careful physical, psychological and social evaluation (ability, function and
motivation) should be made before patients and/or their relatives are taught
massage. The patient's mobility and function must be sufficient to enable them
to undertake the massage, for example the ability to bend the elbow. Some
patients find that doing the massage makes the affected arm ache. If a patient
is unable to perform SLD, a relative or friend can be taught the technique –
but only if this is acceptable to the patient.

The main indications for SLD are:

- as part of lymphoedema management both in the intensive and maintenance phases of treatment

- after a course of MLD
- mild lymphoedema in conjunction with the use of compression garments
- midline oedema, e.g. facial, genital and truncal swelling
- to help soften and improve the elasticity of the skin, particularly when the skin is attached by scarring to underlying tissues
- as an adjunct to pneumatic compression therapy (PCT) (see p.236), both before and after the use of the pump, to assist in the resorption of proteins from the tissues.[2]

The contra-indications which apply to MLD also apply to SLD:

- active cancer (but may be used in advanced cancer; see p.338)
- an acute inflammatory episode (AIE)
- an acute allergic reaction
- cardiac failure
- superior vena caval obstruction
- venous thrombosis in the last 6 months.[3]

Additional contra-indications to SLD include:

- lack of motivation (often because of lack of understanding)
- impaired mobility and function of the upper limbs.

Some patients feel uncomfortable with the idea of massage and on no account should pressure be put on the patient or relatives to do it.

Training of staff

The confidence of the therapist to practise and teach SLD greatly influences the degree to which the patient becomes motivated and skilled in self-massage. To develop this confidence, the therapist needs to undertake training and practise the technique in order to develop expertise. SLD has often been regarded as a mere adjunct to lymphoedema management. Arguably, when SLD is used as an integral part of treatment and time has been devoted to teaching it, the results will be better.

Many courses concerned with the management of lymphoedema include SLD and a few specifically teach SLD. Ideally the therapist should have some training in MLD.[1] It is not sufficient for therapists to be self-taught. They need to have had training and experience of performing the massage to be successful in passing on their knowledge to patients. If several members of staff teach SLD in the same clinic, they need to agree and standardise their technique to ensure consistency.

Teaching

The success with which patients and their relatives learn SLD is dependent on the quality of teaching and on the enthusiasm and effort of the teachers. Learning for the patient should be progressive, both from the point of view of understanding their condition and of becoming skilled in the technique. It is unrealistic to expect patients on their first visit to the clinic to assimilate the movements and the complete massage sequence on their first attempt. If they are overloaded with information at this point, they are less likely to continue with the technique and the therapist's time and effort will be wasted. Patients often find great difficulty in learning and memorising the technique and adhering to the daily treatment regimen.[1]

Most adults learn best by seeing, experiencing and finally practising the massage themselves. By experiencing the massage they are able to feel the movement of the skin and the lightness of the touch (something very difficult just to explain). The massage and the way it is taught are not just a physical exercise, but can also influence patients' psychological wellbeing, by helping them to adjust and feel more comfortable about their condition.

The time taken to teach is variable; 30 minutes or more may be necessary to allow the patient and/or relative to obtain an adequate experience of the massage. If this is not possible, careful planning will be needed and the teaching broken down into short sessions over several visits. This may mean that only the hand movement and one sequence are taught at the first visit. This can then be reviewed, extended and refined at subsequent visits. It is beneficial to get the patient or relative to demonstrate the massage, as this helps in evaluating how the patient or relative is progressing in learning the technique.

Teaching aids

A simple diagram of the upper or lower part of the body with arrows to show the direction of hand movements and numbers to show the sequence of hand positions has proved to be successful with patients and relatives (Figure 13.1). These diagrams can be shared between health professionals if a patient either transfers clinics or sees different therapists within the same clinic. A copy

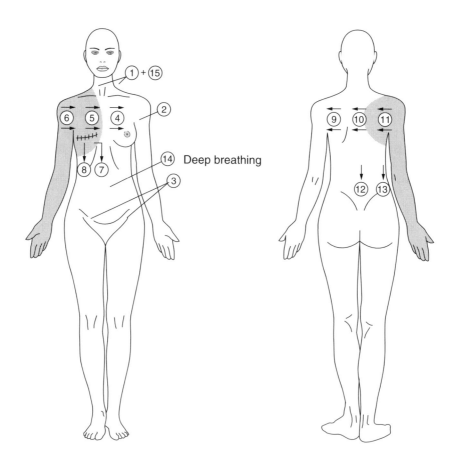

Figure 13.1   Breast cancer-related lymphoedema of the right arm. Shading denotes swelling or at risk quadrant; arrows show the direction of hand movements; numbers show the sequence of hand positions.

should be given to the patient and one kept in the patient's records. This enables the therapist to see what has been taught to the patient in the past and to build on the patient's experience. It avoids patients becoming confused by being taught different techniques. Each time any additional movements or changes are made to the sequence the chart should be updated. There are several videos available showing SLD which are useful for patients to borrow while they are learning the technique. Inevitably there are minor variations in the recommendations but the underlying principles are the same.

Method

Preparation and positioning

The massage should be undertaken in a warm, quiet, comfortable room. Clothing and jewellery on the areas to be massaged should be removed and the patient covered with towels or a blanket. If a relative or therapist is to do the massage, it is important that the couch or bed is at a comfortable height to avoid back strain.

The position of the patient will need to be adjusted according to the patient's preference and take account of any underlying medical condition. If the patient is performing self-massage and the oedema is in the upper part of the body they may choose to be sitting or lying. However, if someone else is doing the massage, it is preferable for the patient to be lying down.

If the oedema is below the waist, ideally the patient should be lying down to avoid compression of the superficial lymphatics in the groin. Whatever position is adopted, the patient and the affected limb should be well supported with pillows.

Details of method

The massage should be light, slow and rhythmic, and should elicit no pain or discomfort. The movements should generally be in the direction of lymph flow towards the nearest functioning regional lymph nodes. It is important that the lymphatics on the unaffected side of the body are treated first to stimulate them and help drain the area before any fluid is moved from the oedematous area. It is generally more beneficial to concentrate the massage on the body rather than on the limb. Indeed, patients are encouraged to wear their compression garments during SLD.

SLD can be done using various movements and at present there is no evidence to suggest one is more effective than the other. However, the more precisely the technique is executed, the better the results are likely to be.

Oil should not be used for this massage as it encourages the hands to slide, and prevents the close skin to skin contact that is required. If the hands become sticky during the massage, a small amount of non-perfumed talcum powder may be used.

The hand movement suggested here is based on a circular movement. The movement comes from the arms with the palm of the hand and fingers being kept straight Each circle is performed with a light pressure for the first half of the circle. Then the pressure is gently released and the skin will bring the hand back. Each movement is performed in the same position several times before moving to another position.

The predominant movement should be of skin rather than the underlying tissue. The amount the skin moves will vary from area to area of the body, and from person to person. The skin should only be moved as far as it will comfortably go. The hands should not slide over the skin as this may create a shearing force and reddening of the skin.

The appendix contains a suggested sequence for SLD for unilateral limb oedema. The sequence will need to be adapted for each patient depending on:

- the site of the oedema
- the patient's mobility
- their ability to learn and to perform the massage
- the time available to them.

They should be encouraged to do the massage at least daily for approximately 15–20 minutes. Any longer than this becomes tedious and can cause strain on the hands and arms. The sequence can also be used by a health professional.

Conclusion

SLD plays a useful role in the management of lymphoedema. Its efficacy depends on the enthusiasm and skill of the teacher, who should have an understanding of the principles of MLD, and the patient.

Acknowledgements

The massage sequence described in this chapter was developed jointly by Sarah Bellhouse (MLD therapist), Angela Williams (ICRF lymphoedema research sister 1991–1997), Karen Jenns (clinical nurse specialist), Karen Hughes (physiotherapist), at the Lymphoedema Clinic, Sir Michael Sobell House, Oxford.

References

1   Mortimer P and Williams A (2000) An evaluation of manual lymphatic drainage for breast cancer related lymphoedema. In press.
2   Leduc A and Leduc O (1996) The physical treatment of the lower limb edema. Multidisciplinary Group of Insufficiency of the Lymph-Venous System.
3   Wittlinger H and Wittlinger G (1998) *Textbook of Dr Vodder's Manual Lymph Drainage, Volume 1: Basic course,* 6th revised English edition. Haug International, Brussels.

Appendix

Self-massage

The shading in Figures 13.2–13.14 in this section denotes the affected limb or area.

Suggested sequence for unilateral arm oedema

1 Deep breathing

Start the session with a breathing exercise. Lying flat on the back with your knees bent, place your hands flat just below the ribs to offer a little resistance. Without arching the back, take a slow, deep breath in through the nose. Your hands should rise on breathing in (abdomen ballooning out). Hold for a count of 2. Then slowly let the breath out through the mouth. The hands should lower on breathing out (abdomen sinking in). The upper chest should not move. Repeat the deep breathing 3–5 times, taking care not to become dizzy.

2 Neck massage

First position

Place your fingers on either side of the neck, keeping the fingers together and straight. The little finger of both hands should be just below the ear lobes. Keeping your hands as near as possible to the perpendicular, take the skin back and then circle down towards the shoulders. Release the light pressure and let the skin bring your hands back to the start position so completing the circle. Repeat the movement 5 times in the same position (Figure 13.2).

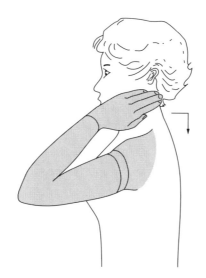

Figure 13.2   Neck massage. First position.

Second position

Move your hands down on both sides of the neck to a second position, so they are approximately half way between the ears and the shoulders. Repeat the movement described for the first position 5 times. The skin will usually move more easily here (Figure 13.3).

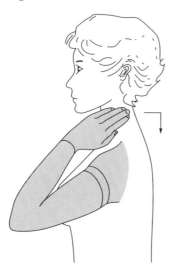

Figure 13.3   Neck massage. Second position.

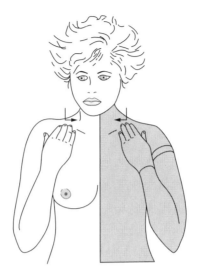

Figure 13.4 Neck massage. Third position.

Third position

Move both of your hands down to the base of the neck to a comfortable position between the collarbone and the large shoulder muscle (trapezius). Relax your wrists and fingers. On both sides, using the pads of your index and middle fingers bring the skin forwards towards the collarbone and then circle in towards the neck. Release the light pressure and let the skin bring your fingers back to the start position so completing the circle. Repeat the movement 5 times in the same position (Figure 13.4).

Repeat all of the neck massage on both sides 3 times.

3 Axillary lymph nodes massage

Working on the *unaffected* side. For comfort and ease, relax your unaffected arm at the side of your body (Figure 13.5).

First position

Place your fingers on the side of the chest about half a hand width below the axilla, keeping your fingers together and straight. Keeping your hands as near as possible to the perpendicular, take the skin towards the back and then circle up towards the axilla. Release the light pressure and let the skin bring your hands back to the start position so completing the circle. Repeat the movement 5 times in the same position.

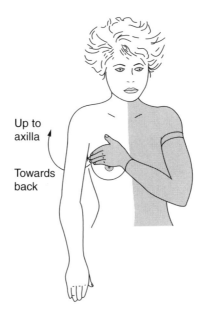

Up to
axilla

Towards
back

Figure 13.5   Axillary lymph nodes massage.

Second position

Move your hand half a hand width lower down the chest wall towards the waist to a second position. Take the skin towards the back and then circle up towards the axilla. Release the light pressure and let the skin bring your hands back to the start position so completing the circle. Repeat the movement 5 times in the same position.

Repeat all of the axillary lymph node massage 3 times.

4 Upper chest massage

Place your fingers of the affected arm, on the front of your chest close to the top of the unaffected arm, keeping the fingers straight and together (Figure 13.6). Take the skin towards the axilla and then circle upwards. Release the light pressure and let the skin bring your hand back to the start position so completing the circle. Repeat the movement 5 times in the same position and do the same movement over all of area 'a' (unaffected side of the upper chest).

Slowly work across your upper chest to the affected side moving from area 'a' (unaffected side of the upper chest) to area 'b' (midline of the upper chest). Then complete the massage for area 'c' (affected side of the upper chest and over the shoulder) changing hands for this last section, as shown in Figures 13.7 and 13.8. Remember to keep the massage movement the same

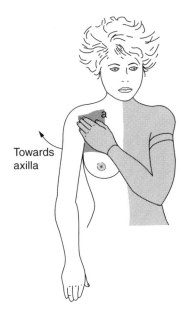

Figure 13.6   Upper chest massage. (a) unaffected side of upper chest.

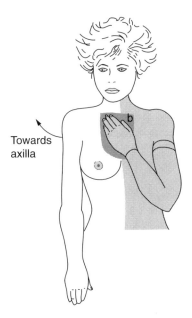

Figure 13.7   Upper chest massage. (b) midline of upper chest.

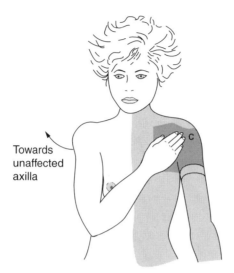

Towards
unaffected
axilla

Figure 13.8 Upper chest massage. (c) affected side of the upper chest and over the shoulder.

as for area 'a' and area 'b'. Pay particular attention to the midline over the breastbone. Repeat all of the upper chest massage 3 times.

5 Deep breathing

Finish the session with the breathing exercise as described at the start of the session. Relax and remain lying down for a couple of minutes before getting up.

Additional sequences for unilateral arm lymphoedema

1 Upper back massage

If someone is able to assist with the massage, then the following can be included after the upper chest massage. Lie down comfortably on your front or unaffected side. Alternatively, you may sit upright ensuring that the upper back is free to be massaged.

Ask them to do the same as the upper chest massage across your upper back starting close to the top of the *unaffected* axilla. Take the skin towards the unaffected arm and then circle downwards. Release the light pressure and let

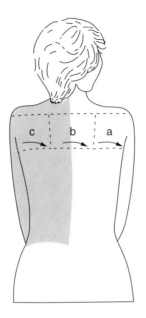

Figure 13.9 Upper back massage.

the skin bring the hand back to the start position so completing the circle. Repeat the movement 5 times in the same position. Slowly work across the upper back to the shoulder of the affected side (area 'c'). Use the same movements on many overlapping positions from area 'a' to area 'b' and area 'c' (Figure 13.9). Again, pay particular attention to the midline over the spine.

2 Groin lymph nodes massage

Place flat hands one either side on the lower abdomen just above the groin creases. Take the skin inwards towards the midline then circle towards the groin. Release the slight pressure and let the skin bring the hand back to the starting position. Repeat the movement 5 times in the same position (Figure 13.10).

3 Lower chest/abdomen massage

This only needs to be done if there is swelling below the breast/scar line. Place the flat hand on the waistline on the affected side of the body in the line of the axilla, keeping the fingers straight and together (Figure 13.11). Take the skin towards the side of the body and then circle downwards towards

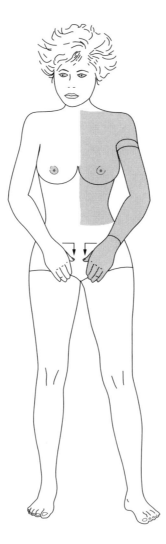

Figure 13.10 Groin lymph nodes massage.

the groin. Release the light pressure and let the skin bring your hand to the start position so completing the circle. Repeat the movement 5 times in the same position and do the same movement over all of the area 'a' then 'b' gradually working from the waistline up to the ribcage. Remember to take the skin down towards the groin.

Finish the session with the breathing exercise as described for the start of the session. Relax and remain lying down for a couple of minutes before getting up.

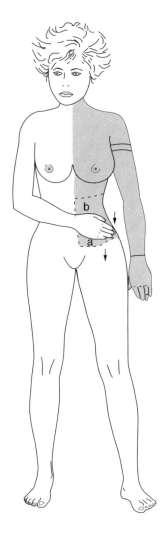

Figure 13.11 Lower chest/abdomen massage.

Suggested sequence for unilateral leg oedema

1 **Deep breathing** – as for arm self-massage; *see* p.223.

2 **Neck massage** – as for arm self-massage; *see* p.223.

3 **Axillary lymph nodes massage** – as for arm self-massage; see p.225.
Work on one side and then repeat for the other side. For comfort and ease,
relax the arm that is not working at the side of your body.

4 Groin lymph nodes massage

Working on the *unaffected* side.

First position

Place your fingers on the inner aspect of the upper thigh, keeping them together and straight. Take the skin towards the inner thigh and then circle up towards the groin. Release the light pressure and let the skin bring your hand back to the start position so completing the circle. Repeat the movement 5 times in the same position (Figure 13.12).

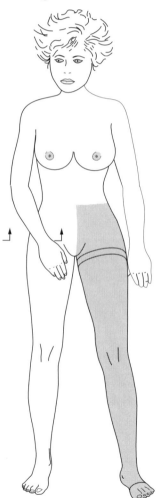

Figure 13.12 Groin lymph nodes massage working on the unaffected side.

Second position

Move your hands to the top of the thigh to a second position. Take the skin towards the inner thigh and then circle up towards the groin. Release the light pressure and let the skin bring your hands back to the start position so completing the circle. Repeat the movement 5 times in the same position

Repeat all of the groin lymph nodes massage 3 times.

5 Lower abdomen massage

Place your fingers, keeping them straight and together, at the far side of the waistline of the unaffected side of the body (Figure 13.13). Take the skin towards the side of the body and then circle up towards the axilla. Release the light pressure and let the skin bring your hand to the start position so completing the circle. Repeat the movement 5 times in the same position and do the same movement over all of the area 'a'. Slowly work across the lower abdomen moving from area 'a' to area 'b' to area 'c'. Use the same movements on many overlapping positions. Repeat all of the lower abdomen massage 3 times.

6 Deep breathing

Finish the session with the breathing exercise as described for the arm self-massage. Relax and remain lying down for a couple of minutes before getting up.

Additional sequences for unilateral leg lymphoedema

Lower back massage

If someone is able to assist with the massage, then the following can be included after the lower abdomen massage. Lie down comfortably on your front.

Ask them to do the same as the lower abdomen massage across your back starting close to the waistline on the unaffected side. Take the skin towards the side of the body and then circle up towards the axilla. Release the light pressure and let the skin bring your hand to the start position so completing the circle. Repeat the movement five times in the same position and do the same movement over all of the area 'a'. Slowly work across the lower back moving from area 'a' to area 'b' to area 'c' as in Figure 13.14. Use the same movements on many overlapping positions. Repeat all of the lower back massage 3 times.

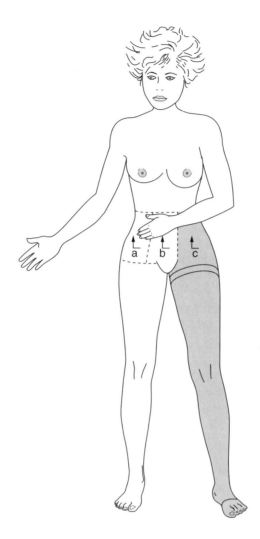

Figure 13.13 Lower abdomen massage.

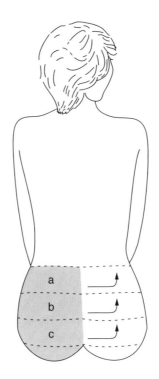

Figure 13.14 Lower back massage.

14   Pneumatic compression therapy

Tracey Bray and Justine Barrett

Pneumatic compression therapy (PCT) may be used to treat primary and secondary lymphoedema in selected cases.[1-4] Although popular in the 1980s, its use has declined considerably, probably because of the benefits obtained with decongestive lymphoedema therapy (DLT). However, recent studies have shown several problems associated with its use in lymphoedema.[5] This chapter discusses the relevant pathophysiology and describes how PCT can complement other aspects of lymphoedema management.

Description

The *Collins Dictionary* gives the following definitions:

- *pneumatic* – concerned with air, gases or wind. A machine or device operated by compressed air

- *compression* – to squeeze together. The act of compression or the condition of being compressed

- *therapy* – the treatment of disorders or disease.

PCT has been described as 'compressing limbs in air bags'.[6] It requires an electric pump which can exert pressures of 30–40mmHg, although some pumps have a pressure range from 20–300mmHg.[7] Older models had an invariable combined inflate and deflate time-cycle, whereas newer ones have variable separate inflate and deflate cycles. Treatment times can now be varied, in contrast to a single on/off option. A polyvinyl chloride (PVC) garment of variable length is fitted onto the arm or leg. It has a lining which can be easily cleaned between patients. When fitted, it is connected by a plastic tube to the pump which cyclically inflates and deflates the garment. Duplex scanning has demonstrated that PCT increases blood velocity.[8] It also increases the resorption of interstitial fluid but does not affect the resorption of proteins.[9]

Garments with multiple chambers generally have several connecting tubes which come together before entering the pump. The individual chambers inflate in a sequential pattern of compression up the limb, creating a peristaltic or ripple effect.[10] The compression always starts distally and moves proximally. The ripple effect of a multichambered sequential pump is much more effective at moving fluid than the simple squeezing effect of a single chamber.

History

PCT has been used for many years to manage swollen limbs. The early machines were adaptations of those used to prevent deep vein thrombosis (DVT) in the legs during surgery. For the purpose of improving lymphatic and venous circulation in the oedematous limb, an automated pneumatic compression unit with a single inflatable chamber was developed.[11,12]

In the 1960s a form of PCT was used to provide a 'pneumatic splint' to reduce arm oedema in postmastectomy patients. Although it helped, the technique was abandoned because suitable, cheap pumps were not available.[13] In the 1970s the use of pumps in physiotherapy departments and at home was advocated because of the reported benefit in patients with swollen arms. Around the same time a method of producing intermittent compression of the leg was developed using an inflatable PVC legging attached to an electric pump and inflated intermittently.[14]

As a result of various studies, the home use of such pumps by patients was encouraged.[13,14] Most pumps were the single chamber variety and were used in conjunction with compression garments. Patients were often told to use the pumps for long periods (4–6 hours), sometimes overnight.

In the UK, pioneering work on pneumatic compression was carried out during the 1970s.[9] Early equipment was bulky because of the size of the compressed air cylinders, but was quickly replaced by a pneumatic system driven by a compressor which supplied air to a single-chambered limb garment with a pressure range of 20–140mmHg. A number of authors have supported the use of PCT as an additional treatment in the management of lymphoedema (*see* p.203).

Types of pumps

There are various makes and models available (Table 14.1). These range from small portable pumps with single or three-chambered garments to larger models with multichambered ones which inflate and deflate sequentially (Figure 14.1). Almost all the pumps use compressed air to squeeze the swollen limb. Functionally, however, they fall into two categories:

- *segmental* (sequential, multichambered) – these have several compartments (3, 5 or 10) which inflate (and compress) in sequence; the pressures here may be graded

Table 14.1   Pumps available for PCT

Number of chambers	Type of compression	Examples[a]
1	Intermittent	Flotron
3	Intermittent sequential	Flotron Plus Flowpac Talley
5	Intermittent sequential (peristaltic)	Flowpress Talley Centromed
10	Intermittent sequential gradient (peristaltic)	Centromed Talley

a   some pumps can be used with different garments from the same manufacturer, e.g. Flowpress garments can be used with Flowpac and Flotron Plus pumps.

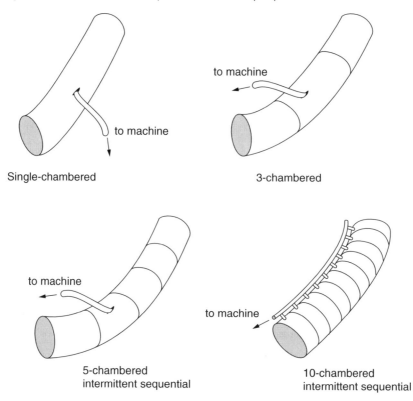

Figure 14.1   Types of intermittent sequential compression garments available for PCT.

- *non-segmental* (single-chambered) – the limb is simply enclosed by a continuous sleeve or stocking and is compressed all at once, and then released.[5]

Mercury is used in a few pumps. This gives a very high but smoothly graded compression. It is claimed that, when used with care, these pumps do not cause complications like traditional PCT pumps and are particularly useful for very fibrotic limbs.[5] As these machines are expensive, they are not widely used.

Indications for PCT

Pitting oedemas generally respond to PCT. It therefore works well in non-obstructive oedemas:

- immobility

- venous incompetence

- lymphovenous stasis

- hypoproteinaemia.[15]

The following limiting factors should be noted:

- high pressures can damage the superficial lymphatics

- single chamber PCT has no direct effect on lymph flow[7]

- PCT may result in genital or truncal swelling

- the patient's lifestyle becomes restricted if the machine is used for long periods[5,16,17]

- patients may become dependent on the machine and overrate its contribution to the total package of care.[18]

Cautions and contra-indications

Cautions

The extent of any cancer should be clarified before using PCT because there is a potential risk of local residual tumour spreading into the veins and lymphatics.[19] The superficial initial lymphatics are delicate and damage can easily occur. PCT can exert pressures up to 300mmHg,[7] and the fragile lymphatics can be broken with consequential disruption of the lymphatic network.[5] Most patients with lymphoedema already have a compromised lymphatic system so that, if used incorrectly, PCT can have a lasting detrimental effect on the limb. Further, if the applied pressure is excessive, there may be bruising as a result of damage to small blood vessels.

The garments used for PCT end at the root of the limb. When a person has an inadequate deep lymphatic system or there is blockage further along the drainage pathway, then the area proximal to the garment becomes overloaded. This can predispose to further fibrosis with the development of a restrictive cuff around the upper part of the limb.[5] Fibrosis is also a risk factor for acute inflammatory episodes (AIE), fistulae and lymphangiosarcoma.[20]

Genital oedema is a major clinical and psychological complication of lymphoedema (see p.331). Sexual intimacy is generally adversely affected. When genital oedema is present, potentially serious lymphocutaneous fistulae can occur.[21] Regardless of the type of pump or the underlying cause of the lymphoedema, nearly half of those treated develop genital oedema with PCT.[21]

Contra-indications

The following are the main contra-indications for PCT:

- arterial deficit, i.e. < 0.8 ankle–brachial pressure index (ABPI)
- AIE
- acute DVT
- pitting oedema associated with cardiac or renal failure
- oedema in adjacent area of the trunk
- active cancer at the root of the limb or in the adjacent quadrant.

Guidelines for the use of PCT

The equipment for PCT comprises:

- pneumatic compression pump
- inflatable sleeve or stocking
- stockinette to protect the skin.

Guidelines for the use of PCT as part of DLT for patients with lymphoedema are detailed in Box 14.A. Limb volumes should be recorded at intervals throughout the programme of treatment to monitor the overall effect.

Box 14.A   Guidelines for PCT

Before PCT

1   For leg swelling check ankle–brachial pressure index (ABPI).

2   Explain the procedure to the patient.

3   Remove jewellery from the part to be treated.

4   Advise patient to empty bladder.

5   Ensure that the patient is in a comfortable lying position with the affected limb supported.

6   In obstructive lymphoedema, the patient or therapist should perform simple lymphatic drainage (SLD) or manual lymphatic drainage (MLD) to stimulate lymphatic flow from adjacent truncal areas.

Actual PCT

1   Apply a cylindrical cotton bandage (stockinette) to the limb.

2   Apply PCT sleeve/stocking to limb, ensuring valves are closed if present (e.g. Flotron).

3   *First session:*
   • familiarise the patient with the treatment
   • set the pressure for 30mmHg for 30min (*possibly only 20mmHg in palliative care*).

   Subsequent sessions:
   • set the pressure to 40mmHg for 30–60min (*possibly 20–30mmHg in palliative care*).

4   Switch on the machine.

5   When treatment is complete switch off the machine and remove sleeve/garment.

After PCT

1   Repeat SLD or MLD.

2   Fit compression garment or apply multilayer lymphoedema bandages (MLLB).

3   Clean PCT sleeve/stocking with soap and water between use by different patients.

4   Limb volumes should be measured at intervals during PCT, e.g. weekly.

Precautions

1   Contact a doctor if:
   • the patient becomes breathless when using the pump, *and stop the treatment immediately*
   • the limb becomes red, hot or painful.

2   Reconsider the use of PCT if swelling develops around:
   • the shoulder or chest wall (with arm oedema)
   • the groin, genitalia or buttock (with leg oedema).

Published data on PCT are generally about prophylactic use in the management of DVT. In relation to lymphoedema, data are not readily available as to what proportion of lymphoedema is treated by PCT, nor of the results and complications.[21] Even so, health professionals need to have an understanding of the benefits and risks of PCT, and of its potential place within a comprehensive lymphoedema management programme. It should be noted that, if support or compression is not applied between treatments, fluid will collect again in the overstretched tissues with a return of the swelling. In a limb which has reduced in size, it takes at least 3 weeks for the skin to regain its elasticity and to maintain the reduced shape without external support.

References

1   Tinkham RG and Stillwell GK (1965) The role of pneumatic pumping devices in the treatment of postmastectomy lymphoedema. *Archives of Physical Medicine and Rehabilitation.* **46**:193–7.

2   Allenby F *et al.* (1973) The use of pneumatic compression in the swollen leg. *Physiological Society.* **February**:65–6.

3   Swedborg I (1984) Effects of treatment with an elastic sleeve and intermittent pneumatic compression in post-mastectomy patients with lymphoedema of the arm. *Scandinavian Journal of Rehabilitation and Medicine.* **116**:35–41.

4   Newman G (1988) Which patients are helped by intermittent external pneumatic compression therapy. *Journal of the Royal Society of Medicine.* **81**:377–9.

5   Casley-Smith JR *et al.* (1996) The dangers of pumps in lymphoedema therapy. *Lymphology,* **29(suppl)**:232–4.

6   Hopkins E (1996) Sequential compression to treat lymphoedema. *Professional Nurse.* **11(6)**:397–8.

7   Twycross R (1997) *Symptom Management in Advanced Cancer,* 2nd edn. Radcliffe Medical Press, Oxford.

8   Moody M (1997) Intermittent sequential compression therapy in lower limb disorders. *Professional Nurse.* **12(6)**:423–5.

9   Leduc A *et al.* (1988) Lymphatic reabsorption of proteins and pressotherapies. In: H Partsch (ed) *Progress in Lymphology – XI.* Elsevier Science, Amsterdam, pp 591–2.

10   Richmond DM (1985) Sequential pneumatic compression for lymphoedema: a controlled trial. *Archives of Surgery.* **120**:1116–9.

11   Brush BF *et al.* (1959) Some devices for the management of lymphoedema of the extremities. *Surgical Clinics of North America.* **39**:1493–8.

12   Yamazaki Z *et al.* (1987) Clinical experiences using pneumatic massage therapy for oedematous limbs over the last 10 years. Paper presented at the 29th Annual Meeting of the International College of Angiology, Montreaux, Switzerland, July 1987.

13   McNair TJ *et al.* (1976) Intermittent compression for lymphoedema of the arm. *Clinical Oncology.* **2**:339–42.

14 Pflüg JJ (1975) Intermittent compression in the swollen legs in general practice. *The Practitioner.* **215**:69–76.

15 Casley-Smith JR (1985) Discussion of the definition, diagnosis and treatment of lymphoedema (lymphostatic disorder). In: JR Casley-Smith and NB Piller (eds) *Progress in Lymphology, Vol X.* University of Adelaide Press, South Australia, pp 1–16.

16 Badger C (1987) Lymphoedema: Management of patients with advanced cancer. *The Professional Nurse.* **January**:100–102.

17 Gray RC (1987) The management of limb oedema in advanced cancer. *Nursing Times.* **73(10)**:504–6.

18 Gillham L (1994) Lymphoedema and physiotherapists: control not cure. *Physiotherapy.* **80(12)**:835–43.

19 Földi M and Kubik S (1989) *Lehrbuch der lymphologie für mediziner und physiotheraputer.* Fischer, Stuttgart and NY.

20 Cancernet (1997) The National Cancer Institute.

21 Boris M *et al.* (1989) The risk of genital oedema after external pump compression for lower limb lymphoedema. *Lymphology.* **31**:15–20.

15   Drug treatment for lymphoedema

Robert Twycross

The emphasis in the management of lymphoedema in the UK and Western Europe is on non-drug treatments. In Australia, there has been a longstanding interest in drug treatment with benzopyrones. In Africa, Asia and South America, however, because the commonest cause of lymphoedema is filariasis, antibiotic treatment should be the norm.

Other drugs which have been tried are diuretics and, in patients with recurrent cancer, corticosteroids. These will be discussed first, mainly because there is no coherent body of evidence about their use – just anecdotes. In contrast, there is an impressive number of randomised control trials of benzopyrones. Reference will also be made to several other drug treatments, including antibiotics for filariasis.

Diuretics

Given that lymphoedema is a failure of lymphatic drainage and is not caused by venous incompetence, systemic fluid retention or right cardiac failure, there is no obvious reason why diuretics should be beneficial. On the other hand, some patients will have one or more of these conditions in association with lymphoedema, particularly in immobile patients with lymphovenous stasis (*see* p.55). Thus a trial of a diuretic should be considered if:

- the lymphoedema has increased since the prescription of a nonsteroidal anti-inflammatory drug (NSAID), a corticosteroid, oestrogen or progestogen

- there is evidence of concurrent cardiac failure

- there is evidence of a significant venous component.

In this latter situation it is possible that limb elevation may well be a better option with less chance of causing systemic hypovolaemia and orthostatic hypotension.

A reasonable trial of diuretic therapy would be furosemide (frusemide) 20mg o.d. or bumetanide 500µg o.d. for 1 week. In congestive cardiac failure, however, the dose will be determined by the severity of the failure and the initial response to treatment, and will be administered concurrently with an ACE-inhibitor, digoxin and/or other appropriate cardiac drugs.

Corticosteroids

If recurrent cancer is the main cause of the lymphoedema, dexamethasone 8mg o.d. PO for 1 week should be considered. However, because cortico-steroids may cause restlessness or agitation, 4mg o.d. may be a safer starting dose in the elderly and the very anxious. There are many sporadic reports of patients benefiting from dexamethasone and a trial of treatment is always worthwhile in cancer patients with worsening lymphoedema and no other obvious exacerbating cause such as an acute inflammatory episode (AIE). By reducing tumour-induced inflammation, the lymphatic obstruction is decreased. If of benefit and no specific oncological treatments are available, dexamethasone 2–4mg o.d. can be continued indefinitely.

Benzopyrones

Benzopyrones are a group of several thousand naturally-occurring sub-stances. About 50 of these have been tested in high-protein oedemas and all have had a beneficial effect. The two main chemical groups are:

- coumarin and its derivatives (coumerols)
- flavone and its derivatives (flavonoids).

The core chemical structure is a benzene ring and a pyrone ring. A pyrone ring is like a benzene ring but with one of the carbon atoms replaced by oxygen. Coumarin contains an α-pyrone ring (Figure 15.1) whereas flavone contains a γ-pyrone ring (Figure 15.2). The α or γ refer to the site in the ring at which an additional oxygen atom is attached.

There are several chemically distinct subgroups of flavonoids, for example flavan and its derivatives (Figure 15.3) and quercetin and its derivatives, in-cluding rutin and the hydroxyethylrutosides (oxerutins) (Figure 15.4). Sodium cromoglicate, used in the management of allergic rhinitis and asthma, is essentially two benzo-γ-pyrone molecules joined together, i.e. double chromone (Figure 15.2). It has also been shown to reduce high-protein oedema.[1]

Coumerols

Most of the known coumerols have been isolated from plants, but some have been isolated from micro-organisms and from animals.[2] The nomenclature is confusing. Coumarin itself has *nine* different chemical names including 1,2-benzopyrone, 5,6-benzo-α-pyrone, 2H-chromen-2-one, coumarinic anhydride.

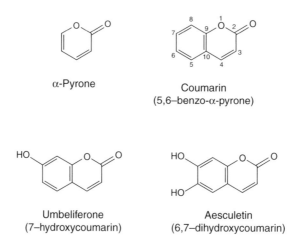

Figure 15.1   Chemical structure of α-pyrone and some of its important derivatives, including benzo-α-pyrone (coumarin).

Many coumerols are known by names derived from the Latin or the collo-quial name of the plant from which they were first isolated or from the place where the plant grows, with the result that the same compound has several botanical names. Equally confusing is the fact that the assigned name may give little or no information as to the compound's structural composition. For example, 7-hydroxycoumarin is also known as *umbeliferone, skimmetin* and *hydrangin.*

The richest sources of coumerols are the Rutaceae and Umbelliferae. The coumerols are secondary products of plant metabolism but their exact role in plant physiology is not clearly understood. Although found in all parts of the plant, the coumerols occur at the highest concentrations in the fruits, followed in decreasing order by the roots, stems and leaves. Coumarin itself occurs in many plants including tonka beans, sweet clover, woodruff, oil of cassia and lavender. It is a relatively simple organic compound and was first synthesised in 1868 by heating O-hydroxybenzaldehyde with sodium acetate and acetic anhydride at 180°C.[3]

Collectively, apart from their effects on high-protein oedema, coumerols have a wide range of pharmacological properties. These include:

- stimulation of plant germination
- antibiotic and pesticidal activity
- anticoagulation.

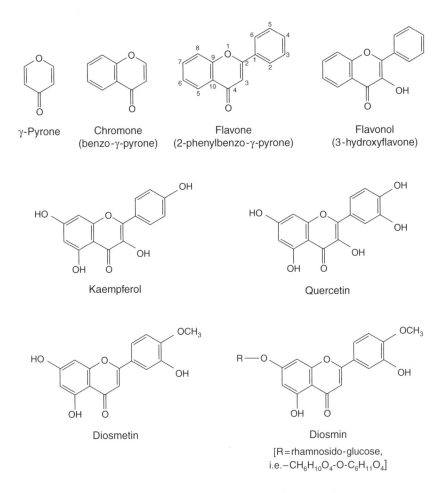

Figure 15.2 Chemical structure of γ-pyrone and some of its more important derivatives, including chromone, flavone and some of the many flavonols.

None of the coumerols has all these properties. Coumarin has a pleasant fragrant odour and in some countries it is used as flavouring for certain recipes. It is also used to enhance the fragrance in some brands of cigarettes. Over 100 000kg per year is used in the USA in soaps, detergents, lotions and perfumes;[1] 7-hydroxycoumarin is also sometimes used in perfumes.

The discovery that spoilt hay made from sweetclover (*Trifolium repens*) was toxic because of an anti-prothrombin action, led to the development of oral anticoagulants. To become anticoagulant, coumarin has to be converted to 4-hydroxycoumarin with the subsequent condensation of two molecules by naturally-occurring formaldehyde. This discovery gave rise to the search for

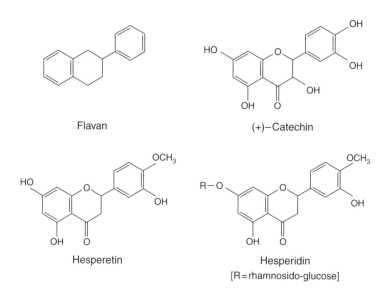

Flavan   (+)−Catechin

Hesperetin

Hesperidin
[R = rhamnosido-glucose]

Figure 15.3 Diagrams of flavan (which lacks the double bond at the 2,3 position and the oxygen at position 4 possessed by flavone) and its derivatives.

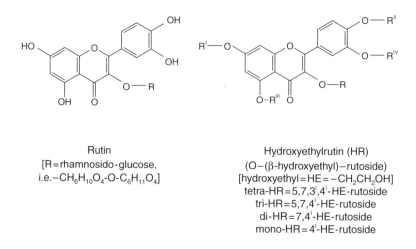

Rutin
[R=rhamnosido-glucose,
i.e.−CH₆H₁₀O₄-O-C₆H₁₁O₄]

Hydroxyethylrutin (HR)
(O−(β-hydroxyethyl)−rutoside)
[hydroxyethyl=HE=−CH₂CH₂OH]
tetra-HR=5,7,3',4'-HE-rutoside
tri-HR=5,7,4'-HE-rutoside
di-HR=7,4'-HE-rutoside
mono-HR=4'-HE-rutoside

Figure 15.4 Diagrams of the quercetin derivative, rutin, and its derivatives (the hydroxyethylrutosides).

similar anticoagulants and poisons for rodents. Most of these are dicoumerols, although the widely used warfarin (3-(α-acetonyl)-4-hydroxycoumarin) is not. On the other hand, most dicoumerols do *not* reduce high-protein oedemas. It should be noted that warfarin and oxerutins (a standardised preparation of rutin-derived flavonoids) do not interact. Oxerutins 1g/day added to warfarin therapy in 12 patients with a deep vein thrombosis had no effect on the activated partial thromboplastin time.[4] A few years ago there was considerable interest in the use of coumarin as an anticancer treatment.[5,6] So far, however, this has not led to any major therapeutic development.

The finding that large doses of coumarin are hepatotoxic in some species has led to its medical use being discontinued in some countries (e.g. Australia and France). Hepatotoxicity appears to be idiosyncratic and therefore unpredictable.[7] In a human toxicology study, 17 out of nearly 2200 subjects (0.8%) developed raised hepatic enzyme concentrations.[7] In some, however, the elevation was associated with metastatic cancer or infective hepatitis, giving a revised figure of $< 0.4\%$. Doses were generally lower than those used clinically, typically 100mg o.d. for 1 month followed by 50mg o.d. for 2 years. None developed permanent liver damage and values returned to normal in 5 people who continued to take coumarin. In clinical studies of patients with lymphoedema receiving 400mg daily for a mean of 15 months hepatotoxicity was reported in 2/1106 cases (0.2%).[8]

In a more recent study, however, 9/140 patients (6%) developed a plasma aminotransferase (AST) concentration more than 2.5 times the upper limit of normal; and in one case the plasma bilirubin rose to 19mg/100ml (330µmol/litre).[9] In all 9 patients, treatment with coumarin was stopped, and values returned to normal. These data are disturbing and suggest that the earlier reports may have underestimated the true incidence of hepatotoxicity. What is not known from this latest study, is whether the AST concentration would have returned to normal (or not progressed) had treatment been continued in the 8 patients who did not become jaundiced.

Be that as it may, after two deaths from hepatotoxicity, the Australian Department of Health cancelled the medicinal licence for coumarin in the mid-1990s and France has done likewise. Hence, even if effective (Box 15.A), coumarin may well not be available much longer. In the future, the focus will be on the oxerutins and other flavonoids. On the other hand, because of greater bio-availability, the use of coumarin–troxerutin combinations allow a reduction in coumarin dose to 25% of the standard 200mg b.d. regimen.[15] Depending on what is the toxic substance – coumarin itself or its metabolites – such formulations could be less hepatotoxic.[16]

Surprisingly, troxerutin (tri-oxerutin) is regarded by the manufacturers as merely an excipient. It is, however, one of the five main constituents of oxerutins (see below) and, although not as potent as mono- and di-oxerutin, it is not inert.[17–19] Its effect will therefore be additive to that of coumarin. At some centres, an alternative mixture (coumarin 60mg, gingko biloba 40mg and melilotus 40mg/day) is used.[20]

Box 15.A   Coumarin

Class of drug: Benzopyrone.

Indications: Lymphoedema.

Contra-indications: Hepatic dysfunction (see Cautions below).

Pharmacology

Coumarin is rapidly and completely absorbed from the gastro-intestinal tract. It is extensively metabolised by the liver and less than 4% reaches the systemic circulation after oral administration. The major metabolite is 7-hydroxycoumarin which, like the parent compound, is biologically active; it accounts for 60–70% of the total dose. The 'area under the curve' for 7-hydroxycoumarin after oral administration of coumarin is about 90% of that after an IV dose. Coumarin is well-absorbed through the skin and it can be detected in the bloodstream for several hours after topical application.[10-12] 7-hydroxycoumarin is conjugated by the liver to a glucuronide, which is then excreted in the urine. Conjugation is mediated by the cytochrome CYP2A6 pathway and there are fast and slow metabolisers.[13] The rate of excretion is dose-dependent; 95% of a 5mg dose is excreted in 4h compared with 95% of a 200mg dose in 10h. With supratherapeutic doses of 1–2g, the amount excreted as 7-hydroxycoumarin-glucuronide drops to 20–40%.

Coumarin and its active metabolite adhere to the endothelium of small blood vessels and decrease vascular permeability to proteins. They also stimulate the local congregation of macrophages in interstitial fluid. The macrophages stimulate proteolysis (fibrinolysis) both chemically and by phagocytosis. This proteolytic activity reduces the potential for protein-induced chronic inflammation and fibrosis and, in lymphoedema, converts a slowly progressive condition into a slowly improving one. Coumarin has numerous other properties including immunomodulation and, in some cancers, an oncostatic, or even oncolytic, effect.[6] Coumarin also inhibits the biosynthesis of prostaglandins and leukotrienes.[14] Various coumarin derivatives, notably warfarin (3-(α-acetonylbenzyl)-4-hydroxycoumarin) and several dicoumerols are anticoagulants; neither coumarin itself nor 7-hydroxycoumarin possess this property.

In some countries, coumarin 15mg is available in combination with troxerutin (trioxerutin) 90mg. The combination modifies the bio-availability of coumarin in a favourable direction. Coumarin is 35% available from the combination preparation compared with 2–6% for plain coumarin tablets.[1,15] Thus plain coumarin 400mg supplies 8–24mg of bio-available coumarin whereas the combination (Lysedem), when taken in typical doses of 2–3 tablets t.d.s. (coumarin 90–135mg), the yield of bio-available coumarin is some 32 and 48mg respectively.

Oral bio-availability: Coumarin 2–6%; 7-hydroxycoumarin about 90%.

Onset of action: Probably rapid but covert for several months in chronic lymphoedema.

continued

Box 15.A   *continued*

Duration of action: The beneficial effects outlast a prolonged course of treatment by weeks or months.

Plasma halflife: Coumarin = about 1h after both IV and PO administration; 7-hydroxycoumarin not known.

Interactions

Patients taking enzyme-inducing anti-epileptic drugs (e.g. carbamazepine, phenobarbital) have an increased rate of 7-hydroxycoumarin-glucuronide formation and urinary excretion.

Cautions

May cause transient elevation of liver enzymes;[9] more serious hepatotoxicity is occasionally seen after several months of treatment, generally with complete recovery after stopping administration. Two deaths from hepatic failure, however, have been reported; as a result, the medicinal licence for coumarin has been rescinded in Australia and France.

Adverse effects

Nausea and/or diarrhoea (reduced from 6% to <1% by enteric-coating). Occasional dizziness, drowsiness, rash, pruritus, muscular aches. Hepatotoxicity is seen in 6% of patients treated for lymphoedema.[9]

Doses and use

The standard oral dose of coumarin in the treatment of lymphoedema is 200mg b.d. No effect will be seen for several months and treatment must be given indefinitely (i.e. for years). Coumarin-troxerutin compound tablets (coumarin 15mg + troxerutin 90mg) are traditionally given in a dose of 2–3 tablets t.d.s. Published data indicate that the two doses are equally effective; this means that the dose can be restricted to 2 tablets t.d.s.[16] Coumarin can also be administered topically on a daily basis as part of skin care.

Supply

Not available in the UK, Australia and France. Availability elsewhere should be checked with the national licensing authority or national formulary.

Tablets coumarin 100mg.

Tablets coumarin 15mg + troxerutin 90mg (e.g. Lysedem, Venalot Depot).

Powder coumarin 10% in sterile talc.

Ointment coumarin 10% in polyethylene glycol.

Flavonoids

These occur widely as pigments in plants. They have been used in various proprietary medications for many years. Although in the past they were extracted from plants, some are now semi- or completely synthetic. Flavonoids possess a wide spectrum of biological activity. From the therapeutic point of view the most important are their anti-oxidant properties. Flavonoids inhibit many different enzymes. Inhibition of cyclo-oxygenase and lipoxygenases seem to be most important, resulting in the diminished formation of pro-inflammatory mediators (prostaglandins (PGs), leukotrienes, reactive oxygen species, nitric oxide). Flavonoids are also antithrombotic because of their ability to scavenge superoxide anions. These anions are strong inhibitors of prostacyclin production. Removal of superoxide anions by flavonoids facilitates the production of anti-aggregatory PGI_2.[21] A deficiency of flavonoids increases capillary fragility and permeability; the flavonoids in lemon skin (citrin) have been shown to correct these. All the benzopyrones which have been tested have been shown to have this property and are sometimes called 'vitamin P' or 'P factors'.

The flavonoids most frequently used therapeutically are the rutin derivatives, mixed O-(β-hydroxyethyl)-rutosides – with the British Approved Name of oxerutins (Box 15.B). Hydroxyethylation of rutin increases its water solubility but also results in a mixture with up to 144 components.[35] Careful control of the process, however, ensures that a standardised combination is produced with four compounds comprising the bulk of the mixture, namely mono-oxerutin (5%), di-oxerutin (34%), tri-oxerutin (46%) and tetra-oxerutin (5%). Some experiments have concluded that mono-oxerutin is the most effective component of oxerutins, whereas others suggest that di-oxerutin is.[17]

More recently, a 'micronised' preparation of two flavonoids (diosmin 90% and hesperidin 10%) has been tested in a pilot study.[36] Micronisation enhances the gastro-intestinal absorption of the two constituent flavonoids, thereby reducing the dose required (500mg b.d.).

Benzopyrones and venous insufficiency

Oxerutins are marketed in the UK as Paroven. It is licensed for use for the relief of the symptoms of oedema associated with chronic venous insufficiency. Two reviews of oxerutins were published in 1992; one brief and the other more comprehensive.[37,38] The former was critical of the rigour of the published trials of oxerutins and stated that evidence for efficacy in chronic venous insufficiency was unconvincing. The more comprehensive review was more positive and concluded that, in patients with either chronic venous insufficiency or diabetes, oxerutins:

Box 15.B   Oxerutins

Class of drug: Benzopyrone.

Indications: Discomfort associated with chronic venous insufficiency (licensed), lymphoedema (unlicensed indication).

Pharmacology

Oxerutins is a standardised mixture of semisynthetic flavonoids, comprising mainly mono-, di-, tri- and tetra-hydroxyethylrutosides. Oral absorption and therefore bio-availability are low. The unabsorbed components are degraded by intestinal flora to aglycones. Peak plasma concentrations are reached 1–6h after ingestion. Excretion is mainly biliary, probably after hepatic metabolism. Only 3–6% of the dose is excreted in the urine. Oxerutins act principally on the microvascular endothelium, reducing permeability for large molecules (e.g. proteins) and capillary filtration rate.

Microvascular permeability: Histamine-induced permeability is reduced by about 40% in healthy volunteers after treatment for 7 days with oxerutins 1.8g/day.[22] In normal and inflamed single frog mesenteric capillaries, permeability was reduced about 50% even though the intercellular gaps in the endothelium persisted.[23,24] A progressive reduction in oedema formation (determined by measuring the increase in leg volume after standing for 1h) was recorded in healthy volunteers during treatment for 3 weeks with oxerutins 1g/day.[25] After a 10-week trial, the effect persisted for some 6 more weeks (Zyma, data on file).

Capillary filtration rate: Reduced by about 20% in healthy volunteers;[26] up to 40% in chronic venous insufficiency and venous hypertension.[26,27]

Microvascular perfusion and microcirculation: Venous partial oxygen pressure, oxygen content and oxygen saturation all improve in patients with chronic venous insufficiency receiving oxerutins, and tissue oxygen extraction is reduced.[28,29]

Erythrocyte function: In vivo inhibition of erythrocyte aggregation was observed in healthy volunteers given oxerutins 2.4g/day for 3 days.[30]

Histamine release from mast cells is inhibited in animals treated with oxerutins.[31]

Prostaglandin production is reduced in dogs.[32]

Free radical scavenging: Studies in rat hepatic microsomal fractions suggest that oxerutins have an anti-oxidant effect and the potential ability to protect against lipid peroxide-induced injury. Oxerutins are potent hydroxyl radical scavengers and inhibit non-enzymatic lipid peroxidation.[33–35] They attenuate nicotine-induced endothelial cell damage.

Oral bio-availability: About 10% of an oral dose is absorbed.

Onset of action: 60–90 min but covert for several months.[27]

continued

Box 15.B   *continued*

Duration of action: The beneficial effects outlast a prolonged course by weeks or months.

Plasma halflife is about 1h after IV administration and 10–25h after oral administration.

Cautions

Oxerutins should not be taken during the first 3 months of pregnancy.

Adverse effects

Few adverse effects have been reported and occur with equal frequency with placebo in controlled trials: nausea, diarrhoea, pruritus, dizziness, headache.

Doses and use

For lymphoedema, 3g/day (i.e. 1.5g b.d. or 1g t.d.s.). Smaller doses have been used in venous insufficiency (0.9–1.2g/day).

Supply

Tablets oxerutins 250mg (Paroven UK).

- improve microvascular perfusion and microcirculation
- reduce platelet aggregation
- have a possible protective effect on the vascular endothelium (Table 15.1).

Further the review concluded that, in trials of up to 6 months, oxerutins significantly improved the symptoms and the signs of chronic venous insufficiency and of venous insufficiency of pregnancy (Figure 15.5). The percentage of patients reporting improvement varies between trials:

- leg pain, 54–82%
- cramps, 59–91%
- tired 'heavy' legs, 64–68%
- restless legs, 35–55%.

Objective measures (leg volume, calf circumference) improved concomitantly. Oedema in chronic venous insufficiency has a relatively low protein content (5–10g/L) compared with chronic lymphoedema (30–35g/L) and will not therefore cause inflammation and fibrosis to the same extent. However, with high venous pressure, fibrinogen is deposited around the capillaries and then polymerises to form an insoluble fibrin complex which traps inflammatory agents, stiffens the vessel wall and modifies perfusion and diffusion. It has

Table 15.1   Vascular effects of oxerutins in the legs of patients with chronic venous insufficiency[38]

Pharmacodynamic parameter	Patients with chronic venous insufficiency (compared with healthy volunteers)	Effect of oxerutins in patients with chronic venous insufficiency[a]
Capillary filtration rate	↑	↓
Venous blood pO_2	↓	↑
Transcutaneous pO_2	↓	↑
Transcutaneous pCO_2	↑	↓
Resting skin blood flow	↑	↓
Veno-arteriolar response	↓	↑
Venous refilling time	↓	↑

a   effects were significant ($p < 0.05$) v placebo or pretreatment.
pCO_2 = partial carbon dioxide pressure; pO_2 = partial oxygen pressure; ↓ denotes decrease; ↑ denotes increase.

been suggested that this impedes oxygen and nutrient exchange, thereby predisposing to ulceration. Benzopyrones have a strong affinity for vein walls[40] and reduce pericapillary fibrin by attracting and activating macrophages to secrete lysosomal enzymes which increase tissue fibrinolysis.[41]

The dose of oxerutins recommended by the manufacturers is 500mg b.d. However, after 3 month's treatment in 30 menopausal women, no difference was noted between 600, 900, 1200 and 1500mg daily and all four doses showed significant benefit compared with placebo.[42,43]

Benzopyrones and lymphoedema

In animals and humans, benzopyrones have been shown to:

- decrease capillary permeability to protein[22]
- increase the number of macrophages in the oedema
- stimulate macrophage-induced proteolysis
- stimulate phagocytosis by macrophages.[44]

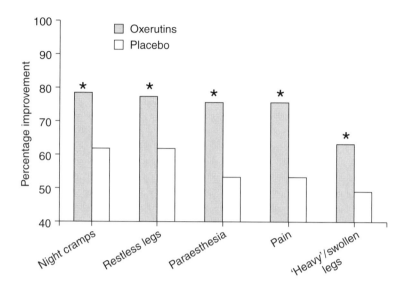

Figure 15.5 Percentage improvement in symptom scores of patients with chronic venous insufficiency treated with oxerutins 1g/day (n = 481) or placebo (n = 115) for 4 weeks; * denotes significant difference (p < 0.05) between treatment groups.[39]

In animals, destruction of the macrophages blocks the proteolytic effect of oxerutins.[45] The breakdown of protein leads to absorption of the resulting amino acids into the vascular system with the concomitant removal of the 'osmotically obligatory-held' interstitial fluid. Continued proteolysis results in the gradual regression of fibrosis. By reducing the protein content of the oedema (including growth factors and cytokines), benzopyrones remove the stimulus for chronic inflammation and fibrosis. AIE become less frequent (see Chapter 9). As a result, comfort and mobility are improved. Even the skin changes of elephantiasis improve in time. Capillary permeability varies according to circumstances. Experiments with a single frog capillary showed that a protein-free perfusate increased permeability and that this was corrected by an albumin-containing perfusate.[46] It has been suggested that the albumin binds reversibly to the luminal surface of the capillary endothelium and thereby increases the hydraulic resistance of the capillary membrane. Oxerutins also reduce the hydraulic permeability in a single frog capillary after this had increased as a result of a protein-free perfusate.[46] The mechanism by which this is achieved is debatable but probably is related to the ability of oxerutins to scavenge free radicals. In contrast, in inflammation, increased capillary permeability is associated with the development of endothelial gaps with associated macromolecular leakiness.

Clinical trials

Benzopyrones may be taken orally or applied topically and, apart from sporadic hepatotoxicity with coumarin, have few adverse effects – principally nausea and diarrhoea in 10–15% – which generally settle spontaneously after several weeks of treatment. The combined results from 1225 patients in 25 open studies of oral benzopyrones gave a mean reduction of oedema of $36 \pm 6\%$ (mean $\pm$ SE) per year.[1] There were no differences between arms and legs. Elephantine legs were less reduced ($15 \pm 6\%$) than grade 1 and 2 lymphoedema ($57 \pm 9\%$; $p = 0.002$).

These results have been confirmed in several randomised double-blind placebo-controlled trials which, with one exception, have shown that benzo-pyrones convert a slowly worsening condition into a slowly improving one (Table 15.2). Typically, the following benefits are seen:

- reduced limb volume

- decreased tissue turgor

- elevated skin temperatures lowered

- reduced bursting pains, tension and heaviness

- increased comfort and freedom of movement.

In one trial, 70% of patients preferred the active drug and 97% noted an increase in wellbeing, compared with 4% when on placebo.[48] Unfortunately, the results are not presented uniformly. Trials 1, 3 and 7 give percentage change in arm volume whereas trials 2, 4, 6, 8 give absolute changes and in trial 5 the results are given as changes in the *ratio* of arm volume (swollen/normal). This makes meta-analysis impossible. However, it is possible to compare increases *v* decreases in arm volumes. When analysed in this way it is apparent that a decrease in arm volume was not achieved with placebo in 7/8 trials (Table 15.3), or in 8/9 trials if trial 8 is regarded as two sequential 6-month trials (*see* Table 15.3, footnote f). On the other hand, a positive reduction was achieved with the benzopyrones in all but one trial, or in 7/9 if trial 8 is regarded as two trials.

It is possible that the exceptional result in trial 8 relates to an order-of-treatment effect. In other words, the benefit seen with placebo was really the delayed impact of a 6-month course of coumarin and the lack of apparent benefit with coumarin related to a slower onset of action in this group of

Table 15.2 Results of randomised placebo-controlled trials of benzopyrones in lymphoedema

Authors	Limb	Background	Subjects[a]	Trial design	Drug[b]	Outcomes			
						Volume	Turgor	Pain	Movement
1 Desprez-Curely et al. 1985[47]	Arm	Postmastectomy lymphoedema of variable duration	92 → 45 / 46	Double-blind, parallel groups (6 months)	Coumarin 135mg+ troxerutin 810mg daily (as Lysedem[c] 3 tablets t.d.s.)	↓[d]	NA[e]	NA	NA
2 Piller et al. 1988[48]	Arm / Leg	Postmastectomy and primary lymphoedema of leg; swelling for >6 months (legs generally much longer). Physical therapy stopped 1 month before trial	50 → 26 (arm) / 14 (leg)	Double-blind, crossover (6 months × 2)	Oxerutins 3g daily (1g t.d.s.)	↓	↓	↓	↑
3 Pecking and Cluzan 1989[49]	Arm	Postmastectomy and postradiotherapy	80 → 39 / 39	Double-blind, parallel groups (9 months)	Coumarin 90mg+ troxerutin 540mg daily (as Lysedem[c] 2 tablets t.d.s.)	↓	NA	NA	NA
4 Casley-Smith et al. 1993[50]	Arm / Leg	Postmastectomy and postsurgical or primary lymphoedema in leg. *Duration of swelling not recorded.* Physical therapy stopped 1 month before trial	36 → 31 / 26 → 21	Double-blind, crossover (6 months × 2)	Coumarin 200mg b.d.	↓	↓	↓	↑
5 Taylor et al. 1993[51]	Arm	Treated breast cancer; long-term physical treatment; stable arm volume for >6 months. *Concurrent maintenance physical therapy*	31 → 22	Double-blind, crossover (24 weeks × 2)	Oxerutins 3g daily	↓	↓	NA	NA

continued

Table 15.2 *continued*

Authors	Limb	Background	Subjects[a]	Trial design	Drug[b]	Outcomes Volume	Turgor	Pain	Movement
6 Mortimer et al. 1995[52]	Arm	Treated breast cancer; swelling for >6 months. *Concurrent maintenance physical therapy*	46 ⟨ 10 / 9	Double-blind, *parallel groups* (6 months)	Oxerutins 3g daily	↓	NA	NA	NA
7 Chang et al. 1996[53]	Leg	Most = filariasis or other infection; some primary, post-traumatic, postoperative	60→60	Double-blind, *parallel groups* (6 months)	Coumarin 400mg daily	↓	↓	↓	↑
8 Loprinzi et al. 1999[9]	Arm	Treated breast cancer; swelling for >1 year. Physical therapy stopped 1 month before trial	138→120 →93	Double-blind, crossover (6 months × 2)[f]	Coumarin 200mg b.d.	No difference	No difference	No difference	No difference

a numbers recruited → numbers completing trial and included in the analysis
b all drugs given PO
c Lysedem tablets contain coumarin 15mg and troxerutin 90mg
d circumference only measured (at wrist, mid forearm, mid upper arm)
e NA = not applicable (i.e. not measured)
f results given only as two 6-month group comparisons.

Table 15.3 Changes in limb volume in randomised placebo-controlled trials of benzopyrones

Authors	Duration of trial (months)	No. of evaluable patients	Placebo	Active drug
1 Desprez-Curely et al. 1985[47]	6	91[a]	↑	↓
2 Piller et al. 1988[48]	12	40	↑	↓
3 Pecking and Cluzan 1989[49]	6	78[a]	↑	↓
4 Casley-Smith et al. 1993[50]	12	52	↑	↓
5 Taylor et al. 1993[51]	12	22[b]	↑	↓
6 Mortimer et al. 1995[52]	6	19[a,b]	↑	↓
7 Change et al. 1996[53]	6	60[a]	→	↓
8 Loprinzi et al. 1999[9]	6 (1)[c]	120	↑	↑
	6 (2)[c]	93	↓	↑

a   group comparisons with approximately half in each of two groups (benzopyrone, placebo); other trials were crossover design (6 months on benzopyrone, 6 months on placebo in random order)
b   compression garments were worn throughout the trial period
c   because the data for the whole 12-month trial was not presented in an integrated form, the crossover design becomes two 6-month group comparisons; (1) refers to the first 6 months and (2) refers to the second 6 months.

patients than those evaluated in other trials. Although this offers an explanation for the discrepancy, it remains surmise and not certainty – and therefore may be wrong. An added difficulty in interpretation is the fact that only about three quarters of the patients evaluated at 6 months were evaluated after 1 year. In other words, the stated mean arm volume at 6 months was *not* the initial mean arm volume of the smaller groups evaluated at the end of the second 6-month period.

In a recent trial of two different doses of coumarin and troxerutin, it was found that coumarin 90mg + troxerutin 540mg daily (Lysedem 2 tablets t.d.s.) was as effective as a dose 50% higher.[16] The trial has been criticised, however, on the grounds that it was not placebo-controlled.[54] The trial which showed no benefit with coumarin 200mg b.d. was cited as showing the continued need for placebo-control.[9] However, 7/7 previous trials of benzopyrones all showed greater benefit with the active drug, a significant finding in itself ($p < 0.05$). In the trial of higher *v* lower dose coumarin, the volume reduction over 12 months was 13% and 15% respectively.[16] Even though volume reductions of 3% and 0.8% were recorded with placebo in the 'placebo-positive' trial,[9] to suggest that reductions of 13–15% do not represent a definite drug effect beggars belief. It should be emphasised that, although the effect of benzopyrones is slow compared with decongestive lymphoedema therapy (DLT) the improvement is achieved without the use of expensive compression garments.[55]

Benzopyrones and DLT

In a review of the results from over 600 patients with arm or leg oedema, pretreatment with oral or topical benzopyrones before DLT improved the mean reduction obtained with DLT by 50% and, with continued benzopyrone treatment after DLT, doubled the mean reduction after 1 year.[55] The greater resolution of oedema after pretreating patients with oral benzopyrones before DLT, and using them topically during DLT, may be related to a partial breakdown of fibrosis in the lymphoedematous limb.

From the data presented in Tables 15.4 and 15.5, it will be seen that the effect of benzopyrones combined with DLT was considerable. Statistical tests were done only on the results from the first two analyses. There was statistically significant benefit from either oral or topical benzopyrone (of the same order of magnitude) and a further statistically significant advantage when both oral and topical benzopyrones were used in combination. The doses used were coumarin 400mg/day or oxerutins 3g/day. Results were comparable and so

Table 15.4 What half the patients can expect to exceed[a]: results with DLT ± benzopyrones in unilateral or bilateral lymphoedema expressed as reduction of limb volume as % of initial limb volume (number of patients in parentheses)

Category of patient	After 4 weeks of DLT	After 1 year on benzopyrones[b]
DLT only	– 11 (356)	– 7.6 (90)
DLT + *oral* benzopyrones	– 15 (111)	– 13 (51)
DLT + *topical* benzopyrones	– 15 (69)	– 11 (24)
DLT + *oral and topical* benzopyrones	– 18 (92)	– 18 (54)

a   the median improvement in each group of patients
b   includes initial month of DLT.

Table 15.5 What three-quarters of the patients can expect to exceed: results with DLT ± benzopyrones in unilateral or bilateral lymphoedema expressed as reduction of limb volume as % of initial limb volume (number of patients in parentheses)

Category of patient	After 4 weeks of DLT	After 1 year on benzopyrones[a]
DLT only	− 6.4 (356)	− 3.1 (90)
DLT + *oral* benzopyrones	− 9.4(111)	− 8.5 (51)
DLT + *topical* benzopyrones	− 9.7 (69)	− 5.3 (24)
DLT + *oral and topical* benzopyrones	− 12 (92)	− 12 (54)

a   includes initial month of DLT.

were merged for the analysis. Topically, benzopyrones were applied in one of two ways:

- coumarin ointment (10% in polyethylene glycol)
- coumarin powder (10% in sterile talc).

The patient population was obtained from consecutive patients treated with DLT mostly by therapists trained by the authors. It should be noted that:

- some therapists performed better than others
- more compliant patients had a better outcome
- elderly patients had a better outcome.

The emphasis was on DLT of course, and it could be claimed that, provided *tablet compliance* is good, a regimen which depends less on the relative merit of the therapist is inherently preferable. Over a whole year benzopyrones alone achieve about 50% of the reduction seen with DLT – and without the added cost and inconvenience of compression garments.

It is not clear why so many patients were not reviewed at the end of 1 year – about 75% in one group. Did they fail to return because they were disappointed/ disillusioned or because the treatment had been so satisfactory that they had no desire to return? In consequence the results at 1 year must be treated with circumspection. That said, it certainly appears that DLT combined with benzopyrone therapy is not only initially better than DLT alone ($p < 0.05$, Wilcoxin 2-sample tests) but continued benzopyrone therapy maintains the

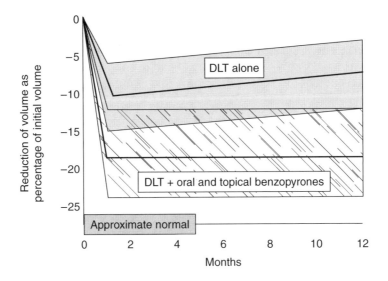

Figure 15.6   Reductions of limb volume as % of initial limb volume, for DLT alone and DLT plus oral and topical benzopyrones; showing the medians (thick lines), and the first (lower) and third (upper) quartiles for each group. The shaded areas between the first and third quartiles contain 50% of the results for each group, with 25% above and 25% below them.[48]

benefit achieved by DLT, particularly if benzopyrones are given both orally and topically (Figure 15.6). In contrast, the lymphoedema in patients treated with DLT alone deteriorated over the subsequent 11 months.

Grape seed extract

Along with extracts from pine bark, lemon tree bark, hazelnut leaves, cherries, blueberries, cranberries and grape skins, grape seeds contain flavonoids called *proanthocyanidins* (formerly oligomeric proanthocyanidin complexes/OPC). The chemical structure of the proanthocyanidins is closely similar to other flavonoids, and their reported properties suggest that there is considerable, possibly complete, functional overlap with coumarin and the oxerutins.[56,57]

The literature on proanthocyanidins stresses their anti-oxidant (free radical scavenging) property and their consequential ability to prevent or minimise many of the degenerative changes associated with ageing by, *inter alia*, stabilising collagen and elastin. As anti-oxidants, the proanthocyanidins are 50 times more effective than vitamin E, and 20 times more effective than vitamin C.[58,59] However, the literature about coumarin and oxerutins comes mainly from Western orthodox medicine and that relating to the proantho-cyanidins from herbal medicine. No reference is made in the respective literatures to any impact by the proanthocyanidins on macrophage numbers and fibrinolytic activity or about coumarin and oxerutins as possible stabilisers of collagen and elastin. Even so, it is probable that these properties are common to all three groups of substances.

A daily dose of grape seed extract 50mg is recommended for general purposes.[56] The same dose of pine bark extract may be used if preferred.[56] 'When greater support is desired', the daily dose can be increased to 150–300mg. In parts of Europe, the proanthocyanidins have been used for many years in patients with varicose veins, and in the management of lymph-oedema (together with DLT). Anecdotal evidence from the UK supports their use in lymphoedema.[59] However, because of recent publicity, it may be impossible to evaluate the benefits of grape seed extract in a properly conducted controlled trial.

Other drugs

Calcium dobesilate and etamsylate are also said to have an impact on high-protein oedema (Figure 15.7).[1,60] This raises the question as to how necessary is the pyrone part of the benzopyrone structure in relation to the reduction of high-protein oedema. Etamsylate is marketed as a haemostatic agent and is said to act by increasing capillary vascular wall resistance and platelet adhesiveness by inhibiting the biosynthesis and actions of PGs responsible for platelet disaggregation, vasodilation and increased capillary permeability. Etamsylate does not affect normal coagulation; administration is without effect on prothrombin time, fibrinolysis, platelet count or function. It is slowly but completely absorbed from the gastro-intestinal tract and excreted in the urine mainly unchanged. Etamsylate is licensed for use in menorrhagia. In the management of surface bleeding, etamsylate can be used together with

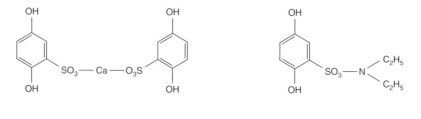

Calcium dobesilate   Etamsylate

Figure 15.7 Diagrams of calcium dobesilate and etamsylate; two non-benzopyrones said to have similar effects to the benzopyrones.

tranexamic acid. The manufacturers of etamsylate have no information on file about its postulated use in lymphoedema.

Unguentum lymphaticum

A herbal cream, unguentum lymphaticum was formulated about 30 years ago to reduce lymphoedema.[61] It contains no benzopyrones but is said to reduce high-protein oedema by similar mechanisms. It is not known which of the herbs are pharmacologically responsible (Table 15.6).

Table 15.6   Unguentum lymphaticum

Constituents	Quantity(g)
Extract of hemlock fruit and herb	4.2
Extract of saffron seed	3.0
Extract of foxglove leaves	2.1
Extract of podophyllum and rhizome	2.1
Extract of hyoscyamus niger leaves	2.1
Extract of marigold flower	0.21
Oil of Peter	8.8
p-Hydroxybenzoic acid methyl ester in 100g of an inert base	0.2

Lymphoedema secondary to filariasis

Over 1 billion people in 73 countries are at risk of contracting lymphatic filariasis (elephantiasis) and there are over 120 million people already affected. To counter this scourge, the World Health Organization (WHO) and SmithKline Beecham signed a Memorandum of Understanding in 1998 whereby SmithKline Beecham will donate albendazole free of charge to WHO for use by governments and other collaborating organisations working for the global elimination of filariasis. SmithKline Beecham will also contribute programme assistance and health education.

Albendazole, already a standard treatment worldwide for intestinal parasites, is 99% effective against the parasite which causes lymphatic filariasis when administered simultaneously with other antiparasitic drugs. Filariasis is carried by mosquitoes and often leads to elephantiasis. The drug regimen needed to interrupt the parasite's life-cycle is one dose annually for 4–5 years to all people in infected areas. SmithKline Beecham's commitment to donating sufficient albendazole to this programme will require several billion doses. WHO recomends that all cases of lymphoedema in filaritic-endemic areas (Africa, Asia, South America) which are not obviously related to cancer or its treatment should be treated with albendazole on the basis that filariasis is the most probable underlying cause. Information on the treatment of filariasis and on anthelmintics generally is available from various sources (e.g. *Martindale: The Extra Pharmacopoeia*).[62]

Clinical trials

Several trials of antibiotic treatment in filaritic lymphoedema have been undertaken. These include:

- diethylcarbamazine (DEC) *v* coumarin *v* coumarin and DEC[63]
- DEC *v* ivermectin *v* placebo.[64]

In the first, a double-blind randomised matched-group trial, there were 40–55 patients per group and patients were observed for 6–45 months (mean 2 years). Patients receiving coumarin had a slow but significant reduction of their lymphoedema whatever the grade – including those classified as elephantiasis. Coumarin alone improved many symptoms and complications, particularly swelling and bursting-pains, inflammation and ulcers. Patients with grade 2 lymphoedema lost 2/3 of their oedema over 2 years; and patients with grade 3–5 lymphoedema lost 1/5.

DEC, an antifilaritic antibiotic, alone gave some reduction of the oedema but this was much smaller than the reduction achieved with coumarin. DEC plus coumarin resulted in *less* reduction than coumarin alone, but was better than DEC alone. Concurrent prescription with coumarin reduced the fever commonly associated with DEC therapy.

In the second study, the therapeutic efficacy and adverse effects of two antifilaritic antibiotics were compared in a randomised controlled trial in 71 men with active filariasis (microfilaraemia +). Patients were kept in hospital for 15 days. Ivermectin caused an abrupt reduction in microfilaraemia to 1.5% of the pretreatment level 12h after the first dose. Microfilaraemia was virtually non-existent on day 14 (0.06% of pretreatment level) but had risen to nearly 10% after 3 months. DEC caused a more gradual drop in microfilaraemia to about 1% on day 14, and 2.4% after 3 months. It is not possible to say whether this related to acquired resistance or drug non-compliance. The incidence of adverse effects was 1% for placebo, 2% for ivermectin (headache and body aches for < 48h), and 3% for DEC (testicular and epi-didymal pain and swelling for up to 7 days). Limb volume was not reported. Filariasis is a curable condition and clearly should be treated with antibiotics so as to prevent progressive lymphatic damage.

Conclusion

The time has come to review thoroughly the benefits of benzopyrones in lymphoedema, possibly by setting up an Expert Committee to examine the evidence from both laboratory and clinical studies. This is now urgent given the fact that at least two countries have withdrawn the marketing licence for oral coumarin. If coumarin goes, will the pharmaceutical industry be willing to market oxerutins instead? It is a matter of concern that many people, par-ticularly those with primary, chronic post-traumatic or chronic postoperative lymphoedema, could be denied a treatment of proven benefit because the tide of professional opinion is presently against it.

References

1   Casley-Smith JR and Casley-Smith JR (1986) *High-protein Oedemas and the Benzopyrones.* JB Lippincott Co, Sydney.

2   Hoult JR and Paya M (1996) Pharmacological and biochemical actions of simple coumarins: natural products with therapeutic potential. *General Pharmacology.* **27**:713–22.

3   Keating GJ and O'Kennedy R (1997). The chemistry and occurrence of coumarins. In: R O'Kennedy and RD Thornes (eds) *Coumarins. Biology, Applications and Mode of Action.* John Wiley and Sons, Chichester, pp 23–60.

4   Eastham RD *et al.* (1972) Warfarin and hydroxyethylrutosides in deep vein thrombosis. *British Medical Journal.* **4**:491.

5   Marshall ME *et al.* (1994) An updated review of the clinical development of coumarin (1,2-benzopyrone) and 7-hydroxycoumarin. *Journal of Cancer Research and Clinical Oncology.* **120(suppl)**:S39–42.

6   O'Kennedy R and Thornes RD (1997) *Coumarins. Biology, Application and Mode of Action.* John Wiley and Sons, Chichester.

7   Cox D *et al.* (1989) The rarity of liver toxicity in patients treated with coumarin (1,2-benzopyrone). *Human Toxicology.* **8**:501–6.

8   Casley-Smith JR and Casley-Smith JR (1995) Frequency of coumarin hepato-toxicity. *Medical Journal of Australia.* **162**:391.

9   Loprinzi CL *et al.* (1999) Lack of effect of coumarin in women with lymphedema after treatment for breast cancer. *New England Journal of Medicine.* **340**:346–50.

10 Ritschel WA and Hussain AS (1988) Transdermal absorption and topical availability of coumarin. *Methods and Findings of Experimental and Clinical Pharmacology.* **10**:165–9.

11   Beckley-Kartey SA *et al.* (1997) Comparative in vitro skin absorption and metabolism of coumarin (1,2-benzopyrone) in human, rat, and mouse. *Toxicology of Applied Pharmacology.* **45**:34–42.

12   Yourick JK and Bronaugh RL (1997) Percutaneous absorption and metabolism of coumarin in human and rat skin. *Journal of Applied Toxicology.* **17**:153–8.

13   Fernandez-Salguero P *et al.* (1995) A genetic polymorphism in coumarin 7-hydroxylation: sequence of the human CYP2A genes and identification of variant CYP2A6 alleles. *American Journal of Human Genetics.* **57**:651–60.

14   Lee RE *et al.* (1981) Inhibition of prostaglandin biosynthesis by coumarin, 4-hydroxycoumarin, and 7-hydroxycoumarin. *Arzneim-Forsch Drug Research.* **31**:640–2.

15   Ritschel WA and Hoffmann KA (1981) Pilot study on the bioavailability of coumarin and 7-hydroxycoumarin upon peroral administration of coumarin in a sustained release dosage form. *Clinical Pharmacology.* **21**:294–301.

16   Burgos A *et al.* (1999) Comparative study of the clinical efficacy of two different coumarin dosages in the management of arm lymphedema after treatment for breast cancer. *Lymphology.* **32**:3–10.

17   Kendall S *et al.* (1993) Effects of hydroxyethyl rutosides on the permeability of normal microvessels in the frog mesentery. *Phlebology.* **Suppl 1**:33–7.

18   Michel CC (1993) Recent findings with O-(β-hydroxyethyl)-rutosides. *Phlebology.* **Suppl 1**:1–2.

19   Rehn D *et al.* (1993) Comparison between the efficacy and tolerability of oxerutins and troxerutin in the treatment of patients with chronic venous insufficiency. *Arzneimittelforschung.* **43**:1060–3.

20   Vettorello G *et al.* (1996) Contribution of a combination of alpha and beta benzopyrones, flavonoids and natural terpenes in the treatment of lymphedema of the lower limbs at the 2d stage of the surgical classification. *Minerva Cardioangiology.* **44**:447–55.

21   Robak J and Gryglewski RJ (1996) Bioactivity of flavonoids. *Polish Journal of Pharmacology.* **48**:555–64.

22   Timeus C (1986) The effect of oral O-(β-hydroxyethyl)-rutosides (HR) versus placebo on vessel wall permeability and selective permeability in the microcirculation of the skin in healthy volunteers. *Phlebology.* **85**:825–7.

23   Michel C *et al.* (1990) Hydroxyethylrutosides (HR) reduce permeability of frog mesenteric microvessels. *Phlebology.* **5(suppl 1)**:3–7.

24   Kendall S *et al.* (1992) Permeability reducing properties of O-(β-hydroxyethyl)-rutosides (Venoruton) and its constituents. Abstract 17th European Conference on Microcirculation, London, July 5–10.

25   Rehn D *et al.* (1991) Time course of the anti-oedematous effect of O-(β-hydroxyethyl)-rutosides in healthy volunteers. *European Journal of Clinical Pharmacology.* **40**:625–47.

26   Cesarone MR *et al.* (1992) Acute effects of hydroxyethylrutosides on capillary filtration in normal volunteers, patients with venous hypertension and in patients with diabetic microangiopathy (a dose comparison study) *VASA – Journal for Vascular Diseases.* **21**:76–80.

27   Roztocil K *et al.* (1977) The effect of hydroxyethylrutosides on capillary filtration rate in the lower limb of man. *European Journal of Pharmacology.* **11**:435–8.

28   McEwan AJ and McArdle CS (1971) Effect of hydroxyethylrutosides on blood oxygen levels and venous insufficiency symptoms in varicose veins. *British Medical Journal.* **2**:138–41.

29   Neumann HAM and van den Brock MJTB (1990) Evaluation of O-(β-hydroxyethyl)-rutosides in chronic venous insufficiency by means of non-invasive techniques. *Phlebology.* **5(suppl 1)**:13–20.

30   Van Haeringen NJ *et al.* (1973) Effect of O-(β-hydroxyethyl)-rutoside on red cell and platelet functions in man. *Bibliotheca Anatomica.* **12**:459–64.

31   Liu WL *et al.* (1992) Effect of O-(β-hydroxyethyl)-rutosides (Venoruton) and its constituents on histamine secretion from isolated rat peritoneal mast cells. Abstract 17th European Conference on Microcirculation, London, July 5–10.

32   Arturson G and Jonsson C-E (1973) Effect of O-(β-hydroxyethyl)-rutosides (HR) and indomethacin on transcapillary macromolecular transport and prostaglandins following scalding injury. *Bibliotheca Anatomica.* **12**:465–70.

33   Rekka E and Kourounakio PN (1991) Effect of hydroxyethylrutosides and related compounds on lipid peroxidation and free radical scavenging activity. Some structural aspects. *Journal of Pharmacy and Pharmacology.* **43**:486–91.

34   Bast A *et al.* (1992) Free radical scavenging connactivity of hydroxyethylrutosides. Abstract 17th European Conference on Microcirculation, London, July 5–10.

35   Van Acker SA *et al.* (1995) Flavonoids as scavengers of nitric oxide radical. *Biochemical and Biophysical Research Communications.* **214**:755–9.

36   Pecking AP (1995) Evaluation by lymphoscintigraphy of the effect of a micronized flavonoid fraction (Daflon 500mg) in the treatment of upper limb lymphedema. *International Angiology.* **14(suppl 1)**:39–43.

37   Anonymous (1992) Paroven: not much effect in trials. *Drug and Therapeutics Bulletin.* **30**:7–8.

38   Wadworth AN and Faulds D (1992) Hydroxyethylrutosides. A review of its pharmacology, and therapeutic efficacy in venous insufficiency and related disorders. *Drugs.* **44**:1013–32.

39   Pulvertaft TB (1983) General practice treatment of symptoms of venous insufficiency with oxerutins. Results of a 660 patient multicentre study in the UK. *VASA – Journal for Vascular Diseases.* **12**:373–6.

40   Neumann HA *et al.* (1992) Uptake and localisation of O-(beta-hydroxyethyl)-rutosides in the venous wall, measured by laser scanning microscopy. *European Journal of Clinical Pharmacology.* **43**:423–6.

41   Quigley FG and Faris IB (1991) Transcutaneous oxygen tension measurements in the assessment of limb ischaemia. *Clinical Physiology.* **11**:315–20.

42   Nocker W and Diebschlag W (1987) Dosis-wirkungsstudie mit O-(Beta-Hydroxyethyl)-rutoside – Trinklosungen. *VASA – Journal for Vascular Diseases.* **16**:365–9.

43   Nocker W *et al.* (1989) 3monatige, randomisierte doppelblinde dosis-wirkungsstudie mit O-(Beta-Hydroxyethyl)-rutoside – Trinklosungen. *VASA – Journal for Vasular Diseases.* **18**:235–8.

44   Piller NB (1980) Lymphoedema, macrophages and benzopyrones. *Lymphology.* **13**:109–19.

45   Casley-Smith JR and Casley-Smith JR (1990) The effects of O-(beta-hydroxyethyl)-rutosides (HR) on acute lymphoedema in rats' thighs, with and without macrophages. *Microcirculation Endothelium Lymphatics.* **6**:457–63.

46   Kendall S *et al.* (1993) Effects of hydroxyethylrutosides on the permeability of microvessels in the frog mesentery. *British Journal of Pharmacology.* **110**: 199–206.

47   Desprez-Curely JP *et al.* (1985) Benzopyrones and post-mastectomy lymph-edemas. Double-blind trial placebo versus sustained release coumarin with trioxyethylrutin (TER). *Progress in Lymphology.* **10**:203–5.

48   Piller NB *et al.* (1988) A double-blind, cross-over trial of O-(beta-hydroxyethyl-rutosides (benzopyrones) in the treatment of lymphoedema of the arms and legs. *British Journal of Plastic Surgery.* **41**:20–7.

49   Pecking A and Cluzan R (1989) Etude de l'action du Lysedem dans le traitement medical des lymphoedemes secondaires aux traitements des cancers du sein. *Phlebologie.* **42**:591–3.

50   Casley-Smith JR *et al.* (1993) Treatment of lymphedema of the arms and legs with 5,6-benzo-[alpha]-pyrone. *New England Journal of Medicine.* **329**:1158–63.

51   Taylor HM *et al.* (1993) A double-blind clinical trial of hydroxyethylrutosides in obstructive arm lymphoedema. *Phlebology.* **8**:22–8.

52   Mortimer PS *et al.* (1995) A double-blind, randomized, parallel-group, placebo-controlled trial of O-(β-Hydroxyethyl)-rutosides in chronic arm oedema resulting from breast cancer treatment. *Phlebology.* **10**:51–5.

53   Chang TS *et al.* (1996) The use of 5,6 benzo-[alpha]-pyrone (coumarin) and heating by microwaves in the treatment of chronic lymphedema of the legs. *Lymphology.* **29**:106–11.

54   Witte CL (1999) The placebo 'arm'. *Lymphology.* **32**:1–2.

55   Casley-Smith JR and Casley-Smith JR (1996) Treatment of lymphedema by com-plex physical therapy, with and without oral and topical benzopyrones: What should therapists and patients expect. *Lymphology.* **29**:76–82.

56   Murray MT (1995) *The healing power of herbs.* Prima Publishing, Rocklin, CA.

57   Duarte NM and Nascimento JM (1998) Pharmacological actions of proantho-cyanidins. *Revista Portuguesa de Farmacia.* **48**:9–12.

58   Taylor GL (1999) Eating for diving fitness: the lesser known antioxidants – part IV: proanthocyanidins. In: *Proanthocyanidins.* www.iantd.com/proanthocyanidins.html. May 1999.

59   Wigg J (1999) A grape success!! *British Lymphology Society Newsletter.* **Issue 25**:7.

60   Casley-Smith JR and Casley-Smith JR (1985) The effects of calcium dobesilate on acute lymphedema (with and without macrophages), and on burn edema. *Lymphology.* **18**:37–45.

61   Veith H and Sichert R (1971) Neue lymphwirksame salbenzubereitung. *Arztliche Praxis.* **23**:633–5.

62   Anonymous (1996) Anthelmintics. In: Martindale: *The Extra Pharmacopoeia,* 31st edn. Royal Pharmaceutical Society, London, pp 103–27.

63   Casley-Smith JR *et al.* (1993) Reduction of filaritic lymphoedema and elephantiasis by 5,6 benzo-α-pyrone (coumarin), and the effects of diethylcarbamazine (DEC). *Annals of Tropical Medicine and Parasitology.* **87**:247–58.

64   Sabry M *et al.* (1991) A placebo-controlled double-blind trial for the treatment of bancroftian filariasis with ivermectin or diethylcarbamazine. *Transactions of the Royal Society of Tropical Medicine and Hygiene.* **85**:640–3.

16 Novel treatments: Transcutaneous electrical nerve stimulation

Alexander Waller and Michaela Bercovitch

Low-level LASER therapy

Robert Twycross

Transcutaneous electrical nerve stimulation (TENS)

The low physical status and short life-span of terminally ill patients make it difficult or impossible to implement regimens such as decongestive lymph-oedema treatment (DLT) (*see* p.97). Further, treatment with benzopyrones is effective only after several months and thus will not benefit such patients.[1] After observing a reduction in swelling in a patient with breast cancer, lymph-oedema and arm pain, we have used transcutaneous electrical nerve stimu-lation (TENS) in over 30 patients with lymphoedema, specifically with the hope of reducing swelling.[2] In this chapter we record our experience while recognising that, given the small numbers involved, it is not possible as yet to come to any definitive conclusion about the value of TENS in lymphoedema.

The use of electricity to relieve pain appears in Egyptian paintings dating from 2500 BC. In 400 BC, Hippocrates described biological sources of electricity such as the electric ray and eel. In the 18th and 19th centuries, galvanic sources were used for the same purpose. Today there are more precise ways to stimu-late nerves and subcutaneous tissue. Electrodes are placed on the body surface and connected to electrical sources generated by batteries. The inspiration for the development of TENS came from the gate-control theory of pain enunciated by Melzack and Wall in 1965.[3] Since then there has been a progressively more widespread use of TENS for pain relief.

TENS equipment

TENS equipment is no longer standardised, for example, some machines have only one electrode. The equipment we use consists of a portable battery-powered stimulator with leads to four square carbon-impregnated rubber

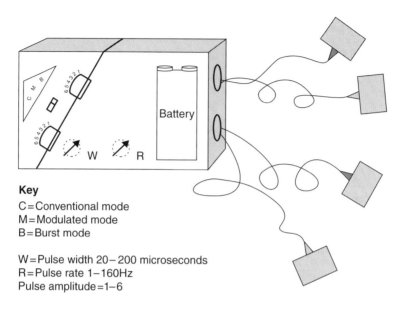

Key

C=Conventional mode
M=Modulated mode
B=Burst mode

W=Pulse width 20–200 microseconds
R=Pulse rate 1–160Hz
Pulse amplitude=1–6

Figure 16.1   The stimulator for TENS.

electrodes 3cm × 3cm in dimension (Figure 16.1). The dimensions of the stimulators vary from the size of a beeper to that of a small portable transistor radio, weight from 50–200g, pulse rate from 1–160Hz, pulse width 20–200 microseconds and one or two channels. A 9V battery provides the power source with a typical battery life of 40–120 hours (but occasionally only 4–16 hours). The guarantee ranges from 0.5–2 years and the cost ranges from £70–250.[4]

Our experience with TENS in lymphoedema

In addition to drug treatment to relieve pain, we routinely use several non-drug methods, including TENS.[5] One patient after mastectomy for breast cancer presented with painful lymphoedema of her left upper limb. In an attempt to relieve her pain, we decided to add TENS to the usual analgesic drug therapy. After 2 days of treatment with TENS (1h t.d.s.), we were surprised to perceive a considerable reduction of the extent of her lymphoedema. After three or four successful treatments with TENS in other patients, we decided to perform formal studies of the possible influence of TENS in relieving lymphoedema in patients with advanced cancer.

First study

The first study in 1995 was a prospective non-randomised open study with the patient living at home and acting as his own control, using the normal limb for comparison. Some patients were already being treated for lymphoedema by standard methods. The circumference of the limb was measured at two points on entry into the study and daily thereafter for 14 days.

Patients received TENS on the lymphoedematous limb for 2 hours daily. One set of electrodes was placed in the middle of the distal part of the lymphoedematous limb, and the second was placed in the middle of the proximal part of the lymphoedematous limb. TENS was applied in the modulated mode at the pulse rate of 100Hz, pulse width of 100 microseconds, and an amplitude adjusted to the patient's level of comfort.

The study was limited to 2 weeks but we speculated that improvement would continue beyond this time and achieve an ultimate mean reduction of about 25% for the upper limb and 30% for the lower limb, with long-term treatment producing an even greater decrease in circumference.

Results

Eighteen consecutive patients with lymphoedema secondary to cancer or its treatment were considered for enrolment. Five patients were excluded because of their reluctance to use the TENS apparatus. Of the rest, 3 patients died and 10 completed the study (Table 16.1).

Over the 2 weeks, we observed a mean decrease of 13% (range 12–18%) in circumference of the lymphoedematous upper limb and 16% in the lymphoedematous lower limb (range 12–20%) (Figures 16.2 and 16.3). Previous treatment of the lymphoedema, if any, was continued throughout the trial. Some of the patients were receiving diuretics, corticosteroids or both without previous physical treatment (Table 16.2).

The decrease of the circumference of both upper and lower lymphoedematous limbs was statistically significant ($p < 0.001$) (Figures 16.4 and 16.5). The circumferences of the lower limbs decreased to a greater extent than the circumferences of the upper limbs, $p < 0.004$ (Figure 16.6). The circumferences of the lower limbs decreased more rapidly than the circumferences of the upper limbs, $p < 0.001$. The use of furosemide (frusemide) and dexamethasone appeared not to influence the extent or rate of decrease in the circumference of the limbs.

The percentage decrease in circumference often differed between the proximal and distal limb measurements – a phenomenon also seen in patients treated by DLT (Figures 16.7 and 16.8). Some of the variability may be because measurements were taken at home by the patient or a family member.

Table 16.1 Characteristics of 10 cancer patients in circumference study

Mean age	54 years (± 12)	
Gender	Male	7
	Female	3
Primary site	Breast	4
	Bladder	3
	Cervix	1
	Colon	1
	Lung	1
Lymphoedematous limb	Arm	6
	Legs	4
Mean duration of lymphoedema	11 months (± 18)	
Previous cancer treatment	Surgery	6
	Radiotherapy	4
Previous lymphoedema treatment		4
Simultaneous treatment	Furosemide (frusemide)	6
	Corticosteroids	2
Duration of treatment	14 days	

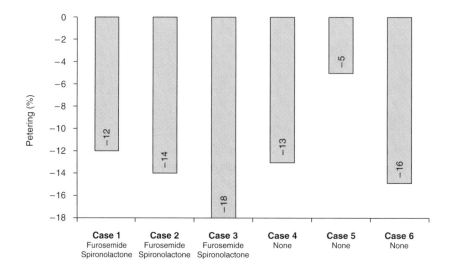

Figure 16.2 Arms: mean circumference petering (14 days).

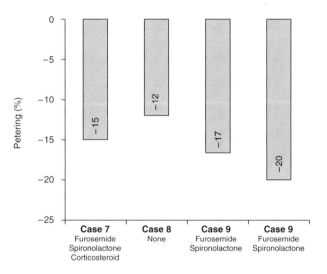

Figure 16.3   Legs: mean circumference petering (14 days).

Table 16.2   Characteristics of 7 cancer patients in volume study

Mean age	57 years (± 8)	
Gender	Male	0
	Female	7
Primary site	Breast	6
	Lung	1
Lymphoedematous limb	Arm	7
	Legs	0
Mean duration of lymphoedema	18 months (± 18)	
Previous cancer treatment	Surgery	6
	Radiotherapy	5
Previous lymphoedema treatment		6
Simultaneous treatment	Furosemide (frusemide)	3
	Corticosteroids	0
Duration of treatment	14 days	3
	28 days	4

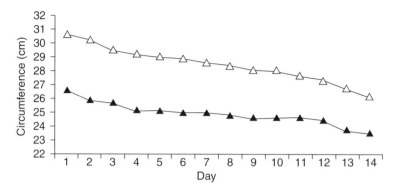

Figure 16.4 General mean circumference decrease for arms *v* time (p < 0.001). ▲–▲ = C1 decrease; △–△ = C2 decrease.

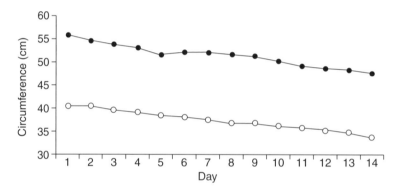

Figure 16.5 General mean circumference decrease for legs *v* time (p < 0.001). ●–● = C1 decrease; ○–○ = C2 decrease.

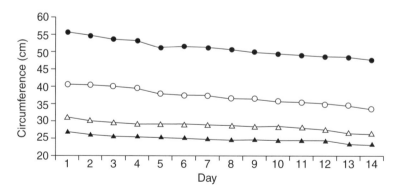

Figure 16.6 General mean circumference decrease for legs and arms (p < 0.004). Legs: ●–● = C1 decrease; ○–○ = C2 decrease. Arms: ▲–▲ = C1 decrease; △–△ = C2 decrease.

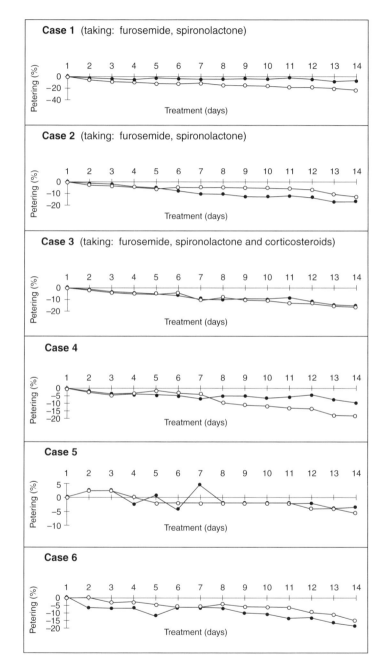

Figure 16.7 Arm circumference petering at two points of measurement for 6 cases. ●–● = decrease of circumference at point 1. ○–○ = decrease of circumference at point 2.

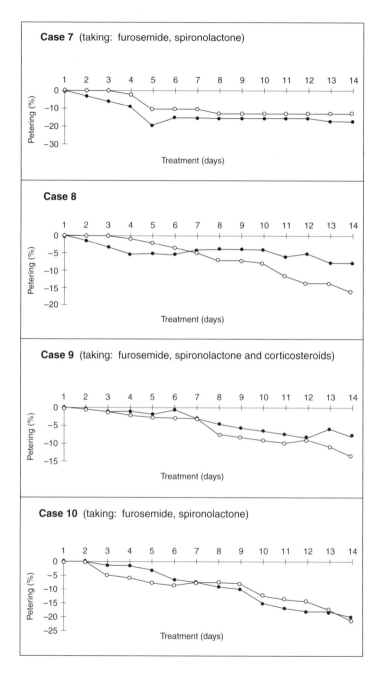

Figure 16.8 Leg circumference petering at two points of measurement for 4 cases. ●–● = decrease of circumference at point 1. ○–○ = decrease of circumference at point 2.

Second study

In the second study (November 1995 – May 1996), the circumference of the lymphoedematous limb and of the unaffected limb was measured on entry into the study and daily thereafter at five points:

- the wrist
- midway between the elbow and the wrist
- the elbow
- the middle of the upper arm
- the shoulder.

Treatment with TENS was continued for 2–4 weeks. Each patient received TENS on the lymphoedematous limb for 2 hours daily (as in study 1). Larger electrodes (4cm × 10cm) were used. As in study 1, one set of electrodes was placed in the middle of the forearm and the second was placed in the middle of the upper arm. We followed 7 consecutive patients with unilateral lymphoedema of the upper limb secondary to cancer or treatment for it. Four patients were withdrawn from the study after 2 weeks because of general deterioration.

The results in the remaining 3 patients (all with arm lymphoedema) were expressed as limb volume calculated from the five measurements of circumference of each limb. In all 3, there was a significant decrease in lymphoedema ranging from 9–36% over the first 2 weeks ($p < 0.001$). The mean volume decrease was 17% for the first 2 weeks and 22% for all 4 weeks of treatment (Figure 16.9). The decrease in volume was significantly greater in the upper arms than in the forearms, $p < 0.001$.

Between 14 and 28 days there was no further significant decrease in limb volumes. Nevertheless, the decrease in volume of the lymphoedematous upper arm was still significantly greater than in the lymphoedematous forearm, $p < 0.001$.

The statistical analysis was performed using analysis of variance.[6] In addition to the patients treated in the two studies, we have treated 15 more patients without performing measurements, sometimes with a spectacular result in relation to a decrease in lymphoedema and pain.

Case history

An 80 year-old man was admitted for symptom relief in July 1996. In 1975 he had been diagnosed as having cancer of the laryngopharynx with regional

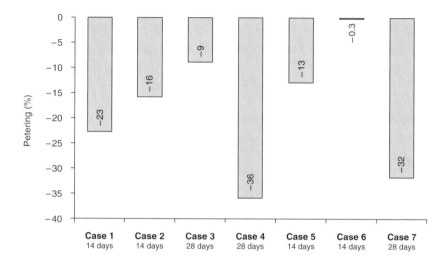

Figure 16.9 Oedema volume petering for all cases (14 and 28 days of treatment).

metastases, and was treated by surgery and radiotherapy. In 1995 cancer of the oesophagus was diagnosed which was treated by surgery, radiotherapy and chemotherapy. In 1997, a gastrostomy was performed because of perforation of the oesophagus.

His symptoms on admission were difficulty in breathing, cough, weakness, dizziness and moderate pain on the left side of the face and neck. On admission we noticed a severe pitting oedema on the eyelids and on the right side of his face and neck (Plate 16.1). He could not see and, because of the tracheostomy, was unable to speak. Diuretics proved ineffective and we decided to use TENS. After 3 days of treatment with TENS using just one channel and two electrodes, we observed an impressive decrease in the facial oedema (Plate 16.2) He was able to open his eyelids and to communicate with the staff by writing (Plate 16.3). After one month, however, his general condition deteriorated and he died peacefully.

Discussion

Although we do not know how TENS diminishes lymphoedema, we may speculate that it stimulates the local microcirculation and promotes better drainage of the lymph, possibly from the superficial system to the deep lymphatic system.[7,8]

We also do not know precisely why the results are better in some people than in others. Our impression is that better results are obtained in patients with a higher proportion of intact lymphatics, and are inversely proportional to the duration of the lymphoedema. However, other variables such as drug treatment (e.g. diuretics, corticosteroids) or the mobility of the patient may be important.

Because of small numbers, we could not stratify according to the grade of lymphoedema. Further, the circumference and volume measurements were not linked to tissue tonometer measurements.[9] Even so, in our patient population, statistically significant benefit was seen with most patients. In the first study, the mean decrease in the circumference of the arms was 13% after 2 weeks, with a best result of 18%. For the legs, the mean decrease was 16%, with a best result of 20%.

In the second study only arms were involved, and the mean decrease in volume after 2 weeks was 17%, with a best result of 23%. After 4 weeks the mean decrease was 22%, with a best result of 33%.

TENS is generally user-friendly and does not require treatment in specialised centres. Further, the cost is minimal compared with other methods (Box 16.A).[10] The method is also relatively straightforward and does not require sophisticated training. There are, however, some contra-indications and potential complications (Box 16.B).

It is frustrating that at present we do not know the precise mechanism of the therapeutic action of TENS in reducing lymphoedema. Nor do we know if other types of oedema (such as that associated with hypo-albuminaemia) also respond to TENS. Further, we do not know the optimal characteristics of TENS (pulse width, frequency, amplitude), the best location of the electrodes, the duration and frequency of treatment, or the ideal size of electrodes. Despite all these unknowns, it is still possible to say that the use of TENS in lymphoedema is promising, but clearly requires further research.

Box 16.A   Advantages and disadvantages of TENS

Advantages

Simplicity.

Does not preclude concurrent physical or drug treatment of lymphoedema and pain.

Low cost compared with DLT.

Disadvantages

Generally less benefit compared with DLT.

Box 16.B Contra-indications and complications of TENS for lymphoedema

Contra-indications

A cardiac pacemaker (particularly a demand pacemaker).

The anterior part of the neck (to avoid stimulating the nerves of the carotid sinus or larynx) which could produce bradycardia and hypotension or laryngeal spasm.

Cognitively impaired and machine-phobic patients.

Local dermatological problems such as a skin rash, infection or ulceration.

Complications

Non-compliance.

Skin reactions:
- burns, irritations
- allergy to electrodes, jelly, tape or gum.

Equipment failure due to faulty leads, stimulator, battery or charger.

Low-level LASER therapy

LASER stands for *light amplification by stimulated emission of radiation* and low-level LASER therapy (LLLT) refers to biomodulation with LASERs which are painless, non-invasive, and do not burn tissue.[11] These LASERs have output powers of 5–500mW and are considered investigational by the Food and Drug Administration (FDA) in the USA and no medical claims of cures are permitted.

The first LASERs were developed in the 1960s from basic principles proposed by Albert Einstein nearly 50 years earlier.[12] Endre Mester is credited as the originator of LLLT. When he began studying LASER therapy, he anticipated that low doses of LASER light would stimulate the growth of cancer cells. What he observed, however, was that LASER did not stimulate cancer cell growth, but it stimulated wound closure.[13]

Common uses for LLLT include the treatment of non-healing wounds, sports injuries and the treatment of acute and chronic pains.[14] The mechanism underlying the effects of LLLT is not fully understood. LLLT possibly increases production of adenosine triphosphate (ATP) by the mitochondria, and so improves cellular respiration and function.[15,16]

With more than 30 years of application and study in both humans and animals, no permanent or long-term adverse effects have been reported with LLLT. The only warning is not to stare directly into the LASER beam, and so prevent retinal injury. LLLT has been used safely with acute injuries and

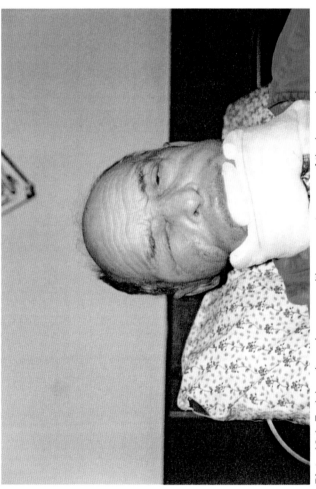

Plate 16.1 Facial oedema in a man with recurrent cancer of the laryngopharynx.

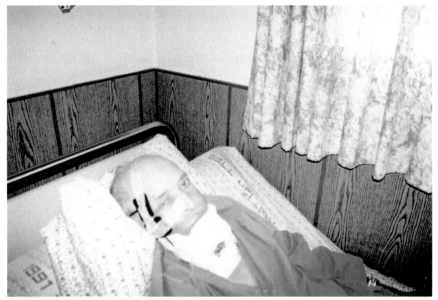

Plate 16.2 Reduction in facial oedema after 3 days with TENS 1h t:d:s.

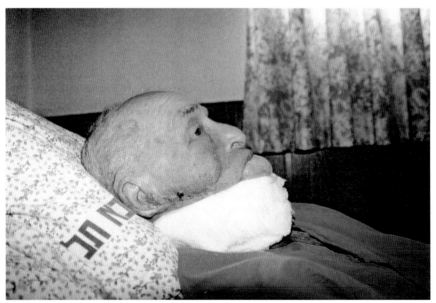

Plate 16.3 Side view showing reduction in oedema after TENS.

fractures, and in children and pregnant women. It does not promote bacterial growth. LLLT is thought to increase lymph vessel diameter and contractility, and to facilitate lymphatic and vascular regeneration (collateralisation) in injured tissues. LLLT stimulates the phagocytic activity of neutrophils and monocytes,[17] releases agents from macrophages which inhibit fibroblasts,[18] activates the immune system,[19] and improves neural function.[20] Studies have demonstrated both microscopically and macroscopically that LLLT enhances the resorption of oedema.[21]

Clinical study

In a study of LLLT in 10 women with unilateral arm oedema after axillary clearance (radical mastectomy) and radiotherapy, all received 16 treatments over 10 weeks.[22] Seven patients were followed up at 1,3,6 and 30–36 months. There was a 42% reduction in upper arm circumference during treatment and a 31% reduction in the months after treatment. For the mid-palm of the hand, there was a 92% reduction after treatment. Other measurement sites showed a circumference reduction of 26–48% with an average overall arm reduction of 45%. Oedema volume reduced 10% with treatment and 29% after treatment.

Whereas the forearm softened during treatment (measured by tonometry), it regressed after treatment. The upper arm, however, showed persistent hardening during and after treatment, a finding which is puzzling. Bio-impedance showed a reduction of approximately 16% in extracellular fluid and 12% in intracellular fluid during treatment, although after treatment the difference was minimal. Subjective parameters uniformly showed improvement with treatment and immediately after treatment, although after 36 months there was a tendency to worsen again. Skin integrity, number of infections, and arm mobility also improved, although with time the improvement abated. The feeling of arm tightness and heaviness was considerably reduced.

References

1   Piller NB (1976) Conservative treatment of acute and chronic lymphoedema with benzopyrones. *Lymphology.* **9**:132–7.
2   Waller A and Caroline N (1996) *Handbook of Palliative Care in Cancer.* Butterworth-Heinemann, Boston, pp 91–6.
3   Melzack R and Wall PD (1965) Pain mechanisms: a new theory. *Science.* **150**:971.
4   Thompson JW and Filshie J (1998) Transcutaneous Electrical Stimulation and Acupuncture. In: D Doyle, GWC Hanks, N MacDonald (eds), *Oxford Textbook of Palliative Medicine,* 2nd edn. Oxford University Press, Oxford, pp 421–37.

5   Twycross R (1994) *Pain Relief in Advanced Cancer.* Churchill Livingstone, Edinburgh.

6   BMDP (1990) *Statistical Software,* WJ Dixon (ed). University of California Press, California.

7   Kaada B (1983) Promoted healing of chronic ulceration by Transcutaneous Nerve Stimulation (TNS). *VASA – Journal for Vascular Diseases.* **12**:262–9.

8   Mortimer PS (1998) The pathophysiology of lymphoedema. *Cancer.* **83**: 2798–802.

9   Gerber LN (1998) A review of measures of lymphoedema. *Cancer.* **83**:2803–4.

10 Casley-Smith JR (1994) *Information about lymphoedema for patients.* The Lymphoedema Association of Australia, Inc.

11 Ohshiro T (1991) *Low Reactive-Level Laser Therapy: Practical Applications.* John Wiley and Sons, New York.

12 Naeser MA and Deuel SK (1999) Review of Second Congress, World Association for Laser Therapy Meeting (WALT). *Journal of Alternative and Complementary Medicine.* **5**:177–80.

13 Mester E *et al.* (1985) The biomedical effects of laser application. *Lasers in Surgery and Medicine.* **5**:31–9.

14 Laakso L *et al.* (1993) Factors affecting low level laser therapy. *Australian Journal of Physiotherapy.* **39**:95–9.

15 Basford JR (1989) Low-energy laser therapy: controversies and new research findings. *Lasers in Surgery and Medicine.* **9**:1–5.

16 Basford JR (1993) Lasers in orthopaedic surgery. Laser surgery: scientific basis and clinical role. *Orthopedics.* **16**:541–7.

17 Karu T *et al.* (1989) Helium neon laser induced respiratory burst in phagocytic cells. *Lasers in Surgery and Medicine.* **9**:585–9.

18 Young S *et al.* (1989) Macrophage responsiveness to light therapy. *Lasers in Surgery and Medicine.* **9**:497–505.

19 Tadakuma T (1993) Possible application of the laser in immunobiology. *Keio Journal of Medicine.* **42**:180–6.

20 Ohshiro T and Fujino T (1993) Laser applications in plastic and reconstructive surgery. *Keio Journal of Medicine.* **42**:191–5.

21 Lievens P *et al.* (1985) The influence of mid laser on the basic motility of blood and lymph vessels. *Medical Laser Report.* **2**.

22 Piller NB and Thelander A (1998) Treatment of chronic postmastectomy lymph-edema with low level laser therapy: a 25 year follow-up. *Lymphology.* **31**:74–86.

17 Surgery and lymphoedema

Tom Carrell and Kevin Burnand

Surgical causes of lymphoedema

Surgery remains a common cause of secondary lymphoedema in the UK, particularly in the management of malignant disease.

The risk of lymphoedema following surgical excision and block dissection of lymph nodes varies with the type of primary tumour and the extent of the lymphatic resection. Inguinal lymphadenectomy for penile and vulval squamous cell cancer is associated with a 15% risk of lymphoedema. This risk increases to > 50% in inguinal block dissection for lower limb cutaneous malignancies.[1] The incidence of secondary lymphoedema of the upper limb after axillary node dissection depends on the level of node clearance, and is about 5%.[2,3] Adjuvant radiotherapy greatly increases these surgical risks.

Rarely, surgery for benign disease is responsible for lymphoedema. Iatrogenic disruption of the femoral lymphatics may occur during groin exploration for recurrent varicose veins and the risk of subsequent lymphoedema has been estimated at 0.5%.[4]

Surgical management of lymphoedema

Despite many attempts over the years to develop surgical techniques to improve limb function and appearance in lymphoedema, < 10% of all patients benefit from surgery. Situations in which surgery may be considered are:

- limb swelling causing marked disability or severe deformity
- lymphoedema caused by proximal lymphatic obstruction with adequate patent distal lymphatics suitable for a lymphatic drainage procedure (about 2% of patients)
- lymphocutaneous fistulae and megalymphatics.

Reduction operations

Numerous operations have been developed in attempts to debulk the limb by removing the oedematous and fibrotic subcutaneous tissues. Only a few have proved successful with acceptable long-term results. Reduction operations are indicated only in the symptomatic relief of gross lymphoedema.

Patients may have unrealistic expectations of the cosmetic result and should be adequately counselled before any decision to operate. Although most commonly performed to reduce lower limb lymphoedema, reduction procedures may be adapted to treat swelling at other anatomical sites, such as genital and eyelid lymphoedema.

Homans' operation

Homans and Auchincloss described a reduction procedure in which the skin on the limb is preserved.[5,6] An incision is made along the length of the affected portion of the limb, anterior and posterior skin flaps are raised and the lymphoedematous subcutaneous tissue is excised down to the deep fascia. The skin flaps are then tailored to an appropriate size, replaced and sutured closed (Figure 17.1).

Because the skin on the affected limb is used to close the defect after debulking, the procedure is only suitable if the skin is in good condition. Each operation typically reduces the limb circumference by a third, and several operations through separate incisions may be required to debulk a limb adequately. Commonly, most of the swelling is below the knee. Initial medial reduction combined with a lateral procedure at a later date produces a good functional result. Thigh and foot swelling can be reduced in a similar fashion.

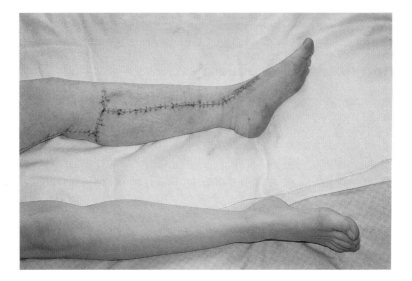

Figure 17.1 A lymphoedematous limb reduced with a good result by a medial Homans' operation.

Thompson's operation

Thompson modified Homans' operation by suturing a denuded skin flap to the deep fascia in the hope that skin lymphatics would then anastomose with deep lymphatic channels.[7] Unfortunately there is little evidence to suggest that this occurs and pilonidal sinus formation and unsightly scarring often complicate the procedure. The operation has largely been abandoned in favour of the simpler Homans' procedure.

Charles' operation

Sir Havelock Charles originally described his reduction procedure for the treatment of tropical elephantiasis.[8] In the operation, all the skin and sub-cutaneous tissue around the calf is excised down to the deep fascia, which may itself then be excised. Split skin grafts are taken from donor sites un-affected by the lymphoedema and applied to the denuded area.

The operation produces a greater reduction in limb circumference than Homans' operation and the ankle and knee areas adjacent to the excision should be tailored to avoid a 'pantaloon' appearance. Although the cosmetic result of the split skin grafts is poor, the operation is generally performed for gross leg swelling with severe lymphoedematous skin changes which contra-indicate Homans' operation (Figure 17.2). Charles reductions can be compli-cated by excessive warty skin and hyperkeratotic scars. These can be shaved off with a scalpel or dermatome but, occasionally, repeat split skin grafts may be required.

Lymph drainage procedures

Many operations have been developed over the years in attempts to connect obstructed lymphatic systems with the venous system. Few have been success-ful with long-term improvement in lymphatic function. About 2% of patients have leg lymphoedema caused by proximal occlusion of the pelvic lymph-atics. If the distal lymphatics remain patent, then a lymph drainage procedure to decompress the obstructed distal system may be of benefit (Figure 17.3). Unfortunately, proximal lymphatic obstruction often leads to occlusion of the distal lymphatics (a process called 'die-back'), rendering the limb unsuitable for drainage procedures. Three operations remain in use today:

- lymphovenous anastomosis
- enteromesenteric bridge by-pass
- omental by-pass

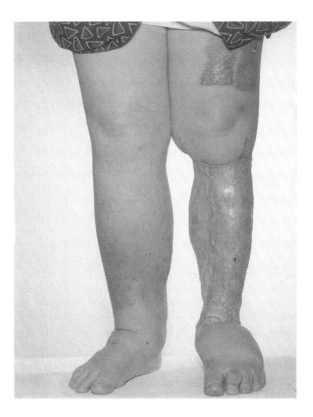

Figure 17.2   A lymphoedematous leg reduced by Charles' operation. Notice the split skin graft donor sites on the thigh.

Lymphovenous anastomosis

Lymphovenous anastomosis of lymphatic vessels to the venous system has been attempted in various forms to drain lymphoedematous limbs.[9–13] The obstructed lymphatic vessels are anastomosed to the femoral vein with the assistance of an operating microscope. Low lymphatic flow rates, the small anastomotic size and luminal fibrosis conspire to give disappointing patency rates. Generally several anastomoses are fashioned in the hope that one or two will remain patent. There have been several reports of good results of lymphovenous anastomosis in the treatment of filariasis, but overall the results are disappointing.[14]

Enteromesenteric bridge by-pass

Kinmonth developed the enteromesenteric bridge by-pass in an attempt to use the rich submucosal lymphatic plexus of the small bowel to drain obstructed

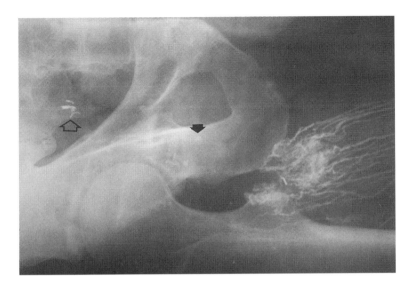

Figure 17.3   A contrast lymphangiogram showing absent pelvic lymphatics causing proximal lymphatic obstruction. The distal lymphatic vessels are still patent and a by-pass procedure could be considered.

leg lymphatics (Figure 17.4).[15] In this procedure, a short length of small bowel is resected and the remaining bowel rejoined by end-to-end anastomosis. The isolated segment is then mobilised on its mesentery, brought down to the groin nodes of the lymphoedematous limb and opened along its antimesenteric border to form a rectangular graft. The mucosa is removed to expose the submucosal lymphatics and the graft applied to the cut surface of the most proximal normal nodes. Lymphatic connections develop between the cut surface of the inguinal lymph nodes and the submucosal lymphatics. Contrast lymphangiography shows lymph drainage to the thoracic duct after a successful procedure.

The operation is suitable only for a small number of patients with proximal obstruction, patent distal vessels and moderate limb oedema. Young patients seem to fare better and good results can be obtained in at least half of these selected patients.[16,17] The procedure carries the risk of complications from the laparotomy as well as the groin incision.

Omental by-pass

Early attempts at similar by-pass procedures with the greater omentum had poor results attributed to the poor lymphatic drainage of the omentum.

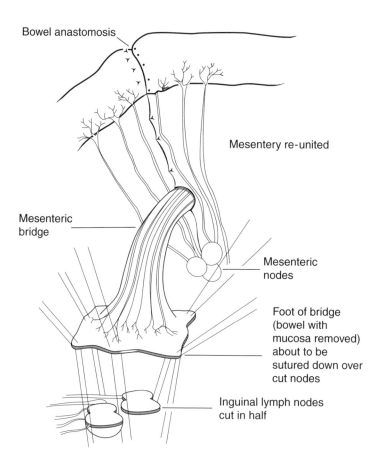

Figure 17.4   A schematic representation of enteromesenteric bridge by-pass.

Recently, improved results have been reported after combined free omental auto-transplants and anastomosis of the lymph nodes to omental veins.[18,19]

Chylous reflux

Patients with megalymphatic disease develop dilated, varicose lymphatic collecting vessels with incompetent valvular function. The consequent incompetent drainage of lymph allows reflux of chyle (intestinal lymph) and may lead to the formation of lymphocutaneous fistulae in the limb. The fistulae appear as vesicles and may leak significant volumes of lymph.

The skin complications of chylous reflux may sometimes be adequately treated by local excision alone. Otherwise contrast lymphangiography may be used to show the megalymphatics and identify the lymphatic vessels feeding the fistulae. These can be ligated to reduce the discharge from the lymphocutaneous fistulae, but at a risk of increasing lymphatic obstruction.

Genital lymphoedema

Lymphoedema of the external genitalia may occur in filariasis and mega-lymphatic chylous reflux. The swelling may interfere with sexual function. LASER treatment can be helpful for removing unsightly lymphangiomas.[20] A debulking operation is often indicated and simple excisions usually produce good results (see p.335).

References

1   James JH (1982) Lymphoedema following ilio-inguinal lymph node dissection. *Scandinavian Journal of Plastic and Reconstructive Surgery.* **16**:167–71.

2   Siegel BM *et al.* (1990) Level I and II axillary dissection in the treatment of early-stage breast cancer. *Archives of Surgery.* **125**:1144–7.

3   Hoe AL *et al.* (1992) Incidence of arm swelling following axillary clearance for breast cancer. *British Journal of Surgery.* **79**:261–3.

4   Ouvry PA and Guenneguez H (1993) Complications lymphatiques de la chirurgie des varices. *Phlebologie.* **46**:563–8.

5   Homans J (1936) *New England Journal of Medicine.* **215**:1066.

6   Auchincloss H (1930) *Puerto Rico Journal of Public Health and Tropical Medicine.* **6**:149.

7   Thompson N (1971) Surgical treatment of chronic lymphoedema of the arm and leg. *British Journal of Hospital Medicine.* **1**:395–408.

8   Charles RH (1912) In: A Latham, TC English (eds) *Elephantiasis Scrotii, A System of Treatment, Vol III.* Churchill, London.

9   Nielubowicz J and Olszewski W (1968) Surgical lymphaticovenous shunts in patients with secondary lymphoedema. *British Journal of Surgery.* **55**:440–2.

10 Degni M (1978) New techniques in lymphatico-venous anastomosis for the treatment of lymphoedema. *Journal of Cardiovascular Surgery.* **19**:577–80.

11 Jamal S (1981) Lymphovenous anastomosis in filarial lymphedema. *Lymphology.* **14**:64–8.

12 Baumeister RG *et al.* (1986) A microsurgical method for reconstruction of inter-rupted lymphatic pathways: autologous lymph-vessel transplantation for treat-ment of lymphedemas. *Scandinavian Journal of Plastic and Reconstructive Surgery.* **20**:141–6.

13 Al Assal F *et al.* (1988) A new technique of microlympho-venous anastomosis. *Journal of Cardiovascular Surgery.* **29**:552–5.

14 Gloviczki P *et al.* (1988) Microsurgical lymphovenous anastomosis for treatment of lymphedema: A critical review. *Journal of Vascular Surgery.* **7**:647–52.

15 Kinmonth JB *et al.* (1978) Relief of lymph obstruction by use of a bridge of mesentery and ileum. *British Journal of Surgery.* **65**:829–33.

16 Hurst PAE *et al.* (1985) Long term results of the enteromesenteric bridge operation in the treatment of primary lymphoedema. *British Journal of Surgery.* **72**:272–4.

17 Fyfe NCM *et al.* (1982) 'Die-back' in primary lymphoedema-lymphographic and clinical correlations. *Lymphology.* **15**:66–9.

18 O'Brien BM *et al.* (1990) Microsurgical transfer of the greater omentum in the treatment of canine obstructive lymphoedema. *British Journal of Plastic Surgery.* **43**:440–6.

19 Egorov YS *et al.* (1994) Autotransplantation of the greater omentum in the treatment of chronic lymphedema. *Lymphology.* **27**:137–43.

20 Novak C and Spelman L (1998) Low energy fluence CO_2 Laser treatment of lymphangiectasia. *Australian Journal of Dermatology.* **39**:277–8.

Further reading

Kinmonth JB (1982) *The Lymphatics: Surgery, Lymphography and Diseases of the Chyle and Lymph Systems*, 2nd edn. Edward Arnold, London.

Browse NL (1986) *A Colour Atlas of Reducing Operations for Lymphoedema of Lower Limb*. Wolfe Medical Publications.

18　Lymphoedema in childhood

Sahar Mansour and Michael Sharland

There are several different causes of lymphoedema in childhood. The management and implications for the child and the rest of the family vary accordingly. A careful evaluation including a detailed history and examination is essential. This chapter will focus on primary lymphoedema of the lower limb. This is by far the most frequent form in childhood. Other forms of lymphoedema are covered in other chapters.

Classification

Lymphoedema can be divided into two groups – primary and secondary. Primary means that there is no obvious underlying cause. There are several different types but probably all related to abnormal development of the lymphatics (Table 18.1). Secondary lymphoedema occurs as a result of damage to the lymphatic system from an identifiable cause. Possible causes of secondary lymphoedema are listed later in this chapter (*see* p.300).

Primary lymphoedema is rare in childhood and adolescence. It affects approximately 1 in 100 000 persons less than 20 years old. The frequency is highest in females, typically during puberty.[1]

History

It is important to differentiate between primary and secondary lymphoedema. This can be ascertained by determining the age of onset, the family history and whether there have been any precipitating factors. The type of primary lymphoedema is determined by the age of onset and the associated features.

Age of onset

Primary lymphoedema is always due to a congenital abnormality of the lymphatics, but may not present until later in life. In 1934, Allen classified primary lymphoedema by the age of presentation. Lymphoedema at birth was called *congenital lymphoedema* and presentation after birth was termed *lymphoedema praecox*.[1] Later, Kinmonth described patients with presentation of lymphoedema after the age of 35 years as *lymphoedema tarda*.[2] Diagnostically it is more helpful to think of lymphoedema presenting before 3 months of

Table 18.1   Congenital lymphoedema

Type	Onset	Associated features	Inheritance
Early onset			
Milroy's disease	Birth–10 years	None	AD[a]
Lymphoedema with recurrent cholestasis	Birth–10 years	Neonatal cholestasis Cirrhosis of liver	AR[b]
Lymphoedema with intestinal lymphangiectasia	Infancy	Diarrhoea, vomiting, failure to thrive, hypoproteinemia, chylous effusions, lymphangiectasia	AD
Lymphoedema with yellow nails	Birth or any age	Dystrophic nails Pleural effusions	AD
Noonan's syndrome	Birth	Congenital heart defect Dysmorphic facies Webbed neck Short stature	AD
Turner's syndrome	Birth	Co-arctation of aorta Short stature Horseshoe kidney	Chromosomes 45XO Sporadic
Late onset			
Meige's syndrome	Puberty	None	AD
Lymphoedema with recurrent lymphangitis	Childhood or puberty	Lymphangitis	AD
Lymphoedema with distichiasis	Puberty or later	Distichiasis Congenital heart defect	AD

a   AD = autosomal dominant
b   AR = autosomal recessive.

age as congenital lymphoedema and lymphoedema presenting between 4 months and 20 years as praecox.[1] The age of onset tends to be consistent within families. The age of onset of the same condition may vary between families (Table 18.1).

Family history

Most forms of primary lymphoedema are caused by genetic factors. Some, but not all, are inherited. The family history generally indicates whether the lymphoedema has been inherited. Most inherited lymphoedema is inherited in an autosomal dominant pattern. There are only a few exceptions, such as lymphoedema with recurrent cholestasis, which appear to be inherited as an autosomal recessive. Some autosomal dominant genes may occur as new mutations so there may be no family history of lymphoedema but the nature of the lymphoedema and the associated findings indicate that these are genetic forms. It is important to identify these because of the significant risk to future offspring.

Approximately 10% of children of index patients and 10% of siblings are also affected. The fact that the offspring and sibling risk is equal supports an autosomal dominant mode of inheritance in many families with primary lymphoedema.[3] The risk is, however, considerably less than 50%, suggesting that some cases may be new dominant mutations and that the expression of the disorder is variable. Other factors may be important in determining the severity of the lymphoedema. Some forms of primary lymphoedema are not inherited.

Associated features

Children may present with one of the associated features (Table 18.1). For example families with lymphoedema-distichiasis syndrome may have evidence of distichiasis (ingrowing eyelashes) for many years before the onset of lymphoedema (Figure 18.1). The total incidence of other malformations is about 20%.[4] A greater proportion of individuals with congenital lymphoedema have associated malformations (25%) than lymphoedema praecox (8%).[1]

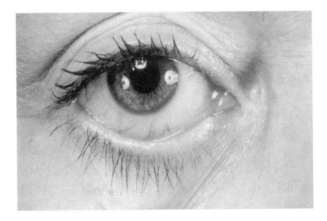

Figure 18.1   In-growing eyelashes (distichiasis) on the lateral side of the upper eyelid. The aberrant eyelashes are frequently finer and more difficult to see.

Many of the conditions which result in lymphoedema have a higher incidence of congenital heart disease. This is particularly true if there is an abnormality in the thoracic duct. The development of the heart occurs at the same time and in close proximity to the development of the thoracic duct. Consequently this association is not too surprising. Other features appear to have no relation to the development of the lymphatic system, for example, one autosomal dominant condition is associated with yellow dystrophic nails.

Precipitating factors and expression

Primary lymphoedema may occur spontaneously but there is often a precipitating factor such as:

- puberty
- pregnancy or the oral contraceptive pill
- minor trauma
- infection.

These are all events which would not cause lymphoedema in an unaffected person. The severity of the lymphoedema varies even within families, although most individuals carrying the gene have at least a minor degree of lymphoedema. In most genetic forms of lymphoedema, the severity is greater in females. Congenital primary lymphoedema and lymphoedema praecox are also more common in females (2 : 1 and 4 : 1 respectively).[5] In lymphoedema-distichiasis syndrome, however, males are generally more severely affected.

Congenital lymphoedema

Congenital lymphoedema has several genetic causes. Lymphoedema of the legs at birth (Figure 18.2) is most commonly:

- Milroy's disease (hereditary lymphoedema)
- Noonan's syndrome
- Turner's syndrome/gonadal dysgenesis.

Milroy's disease

Milroy's disease accounts for only about 5% of all cases of primary lymphoedema.[4] The term is restricted to lymphoedema which is congenital and

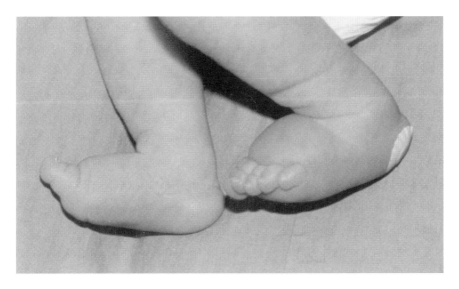

Figure 18.2   Lymphoedema at birth often presents with swelling of the dorsum of the feet.

hereditary. It is an autosomal dominant condition but there is a predominance of affected females suggesting variable expression with increased expression in females. Lymphography shows lymphatic hypoplasia (distal or proximal) or aplasia and abnormalities of the lymph nodes (fibrosis). The type of abnormality seems to be consistent within families. Often there is asymmetry in the degree of swelling.

Noonan's syndrome

One of the features of this autosomal dominant condition is congenital oedema of the feet. Affected individuals have short stature, mild to moderate learning difficulties and a characteristic facies with ptosis, hypertelorism (abnormal distance between the eyes) and low-set ears (Figure 18.3). Heart abnormalities, particularly pulmonary stenosis and cardiomyopathy, are common. Many different presentations of lymphatic vessel dysplasia have been reported in Noonan's syndrome. Lymphoedema of the legs, typically the feet, is the commonest presentation. This generally occurs at birth but sometimes later. Rarely, patients with this condition may present with intestinal lymphangiectasia, pulmonary lymphangiectasia and hydrops foetalis. Increased nuchal translucency in the first trimester of pregnancy has been associated with Noonan's syndrome. A webbed neck is present in 60% of affected individuals. Lymphangiography in this condition has shown various abnormalities,

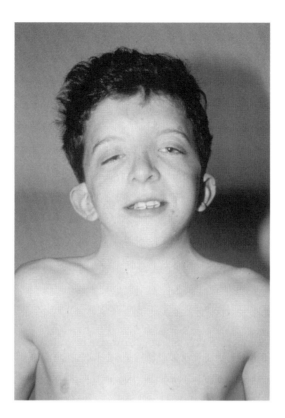

Figure 18.3 The classical features of Noonan's syndrome – bilateral ptosis, hypertelorism, low-set posteriorly rotated ears and some webbing of the neck.

including aplasia or hypoplasia of the lymphatic vessels, restricted lymphatic flow and lymphangiectasis.

Turner's syndrome and gonadal dysgenesis

Turner's syndrome is caused by the absence of one X chromosome. This may be present in all cells or found as a mosaic and occurs as a new event (it is not inherited). The most characteristic features are short stature and streak ovaries resulting in primary amenorrhoea. Neonates born with this condition frequently present with a webbed neck and one third has peripheral lymphoedema, mainly of the feet and legs but occasionally of the hands. Lymphography generally shows distal lymphatic hypoplasia. Turner's syndrome is also associated with congenital heart disease, particularly co-arctation of the aorta or pulmonary stenosis.

Other causes of gonadal dysgensis (e.g. androgen receptor insensitivity) may also present with peripheral oedema of the lower limbs or feet. These are inherited as X-linked conditions. When associated with gonadal dysgenesis, spontaneous regression of the lymphoedema frequently occurs within a few years.

Late onset lymphoedema

Some primary lymphoedemas present later during childhood, more commonly at puberty. The most common syndromes with primary lymphoedema of late onset are:

- Meige-lymphoedema praecox
- lymphoedema-distichiasis
- yellow nail syndrome.

Meige-lymphoedema praecox

Meige-lymphoedema praecox is the commonest cause of primary lymphoedema. Sometimes it is simply called primary lymphoedema. The lymphoedema in Meige's syndrome generally occurs at puberty and typically involves the feet and ankles. This condition is inherited in an autosomal dominant pattern and there are generally no associated features. There is variable expression with increased severity in females. Lymphography shows either distal or proximal hypoplasia of the lymphatics, but the abnormality tends to be consistent within a family. This suggests that there may be more than one gene causing this abnormality.

Lymphoedema-distichiasis

Lymphoedema-distichiasis is an autosomal dominant condition which is rarer but more distinctive. Families with this condition develop lymphoedema at puberty or later. The males are often more severely affected but, again, expression is variable. The first presenting feature is generally distichiasis (in-growing eyelashes) which is present from early childhood. The aberrant eyelashes arise from the posterior lid margin in the position of the meibomian glands. They may cause recurrent conjunctivitis, irritation and photophobia. Affected individuals may pluck the eyelashes out or resort to electrolysis.

Lymphoedema-distichiasis is also associated with an increased incidence of congenital heart disease, sinus bradycardia (generally intermittent), ptosis of the eyes (often unilateral), cleft palate, neck webbing and spinal extradural cysts.

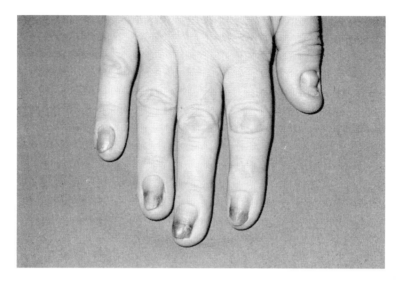

Figure 18.4   Yellow dystrophic nails associated with yellow nail syndrome.

The lymphoedema generally only affects the lower limbs and is frequently associated with varicose veins. Lymphography, unlike in other forms of primary lymphoedema, shows bilateral hyperplasia of the lymphatics and partial or complete obstruction at the level of the thoracic duct.

Yellow nail syndrome

Yellow nail syndrome is a rare autosomal dominant condition (Figure 18.4). The peripheral lymphoedema of the legs is associated with slow growing, yellow-brown dystrophic nails. It is associated with chronic pulmonary problems such as recurrent bronchitis, bronchiectasis and chylothorax. Concomitant humoral and cellular immune deficiency may result in recurrent infections. The onset of the lymphoedema may be at birth (10%) or any time during childhood or adulthood. The lymphoedema may affect the face, vocal cords or genitalia. Rarely, like Noonan's syndrome and Turner's syndrome, this condition may present in the foetus as 'non-immune foetal hydrops'.[6]

Secondary lymphoedema

Secondary lymphoedema is rare in childhood. Causes include:

*   trauma to lymph pathways (including surgery)
*   malignant disease (intra-abdominal or rhabdomyosarcoma)

- filariasis (rare in the UK)
- infections and inflammations (e.g. chronic eczema)
- radiation.

If there has been a significant precipitating factor and no family history, the lymphoedema is probably secondary. Secondary lymphoedema is typically unilateral and in some cases is curable.

Apart from filariasis, infections are more often a complication of pre-existing lymphoedema than the cause of it. Multiple recurrent infections resulting in chronic lymphoedema may occur in patients with chronic eczema of the limbs causing breaches in the epithelial barriers of the skin. The most common organisms are Streptococci and Staphylococci. Lymphangitis causes damage to the lymphatic vessels and the resulting protein-rich lymphoedema is prone to further infections, thereby exacerbating the situation.

Examination

The examination of a child or young person with lymphoedema is much the same as an adult (see p.97). The swelling may vary from mild, painless swelling of the ankle to huge swelling of the whole leg. The swelling is often said to be firm and non-pitting but frequently it is pitting, particularly in the early stages. The swelling is sometimes slowly progressive but may remain unchanged for many years.[1] In the later stages the skin becomes thickened with warty changes at the base of the toes. Ulceration is not a feature.

There may, however, be associated features which give an indication as to the underlying cause. Clues to genetic causes include:

- varicose veins and other abnormalities of development, e.g. congenital heart defects or arrhythmias
- distichiasis
- yellow nails
- malabsorption.

Investigations

A careful clinical history and physical examination will lead to a diagnosis in most patients with primary lymphoedema. Investigations are directed by the clinical findings. If in doubt about whether the swelling is lymphoedema, a lymphangiogram may be helpful. However this is an invasive technique, may be painful and, if possible, should be avoided. Lymphangiography is associated with complications such as wound infections at the cut-down site, pulmonary complications and idiosyncratic hypersensitivity reactions.

Unilateral lymphoedema, particularly with onset after birth and with no family history must be investigated for an underlying cause. This would include pelvic ultrasound or radiological imaging (CT or MRI) to exclude obstructions or malignant disease.

A neonate with bilateral lymphoedema of the dorsum of the feet and neck webbing should have their chromosome karyotype examined for Turner's syndrome, and an echocardiogram to exclude co-arctation of the aorta (Turner's), pulmonary stenosis or cardiomyopathy (Noonan's). A neonate with isolated leg lymphoedema and a family history will probably have Milroy's disease.

Radiological appearance

Primary lymphoedema may be classified according to the underlying lymphatic abnormality.

Hypoplasia/aplasia of the lymphatics

This is the commonest abnormality found in primary lymphoedema (about 80%). There is a deficiency in the number and size of the lymphatic channels. Most primary lymphoedemas, including all those with gonadal dysgenesis (e.g. Turner's syndrome), show this abnormality. Distal hypoplasia is more common in females and presents with mild symmetrical below-knee swelling. Proximal hypoplasia presents with leg swelling which is often more acute in onset, unilateral and has an equal sex distribution.[5]

Bilateral hyperplasia

An increase in the number and size of the lymphatic vessels on both sides is typical of the changes seen in lymphoedema-distichiasis syndrome.[7] This is often associated with absence or obstruction of the thoracic duct.

Megalymphatics

Megalymphatics are generally unilateral. The lymphatics are very dilated and numerous in the lower limb and/or abdomen. Clinically this finding is often associated with capillary haemangiomas on the trunk or at the root of the affected limb. There is generally no family history and, unlike other causes of primary lymphoedema, the sex distribution is equal. Megalymphatics are probably due to a malformation during embryological development *in utero* rather than a genetic disorder.

Management

Management in childhood is similar to the management of an adult with lymphoedema. If an underlying cause is identified, the first line of management is to treat this. Skin care and exercise are appropriate at all stages. It is important to control potential causes of secondary bacterial infection by good skin hygiene, adequate treatment of athlete's foot (tinea pedis), chronic eczema, infections, and the care of any incidental wounds. Exercise may reduce swelling, particularly while wearing compression garments. The affected person should avoid standing for long periods of time.

Symptomatic relief can be provided by stockings, elevation and control of infections. The best treatment in childhood is compression garments, particularly if the swelling is mild–moderate (*see* p.165). There is no reduction of swelling with diuretics. Surgery should be avoided in children, as the swelling frequently does not reach a stable state until adulthood. The surgery may result in a reduction in the size of the swelling but at the price of significant scarring.

However, when treating a child, other factors need to be taken into consideration. The treatment must be appropriate to the child and the parents' needs. There is some debate as to when the child should be treated; some congenital and primary lymphoedemas may resolve with little or no intervention. The age of the child, the attitude of the parents and the degree of swelling are all important considerations.

Infants

Infants may benefit from lymphatic massage of the affected limb, and the parents can be taught how to perform this. If the lymphoedema is severe or causing some unbalance, the infant may benefit from bandaging during the day or night. Compression garments are not often used at this age as the child is growing rapidly, making it difficult to obtain correctly fitting garments.

Early childhood

By the time the child is 3–4 years old compression garments can be considered. At this age children are able to say if they feel discomfort, and they are growing less rapidly. Careful measurement and fitting of stockings is essential to avoid increasing swelling in the feet. Good shoe fitting is important and may help to control foot swelling.

Teenagers

The major problem of wearing compression stockings in late childhood and adolescence is a cosmetic one. Children do not want to look different and are keen to disguise any disabilities. It may improve compliance if the stockings are a more acceptable colour or disguised by leggings or trousers. This is particularly important in physical exercise classes. The child can benefit most by wearing the stockings during exercise but this may be the time when the stockings are most exposed. Teenagers and their parents frequently ask to meet others of the same age with similar problems, and it may help to put them in touch with the Lymphoedema Support Network (see p.8).

Complications can occur at any stage. Secondary infections should be rapidly treated (see p.130). Many patients comment that the swelling has permanently increased with infections. Varicose veins may occur in association with, rather than as a result of, the lymphoedema. If these are painful or unsightly, surgery may be required even as early as adolescence. Other associated features may require attention by the appropriate specialist department, for example cardiology for congenital heart defects and ophthalmology for distichiasis.

Psychological aspects

It is very important to remember the psychological effect of the lymphoedema and its treatment. The unsightly appearance of the swelling can be distressing, particularly for an adolescent. Lymphoedema may affect job prospects and limit exercise, leisure (including travel) and daily activities.[1] It can make finding comfortable shoes and clothes far more difficult.

Genetic considerations

Many primary forms of lymphoedema are inherited in an autosomal pattern with variable expression or occur as sporadic new mutations, either germline or mosaic. Understanding the mode of inheritance in each situation allows the clinician to give accurate recurrence risks and look for any of the associated features or complications. If the family history suggests that a person is likely to develop lymphoedema, it is important to educate the family about the risk and introduce preventive measures, for example TED stockings, leg elevation, movement during long flights, avoidance of secondary infections (*see* pp 118 and 134).

Recent linkage studies have located the genes for Milroy's disease,[8] lymphoedema-distichiasis[9] and Meige's late onset lymphoedema in some families. Linkage has also been found for some of the syndromes which feature lymphoedema, for example Noonan's syndrome. Hopefully, as more genes are identified, our understanding of the mechanisms involved in the normal and abnormal development of the lymphatic system will be enhanced – and management improved accordingly.

Acknowledgements

We should like to thank Eunice Jeffs, lymphoedema nurse specialist at St George's Hospital, London for her advice about management of lymphoedema in childhood. The figures were kindly provided by Dr Peter Mortimer, Department of Dermatology, and Professor Patton, Department of Clinical Genetics, St George's Hospital, London.

References

1   David M *et al.* (1985) Primary lymphoedema in children and adolescents: A follow-up study and review. *Pediatrics.* **76**:206–18.
2   Kinmonth JB *et al.* (1957) Primary lymphoedema: clinical and lymphangiographic studies of a series of 107 patients in which the lower limbs were affected. *British Journal of Surgery.* **45**:1–10.
3   Dale RF (1985) The inheritance of primary lymphoedema. *Journal of Medical Genetics.* **22**:274–8.
4   Kinmonth JB (1982) *The Lymphatics: Surgery, Lymphography, and Diseases of the Chyle and Lymph Systems.* Edward Arnold, London.
5   Wright NB and Carty HML (1994) The swollen leg and primary lymphoedema. *Archives of Disease in Childhood.* **71**:44–9.
6   Govaert P *et al.* (1992) Perinatal manifestation of maternal yellow nail syndrome. *Pediatrics.* **89**:1016–8.
7   Dale RF (1987) Primary lymphoedema when found with distichiasis is the type defined as bilateral hyperplasia by lymphography. *Journal of Medical Genetics.* **24**:170–1.
8   Evans AL *et al.* (1999) Mapping of primary congenital lymphoedema to the 5q35.3 region. *American Journal of Human Genetics.* **64**:547–55.
9   J Mangion *et al.* (1999) A gene for lymphoedema-distichiasis maps to 16q24.3. *American Journal of Human Genetics.* **65**:427–32.

19 Lymphoedema of the head and neck

Simon Withey, Paul Pracy and Peter Rhys-Evans

The term lymphoedema is used, often inaccurately, to describe swelling in the head and neck whatever the cause. Most postoperative and postradiation swelling is simple oedema, secondary to trauma or inflammation, in which the lymphatic component is only minor. Most of these swellings resolve as the inflammation settles and collateral venous and lymphatic channels open. No specific treatment is required in these cases.

The rare cases of progressive lymphoedema present a much more challenging problem. There are few reported cases and only anecdotal information regarding management. Each patient should therefore be treated according to their symptoms with management tailored to their specific needs. Many patients have a relatively short life expectancy and aggressive treatment may not be in their best interest.

Pathophysiology

An increase in extracellular fluid sufficient to cause swelling is called oedema. Although the lymphatics have a responsibility for controlling extracellular fluid volume and compensating for an increase in capillary filtration pressure, they are not responsible for all cases of oedema. Strictly, lymphoedema is extracellular swelling as a result of lymphatic failure, together with normal capillary filtration (*see* p.11). The cause of extracellular fluid swelling in the head and neck is varied, often mixed and difficult to determine.

The head and neck contains an estimated 150–300 lymph nodes, representing one third of the lymph nodes of the body. This is indicative of the massive lymphatic drainage within the region. The potential for lymphatic flow is such that the system can compensate after the loss of a relatively large proportion of lymphatic channels. However there remains a crucial point beyond which the system is unable to cope and, once this is reached, the result is lymphoedema.

In the head and neck the most minor abnormality may be cosmetically distressing. Primary lymphoedema of the head and neck has been reported on few occasions, and, although it is aesthetically disfiguring, it rarely has serious consequences for the health of the individual. Secondary lymphoedema has several causes, and ranges from minor degrees of eyelid swelling to life-threatening oedema. It is the combined effects of surgery and radiotherapy which account for the most pernicious effects of lymphatic obstruction.

Anatomy

Management of the cervical lymph nodes is integral to the treatment of patients with tumours of the head and neck. The spread of cancer to the cervical lymph nodes results in a 50% decrease in survival[1] and the best possible chance of cure for these patients is treatment with radical surgery, often in combination with radical radiotherapy.

The architecture of the lymphatics within the head and neck is similar to other regions of the body. There are no lymphatics within the epidermis but the area is drained by a valveless dermal plexus of non-contractile vessels.[2] These connect with deeper collecting lymphatics which have smooth muscle walls, valves, and a peristaltic action. Lymph is propelled from one segment of the muscular lymphatic vessel to the next, and each segment is isolated by a proximal and a distal valve. These muscular segments, or lymphangions, contract under the influence of a stretch-sensitive pacemaker; as they do, the lymph is propelled through the proximal valve into the next lymphangion. The flow between lymphangions takes a predictable route, unlike the flow in the unvalved dermal lymphatics which may be in both directions. It is into these vessels that the majority of the collateral channels open, and so allow drainage from otherwise compromised areas.[3,4]

The head and neck lymphatic flow is through two interconnecting levels of lymphatics (Figure 19.1). Superficial vessels drain the skin and a deep system of lymphatics drains the lymph from the mucosal linings of the respiratory and digestive tracts. Flow from the skin and the superficial tissues is to a ring of primary lymph nodes which includes the occipital, post-auricular, pre-auricular, parotid and facial nodes. These drain in turn into the deeper nodes which lie adjacent to the internal jugular vein. The deep structures of the head and neck drain directly to the deep cervical nodes which extend from the base of the skull to the root of the neck. The efferent lymphatics then pass via the jugular trunk to the thoracic duct on the left side of the neck and to the right lymphatic duct on the right.

The metastatic spread of head and neck cancers is reasonably predictable.[5–7] The more lateral lesions spread first to ipsilateral lymph nodes and surgery may be confined to one side of the neck. Midline tumours and those of the tongue and nasopharynx have a greater tendency to spread bilaterally and more often require bilateral treatment of the neck.

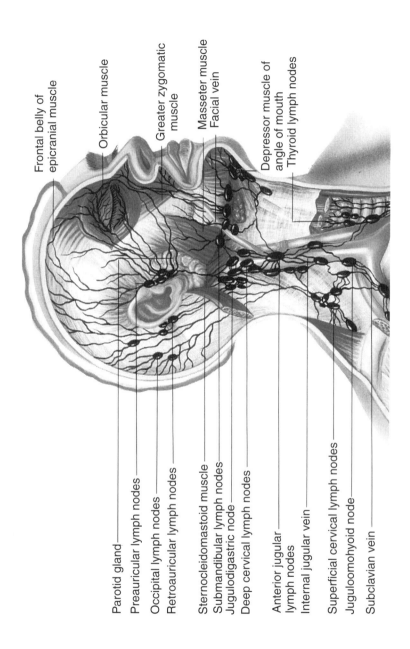

Frontal belly of epicranial muscle

Orbicular muscle

Greater zygomatic muscle

Masseter muscle
Facial vein

Depressor muscle of angle of mouth
Thyroid lymph nodes

Parotid gland
Preauricular lymph nodes
Occipital lymph nodes
Retroauricular lymph nodes

Sternocleidomastoid muscle
Submandibular lymph nodes
Jugulodigastric node
Deep cervical lymph nodes

Anterior jugular lymph nodes
Internal jugular vein

Superficial cervical lymph nodes
Juguloomohyoid node
Subclavian vein

Figure 19.1   Lymphatics of the head and neck.

In an attempt to explain the pathways of metastatic spread taken by tumours of the upper aerodigestive system, the Memorial Sloan Kettering Cancer Centre subdivided the regional lymph nodes into several groups or levels (Figure 19.2). Level 1 includes the contents of the submandibular and submental triangles. The nodes lying along the internal jugular vein and beneath the sternomastoid muscle are divided into three groups and labelled levels 2–4. Levels 2 and 3 are separated by the carotid bifurcation and the hyoid bone, and levels 3 and 4 merge at the level of the omohyoid muscle. Level 5 includes the contents of the posterior triangle. Level 6 and level 7 represent the paratracheal and superior mediastinal nodes respectively.

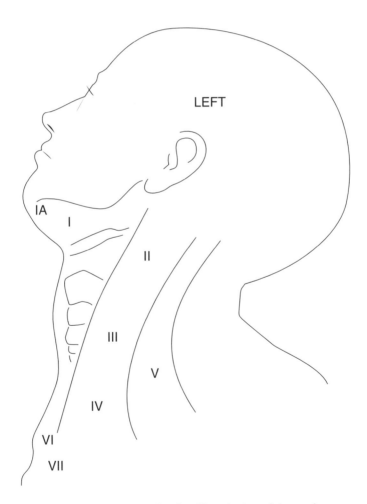

Figure 19.2   The Sloan Kettering levels of lymphatics of the neck.

Surgery remains the main treatment for patients with palpable nodal metastasis of the neck. If multiple nodes are involved or if there is extra-capsular spread of tumour, the rate of recurrence is reduced by additional treatment with radiotherapy.[1] For maximal effect radiation therapy should be started as soon as possible after surgery, and high doses are required in attempts to sterilise the field.[8]

Primary lymphoedema

Individual reports of primary lymphoedema of the head and neck have been published but the condition is extremely rare.[9] Primary oedema of the head and neck may be subdivided, as elsewhere, into *congenita, praecox* and *tarda* (*see* p.23). It is most frequently seen concurrently with arm oedema, sug-gesting that there is a widespread congenital lymphatic insufficiency.[10] Many patients, particularly women, complain of minor facial oedema, worse in the morning and at the time of their menses, in addition to limb oedema.[11] Head and neck lymphangiography has been performed on few patients because of the wish to avoid surgical exploration of the face. It is assumed, however, on the basis of limb lymphangiography on these patients, that the majority have aplasia or hypoplasia of the lymphatics.[11]

Primary oedema of the head and neck is generally disfiguring rather than disabling. In the early stages oedema is generally worse in the morning and patients may be helped if they sleep in a sitting position. Antibiotics should be given prophylactically to those patients who have recurrent acute inflammatory episodes (AIE) (*see* p.137), and to all patients for an established episode. Manual lymphatic drainage (MLD) will help collateral lymphatics clear areas of stagnation and should be offered to all patients who have trouble-some swellings. Patients with head and neck lymphoedema are generally able to perform their own simple lymphatic drainage (SLD) after a short time.

Secondary lymphoedema

Lymphoedema secondary to scarring

Tissues may become oedematous when a critical number of lymphatics are damaged. If a crescentic trapdoor facial flap is created, either surgically or traumatically, and the direction of the valved lymphatics in the base of the flap is afferent then drainage must rely on the valveless dermal vessels. This tendency to swell is compounded by a three-dimensional scar contracture around the flap which results in 'mushrooming' and stiffening of the central tissue.[12] The lymphatic component of such 'pin-cushioned' flaps may improve after several months as dermal lymphatic collaterals develop. Treatment of such scars should start with regular MLD to stimulate these channels. If the scar contracture is felt to make a significant contribution to the problem then scar revision should be considered.

Lymphoedema secondary to recurrent infection and inflammation

Elephantiasis nostras

This is a rare condition which may result in persistent swelling of the lips secondary to recurrent attacks of bacterial infection and lymphangitis.[13,14] Prophylactic penicillin reduces the incidence of repeat infections (see p.137). Elevation of the head while sleeping and the application of pressure to the area in the form of a fitted mask have been suggested.[15] When the swelling becomes refractory to conservative measures, surgical treatment by wedge resection will improve the appearance.

Cheilitis granulomatosa

This is another uncommon condition in which there is progressive chronic swelling of the face and lips. The swelling may be associated with fissuring of the tongue and intermittent facial paralysis, a triad known as the Melkersson-Rosenthal syndrome. Because the condition is frequently found in association with granulomas, some authors have suggested that cheilitis granulomatosa may be a variant of a chronic inflammatory condition such as sarcoidosis, tuberculosis or Crohn's disease. It is most likely, however, that it represents a distinct pathological entity of unknown cause.[13]

Secondary to acne and rosacea

Persistent localised facial oedema can be the consequence of skin disease. In acne vulgaris and rosacea, persistent facial oedema is thought to result from chronic inflammation and prolonged lymphatic stasis.[16] As in the case of elephantiasis nostras, infections may cause progressive damage to lymphatic drainage by intraluminal obliteration of the dermal lymphatic vessels.[17] A similar situation has been reported following persistent head lice infestation with the patient developing lymphoedema of the earlobe.[18]

Nasal lymphoedema

Although the nose may become lymphoedematous as part of generalised facial lymphoedema, localised nasal lymphoedema is most commonly seen in association with a rhinophyma. Rhinophyma is a condition combining sebaceous hyperplasia and infection. The recurrent inflammation causes blockage and obliteration of the lymphatics with resultant swelling. In its early stages the treatment is medical with anti acne antibiotics or retinoids but, once chronic lymphatic insufficiency is present the management is surgical. Tangential excision or dermabrasion are the procedures of choice.

Eyelid oedema

Chronic lymphatic insufficiency of the eyelids causes a conspicuous and disfiguring deformity which typically follows trauma, infection or recurrent inflammation (Figure 19.3). Traumatic lymphatic damage may be either

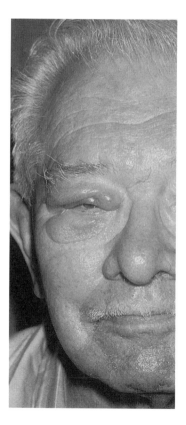

Figure 19.3   Eyelid lymphoedema.

directly to the initial lymphatics following contusion of the lid or to the efferent temporal lymphatics of the lid.[19] Recurrent AIE, including dermatomyositis, and recurrent attacks of contact dermatitis or angioedema may cause an obliterative fibrosis within the lymphatics.[10]

Eyelid oedema should initially be managed with MLD and conservative measures. Surgery may be recommended to preserve vision in patients with severe upper lid oedema and pseudoptosis or in rare cases of complete palpebral obliteration. It may not be necessary to remove much of the subcutaneous tissue of the lids, as the scarring following surgery tends to eliminate spongy areas of low tissue tension where fluid may accumulate.[11] However, if fluid re-accumulates, then consideration should be given to complete excision of the subcutaneous tissues. There have been reports of fluid re-accumulation within full thickness grafts of the eyelid successfully treated by re-excision and application of a split thickness graft.[20] Cosmetic treatment to areas of recurrent idiopathic oedema of the lids and malar eminences constitutes a difficult problem. Blepheroplasty may worsen the oedema, particularly in cases of malar oedema.[21] The use of buried de-epithelialised dermal flaps to relieve eyelid lymphoedema has been advocated,[19] a technique paralleling Thompson's buried dermal flaps for lymphoedema of the extremity.[22] Single laterally based flaps are used for draining the upper lid, and bilateral flaps to drain the lower lid.

The yellow nail syndrome is a distinct entity consisting of thickened yellow nails with a hump in the longitudinal axis of the nail associated with lymphoedema. A case of eyelid oedema associated with yellow nail syndrome has been successfully treated by skin grafting.[23]

The bulbar conjunctiva contains a broad network of anastomosing vessels that drain to the upper and lower fornices, and the palpebral conjunctiva drains toward the retrotarsal lymph network of the lid.[19] Eyelid lymphoedema may thus extend onto the conjunctiva. Two patients with widespread lymphatic disease in whom considerable cosmetic deformity was caused by the gross distension of the conjunctival lymphatics have been reported.[11]

Lymphoedema secondary to surgery and radiotherapy

After extensive surgery and radiotherapy there may be a critical reduction in the number and volume of lymphatic vessels draining the head and neck with subsequent accumulation of a protein-rich fluid in the interstitial space. However, because of the potential for extensive collateral flow, swelling is typically minimal and short-lived. Blockage of the collaterals is generally the result of recurrence after surgery and radiotherapy or fibrosis exacerbated by recurrent AIE. In the most extreme cases the resultant swelling may give rise to a classical appearance which has been described as 'pumpkin head oedema' (Figure 19.4).

A unilateral neck dissection involves removal of some or all of the deep lymph nodes on one side of the neck as well as the creation of a skin incision at one or possibly two levels around a quarter of the circumference of the neck. When the procedure is combined with radiotherapy many of the lymphatics which have survived surgery, particularly those of the dermis and the mucosa of the aerodigestive system, will be obliterated by the subsequent fibrosis. This sequence of events may almost completely obliterate the lymphatic outflow from one side of the head and neck. Despite this dramatic reduction in outflow channels for the lymph, unilateral neck dissection rarely causes more than transient oedema.

Patients treated with bilateral neck dissections and radical radiotherapy are at the greatest risk of developing significant lymphoedema. In these patients the anterior and lateral lymphatic channels have been removed surgically and the

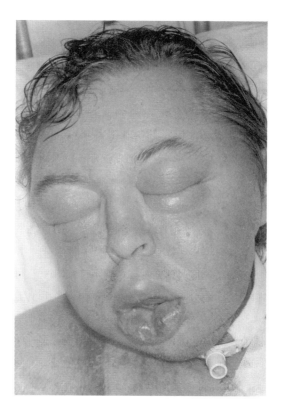

Figure 19.4   Pumpkin head oedema. Reproduced with permission.

dermal lymphatics within the skin flaps have been transected by a surgical incision and subsequently damaged by the radiotherapy. Even after such extensive damage lasting lymphatic obstruction is relatively rare. Dermal lymphatics open and the drainage channels of the posterior triangle, together with those of the oral and pharyngeal mucosa, will assist in drainage.

The chances of developing problems are increased by unusually high doses of radiotherapy, recurrent AIE and scar contracture; the last two are often the 'final straw' which precipitates delayed oedema. The situation may be exacerbated by an increase in the venous pressure of the head and neck in patients who have also had bilateral internal jugular vein ligation. In these cases an increase in the filtration pressure will result in a considerable increase in the interstitial fluid volume overwhelming the lymphatic 'safety valve' and resulting in combined venous and lymphatic swelling.[10] Generalised lymphoedema of the head and neck results in the skin becoming thickened and stiff. In severe cases the tongue and oropharynx swell and this may necessitate tracheostomy and/or feeding via an enterostomy tube. Embarrassed by their disfigurement and often unable to speak because of gross tongue swelling, these patients may become increasingly isolated. This is exacerbated by reduced hearing secondary to oedema of the external auditory meatus and an inability to see through swollen closed eyelids.

Lymphoedema following surgery and radiotherapy does not always present such a dramatic and disastrous picture. A temporary lymphoedematous swelling is frequently seen in the subcutaneous tissues above the scar of a patient following a neck dissection. This swelling probably results from a mixture of lymphatic and venous insufficiency and begins to improve as soon as superficial veins and lymphatics connect across the wound. A similar collection of fluid is frequently seen in the submental area; this so-called dewlap is a characteristic of patients who have undergone bilateral neck dissections and those treated by surgery or radiotherapy for laryngeal tumours. Although the swelling will tend to improve, these patients will frequently complain of a brawny thickening of the tissues.

Management

The treatment of localised lymphoedema within the head and neck has been discussed in the previous section. Much improvement of regional oedema can be achieved with simple conservative treatment of the skin, avoidance and treatment of infection, and massage to open the collateral lymphatics. Once lymphoedema is established and the oedema has become 'solid' the condition is incurable.[10] Under these circumstances surgery may be used to debulk the tissue but has little else to offer.

Most cases of generalised lymphoedema of the head and neck follow complex surgical procedures and radiotherapy. In the first months after surgery some improvement can be expected as collateral channels open. When the lymphoedema develops later it suggests that compensatory mechanisms of drainage have failed, either as a result of recurrent tumour or because frequent AIE and fibrosis have blocked the remaining lymphatics, or sometimes as a consequence of scar contracture.

Many patients with severe progressive generalised post-surgical oedema of the head and neck will need to be treated with a tracheostomy tube and fed via an enterostomy. They may gain some symptomatic relief from custom-made collars to provide support for the ever increasing weight of the head. The collar may also help to ensure that any remaining lymphatic channels are not obstructed further due to an awkward position of the neck. In cases of 'pumpkin head' oedema, the swelling will eventually become so severe that the soft tissue of the external auditory meatus will swell and block the ear. These patients should be offered a bone conducting hearing aid, although great care should be taken with the fitting of these devices as dermal abrasions and pressure sores may develop. If the eyelids are swollen and obstruct vision, a blepharoplasty incision may be used to remove all subcutaneous tissues from the eyelids. The thinned flaps are then draped back over the eyelids, if oedema fluid recollects the upper lid skin may be replaced by a split thickness graft and the lower by a full thickness graft.[20]

Education

The patient needs a clear understanding of how and why the problem has arisen and how it is likely to progress. They must be aware of the importance of scrupulous hygiene and should understand the aims and limitations of the treatment. In the severe post-surgical cases, the condition is not curable and there may be no potential for collateral flow and spontaneous improvement. Although these patients may have been cured of their disease they will then be subjected to a lifetime of treatment for this unfortunate iatrogenic condition.

Investigations

The most likely cause of delayed oedema of the head and neck after surgery and radiotherapy is recurrent disease and this should be looked for in all such cases. The patient should have repeat scans. Interpretation of scan images is often difficult because of the anatomical disruption of previous surgery and subsequent tissue inflammation. MRI with STIR sequences and positron emission tomography (PET) have proved useful.

Hygiene

In the management of any case of lymphoedema it is essential to minimise the risk of AIE. All patients should receive advice on oral hygiene and skin care, although this in itself may be difficult because of inaccessibility of the mouth and poor vision. Patients who suffer recurrent AIE or severe swelling should receive prophylactic antibiotics in the form of phenoxymethylpenicillin 500mg daily (see p.137). Antifungal therapy should be given because of the high risk of oral candidiasis.

Drug treatment

Attempts to treat pure lymphoedema with diuretics are both physiologically unsound and unhelpful. In cases of post-surgical head and neck oedema the picture may be mixed, with a combination of lymphatic and venous components. In this situation diuretic therapy may help settle the venous swelling by reducing the capillary filtration pressure.[24]

Benzopyrones are said to act in part by increasing macrophage proteolysis and improving the contractile properties of the collecting lymphatics (see p.245). The exact role of the benzopyrones remains unclear, but those who champion their use claim a clinically significant reduction in oedema in most patients. Patients' symptoms and AIE were reduced during the periods of treatment in many cases.[25]

If recurrent disease is suspected as the cause of the lymphoedema, consideration may be given to the use of chemotherapy. Recurrent tumour will provoke lymphoedema as a result of lymphatic blockage by malignant cells. The local inflammatory response to the tumour will exacerbate the problem by causing an obliterative fibrosis. Cytotoxic agents act both by clearing malignant cells from the lymphatics and by reducing the local inflammatory response to tumour. However, many of these patients are in the terminal stages of their illness and the adverse effects of the chemotherapy may outweigh any palliative benefit.

Manual lymphatic drainage

MLD is the most effective method of reducing limb oedema and has been used in the head and neck with good effect.[26,27] Complete lymphatic obstruction is not compatible with life and one must assume that even in the worst cases of head and neck lymphoedema some lymphatic channels are open. It is known that normally functioning lymphatics increase their output if subjected to mild mechanical stimulation. Once the normal lymphatics have been stimulated, oedema fluid can be gently pushed from the lympho-static areas towards any functioning vessels. Care must be taken with the massage as excessive vigour can damage normal lymphatics.[25] In the man-agement of lower limb lymphoedema, after MLD, the leg is bandaged in an attempt to reduce the filtration pressure gradient. This is obviously impractical in the head and neck but some have suggested using elasticated compression garments as used in the management of burns patients.

There is an increased risk of disseminating tumour if MLD is used in the presence of recurrent disease but, in a hopeless situation where any allevi-ation of swelling will be an improvement, this should probably not cause undue concern.[28]

Transcutaneous electrical nerve stimulation (TENS)

TENS has been reported to improve the swelling of patients with both peripheral and head and neck lymphoedema (see p.271). It is thought that the technique works by stimulating the contractile muscular lymphatics and also influencing the extrinsic muscular compression of the lymphatic chan-nels. It provides a simple non-invasive technique and is worth considering in moderate or severe cases of oedema which do not resolve spontaneously after 2–3 months. It may be used in conjunction with MLD.

Surgery

In severe head and neck lymphoedema, except in the case of obstructed vision, surgery is very much a final option. In the most severe cases the surgeon will be operating in a field that has been severely damaged by previous surgery and radiotherapy; healing will be poor and tissue planes non-existent.

Many of the procedures which are used in the alleviation of limb lymph-oedema are not suitable for use in the head and neck and the main hope lies in the introduction of a new drainage channel. Microsurgical reconstructive procedures have shown some promise in the management of peripheral oedema but they are unlikely to have a place in the management of head and neck oedema because surrounding tissues will have been too severely damaged.

The most promising procedures in these difficult situations are the use of flaps, containing axial lymphatics, in an attempt to re-establish lymphatic flow. The omentum has a rich lymphatic supply with a number of collecting lymphatics running parallel to the gastro-epiploic vessels.[29] Reports suggest successful reduction of swelling using the omentum in limb oedema, but list a high complication rate such as hernias and intestinal obstruction.[30] Although there have been no reports of omental by-pass in head and neck lymph-oedema, the technique may have some potential.

In 1935 Gilles reported the use of a 'plastic operation in the treatment of lymphoedema'. A skin flap was raised from the medial side of the arm of a patient with lower limb lymphoedema praecox. The distal end of the flap was inset into the upper thigh. Three months later the flap was divided and the proximal end was inset below the axillary lymphatics. Follow up at 15 years showed no recurrence of the lymphoedema.[31] Clodius has used a similar tech-nique for reducing lower limb oedema, this time using the axial lymphatics of the groin flap from the contralateral side.[32] If these flaps are raised in an attempt to reduce head and neck oedema they should contain axial lymphatics that are not dilated and the lymphatic outlet should be as close as possible to the axilla.[28] We have recently used a tubed deltopectoral flap to drain the left side of the face of a patient with 'pumpkin head oedema'. Three weeks after the de-epithelialised segment was inset into the cheek the patient was able to open his eye for the first time in 3 months. Such flaps will not cure the lymphoedema but may provide some relief for a patient who suffers from progressive head and neck lymphoedema.

References

1   O'Brien CJ et al. (1986) Neck dissection with and without radiotherapy – prog-nostic factors, patterns of recurrence and survival. American Journal of Surgery. **152**:456–63.

2   Kobayashi MR and Miller TA (1987) Lymphedema. Clinics in Plastic Surgery. **14**:303–13.

3   Ryan TJ (1995) Mechanical resilience of skin: A function for blood supply and lymphatic drainage. Clinics in Dermatology. **13**:429–32.

4   Leemans CR (1992) The value of neck dissection in head and neck cancer. Doctorate thesis. Vrije University, Drukkneij Elinwijk, Utrecht.

5   Lindberg R (1972) Distribution of cervical lymph node metastasis from squamous cell carcinoma of the upper respiratory and digestive tracts. Cancer. **29**:1446–9.

6   Byers RM et al. (1988) Rationale for elective modified neck dissection. Head and Neck Surgery. **10**:160–7.

7   Shah JP (1990) Patterns of cervical lymph node metastasis from squamous car-cinomas of the upper aerodigestive tract. American Journal of Surgery. **160**:405–9.

8   Medina JE et al. (1999) Management of cervical lymph nodes in squamous cell carcinoma of the head and neck. In: LB Harrison, RB Sessions, WK Hong (eds) Head and Neck Cancer: A Multidisciplinary Approach. Lippincott-Raven, Philadelphia, pp 353–78.

9   Parsa FD and Sickenberg M (1989) Lymphoedema of the face. *Annals of Plastic Surgery.* **23**:178–81.

10 Mortimer PS (1995) Managing lymphoedema. *Clinics in Dermatology.* **13**: 499–505.

11 Kinmonth JB (1982) *The Lymphatics: Surgery, Lymphography and Diseases of the Chyle and Lymph Systems*, 2nd edn. Edward Arnold, London.

12 Jackson IT (1985) *Local Flaps in Head and Neck Reconstruction.* CV Mosby, St Louis.

13 Cranberg JA *et al.* (1990) Angioedema, elephantiasis nostras and cheilitis granulomatosa. *Allergy Proceedings.* **11**:79–82.

14 Castellani A (1960) Elephantiasis nostras and elephantiasis tropica: a comparative study. *Tropical Medicine and Hygiene.* **63**:216.

15 Beninson J (1971) Successful treatment of elephantiasis nostras of the lip. *Angiology.* **22**:448–55.

16 Harvey DT *et al.* (1998) Rosaceous lymphoedema: A rare variant of a common disorder. *Cutis.* **61**:321–4.

17 Harwood CA and Mortimer PS (1995) Causes and clinical manifestations of lymphatic failure. *Clinics in Dermatology.* **13**:459–71.

18 Mahzoon S and Azabeh B (1983) Elephantiasis of external ears: a rare manifestation of pediculosis capitis. *Acta Dermato-Venereologica (Stockholm).* **63**: 363–5.

19 Stricker M (1977) The palpebral lymphedema. In: L Clodius (ed) *Lymphoedema.* Georg Thieme, Stuttgart.

20 James JH (1978) Lymphedema of the eyelids. *Plastic and Reconstructive Surgery.* **61**:703–6.

21 Rees TD *et al.* (1990) Blepharoplasty and facialplasty. In: JG McCarthy (ed) *Plastic Surgery.* WB Saunders, Philadelphia, pp 2320–414.

22 Thompson N (1969) The surgical treatment of advanced post mastectomy lymphoedema of the upper limb. With the late results of treatment by the buried dermis flap operation. *Scandinavian Journal of Plastic Surgery.* **3**:54.

23 Maisels DO and Korachi AOA (1985) Lymphoedema of the eyelids in the yellow nail syndrome. *British Journal of Plastic Surgery.* **38**:93–6.

24 Mortimer PS (1997) Therapy approaches for lymphoedema. *Angiology.* **48**:87–91.

25 Casley-Smith JR (1977) The structural basis for the conservative treatment of lymphoedema. In: L Clodius (ed) *Lymphoedema.* Georg Thieme, Stuttgart.

26 Einfeldt H and Lange G (1989) Das 'tertiare' lymphodem- procedere in der lymphdrainagetherapie. *Zeitschrift Lymphologie.* **13**:57–61.

27 Ruger K (1993) Das kopflymphodem in der klinischen praxis. *Zeitschrift Lymphologie.* **17**:6–11.

28 Einfeldt H *et al.* (1986) Therapeutische und palliative lymphdrainage zur odemtherapie im gesichts-und halsbereich. *HNO.* **34**:365–7.

29 Clodius L (1990) Lymphedema. In: JG McCarthy (ed) *Plastic Surgery.* WB Saunders, Philadelphia, pp 4093–117.

30 Goldsmith HS (1974) Long term evaluation of omental transposition for chronic lymphoedema. *Annals of Surgery.* **180**:847–9.

31 Gilles HD (1950) The lymphatic wick. *Proceedings of the Royal Society of Medicine.* **43**:1054–6.

32 Clodius L *et al.* (1982) The lymphatics of the groin flap. *Annals of Plastic Surgery.* **9**:447–58.

20 Breast lymphoedema

Marilyn Kirshbaum

In women with breast cancer, ipsilateral arm swelling is the most frequently recognised feature of lymphatic dysfunction. Consequently, the physical[1-4] and psychological[5-8] aspects of lymphoedema of the arm in women are well-documented. There is a small number of men with swelling of breast tissue subsequent to cancer treatment, and their physical and psychosocial needs require specific attention. This chapter will focus on the issues associated with breast lymphoedema in women.

Description

Breast lymphoedema presents as swelling of all of the breast or part of it. It is the result of disruption of the lymphatic drainage of the breast and axilla. This can be caused by radiotherapy, surgery and/or recurrent cancer. Sometimes, infection is also a causal factor.

The patient may describe discomfort as 'heaviness', a 'tight feeling' or mention that she feels 'lopsided'. The swelling is typically most marked in the lower part of the breast below the scar because of the pooling of lymph. Truncal oedema is recognised by the prominent indentations made by the straps of undergarments. Skin changes such as redness and discolouration may be present. However, these may be complications of breast cancer treatments rather than caused by the lymphoedema.

The upper outer quadrant of the breast sometimes appears to be affected but this more commonly reflects postradiation scarring. It tends to be a well-defined area with skin changes such as *peau d'orange* caused by fibrotic tethering and local collections of lymph. It does not pit on pressure and is often tender to palpate.

The lymphatic drainage of the breast

Lymph from the breast is drained through a system of nodes which feeds into the subclavian lymph trunk and into the venous system at the junction of the subclavian and internal jugular veins.[9] The nodes comprise five groups:

- pectoral – along the inferior border of the pectoralis minor muscle
- subscapular – along the subscapular artery and veins

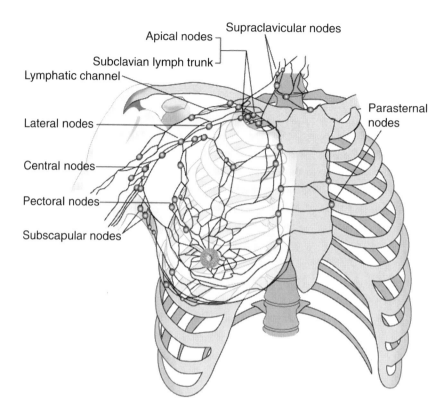

Figure 20.1   Nodal groups involved in lymphatic drainage of the breast.

- lateral – along the distal part of the axillary vein
- central – embedded in axillary fat
- apical – along the axillary vein between the clavicle and pectoralis minor (Figure 20.1).

The diffuse network of lymphatics which drain the breast can be divided into two sets of pathways:

- dermal
- parenchymal.

The dermal network consists of superficial vessels which drain the skin of the breast. The skin from the lateral part of the breast is drained by lymphatic vessels which lead to the axillary nodes (Figure 20.2). Lymphatics from the upper part of the breast connect with the lower and deeper supraclavicular

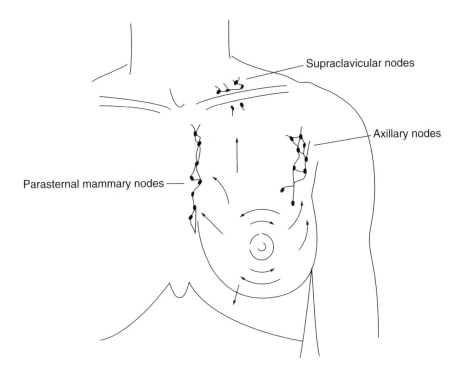

Figure 20.2 Lymphatic drainage from the breast.

nodes, and skin lymphatics over the medial part of the breast connect with the parasternal mammary nodes near the internal thoracic (mammary) artery. Breast cancer may spread through the dermal lymphatic network on the affected side and present as cutaneous nodules. The cancer can also spread between the breasts through the shared midline pathway; this sometimes progresses to bilateral disease.[10]

The deeper lymphatic vessels of the parenchyma of the breast lead mainly to the anterior axillary nodes via the axillary tail. Other pathways lead to the posterior axillary nodes, parasternal nodes and axillary vein.

Cancer treatments

The most common treatments associated with breast lymphoedema are:

- breast surgery
- axillary node surgery
- radiotherapy.

Some women receiving adjuvant hormone therapy gain weight and retain fluid, thereby exacerbating the problem.

Breast and axillary node surgery

Surgery is often a potentially curative treatment modality for breast cancer.[11] After confirmation of the diagnosis, excision of a breast cancer is performed by either lumpectomy, quadrantectomy or mastectomy. Axillary surgery involving level I, level II or level III dissections of the lymph nodes is often necessary to determine the presence and extent of metastatic spread and guide further treatment decisions (Figure 20.3).[12] Generally, the higher the level of dissection, the greater the number of lymph nodes removed and the greater the morbidity.[13]

The most common complications associated with breast and axillary node surgery have been identified as:[13–15]

• haematoma/seroma

• wound infection

• limitation of arm movement

• breast, axillary and arm numbness and pain (see p.68)

• breast lymphoedema

• lymphangitis/lymphoedema of the arm.

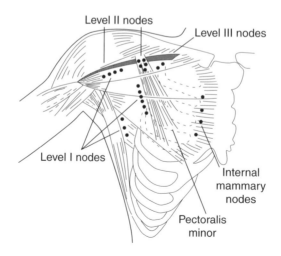

Figure 20.3   Levels of axillary lymph nodes.

Fluid accumulation presenting as a haematoma or seroma is the complication of breast and axillary surgery which causes the most concern because it predisposes to the other complications listed above. Some damage to vulnerable breast tissue and blood and lymphatic vessels is unavoidable during breast and axillary surgery whatever the skill and experience of the surgeon. During surgery, blood and lymphatic vessels are transected. It is inevitable that blood and lymph will leak into the operative area despite seroma prevention practices such as internal suturing, cauterisation and closed suction drains.

Recognition that fluid accumulation is a serious problem is the first step towards improvement.[15,16] Attention and time should be given in the operating theatre to inspecting the surgical area carefully before suturing the skin and to stopping any uncontrolled bleeding. After surgery, movement of the arm on the affected side acts as a pump which forces lymph into the empty axilla.[15] The respiratory movements of the chest wall and movement of the shoulder thereby delay skin flap adherence and increase fluid accumulation. Closed axillary suction should be continued until the daily amount extracted is < 20ml.[16] Early discharge from hospital could increase the likelihood of seroma formation, and ultimately the development of lymphoedema.

Sentinel lymph node biopsy

Routine axillary lymph node dissection has recently come under scrutiny with the hope of reducing morbidity. A surgical procedure called sentinel node biopsy has been used to stage patients with melanoma[17] and is now increasingly being used with breast cancer patients so as to avoid unnecessary axillary dissections and the associated morbidity. The sentinel lymph node is the first lymph node in the lymphatic drainage area to receive lymph from the tumour site.[18] It is now thought that, if breast cancer cells spread to the axilla, they must first pass through the sentinel lymph node. Hence, if the sentinel lymph node is cancer-free, metastasis through the lymphatics to the axillary nodes has not occurred and further axillary surgery is unnecessary.

The sentinel node is identified by lymphatic mapping using one of several blue dyes with or without radioactive markers or lymphoscintigraphy. However, despite numerous reports, there is not yet a consensus about the most reliable technique.[19,20] Recent research using immunohistochemistry resulted in the detection of micrometastases in 14% of a group of 52 patients who were thought to be clear when tested with patent blue-V dye.[21] There were, however, one or two people in whom the sentinel node was negative but another node was positive. Despite the small possibility of a false negative result, sentinel node biopsy is clearly a promising procedure and will obviate the need for a full axillary dissection in many women with breast cancer.

Radiotherapy

Most women who have radiotherapy to the breast or chest wall experience some local swelling. It generally resolves spontaneously within 3 months and is not seen as a major problem by either oncologists or most women.[14] Some women, however, continue to experience swelling and discomfort. This can be extremely distressing because, despite conservative surgery, they are left with a swollen uncomfortable breast. Possible predisposing factors to the development of lymphoedema include:

- the dose of radiation

- a severe skin reaction

- radiation-induced fibrosis.

Radiation dose

When the breast is irradiated, all parts of the breast do not receive an equal dose. On average, there is a 10% discrepancy between different areas of the breast. The dose received at the extremes of the latitudinal field are greater, thus causing more damage to lymphatics. Larger breasts also receive higher doses of radiation at the extremes of the latitudinal field as a result of radiation scatter (Figure 20.4).

Lateral wedges are routinely used to compensate for longitudinal dose variations. Medial wedges, which need to vary in size according to individual breast size, can compensate for latitudinal dose variations[22] but are not commonly used in the UK.

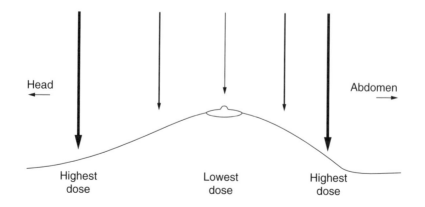

Figure 20.4   A cross-section of the breast showing the distribution of radiation given to the breast as a result of radiation scatter.

The severity of skin reactions

Adverse effects of adjuvant breast radiotherapy on the skin include erythema, pruritis, dry desquamation, moist desquamation, telangiectasia, photosensitivity, fibrosis and hyperpigmentation.[23] These are either early acute (transient) effects or late (chronic) radiation effects. The severity of these reactions has been shown to be dependent on a combination of dose–time–volume factors such as:

- total radiation dose

- fractionation schedule

- energy of the radiation used

- volume of the normal tissue included in the treatment field

- the radiosensitivity of the normal tissue involved.[24]

Many predictive factors relate to individual characteristics such as age, co-existing disease, drug therapy, nutritional status, smoking, infection and ultra-violet light exposure.[25] Breast lymphoedema may be associated with similar causal factors.

Radiotherapy to damaged breast tissue causes more fibrosis

The effects of breast surgery may result in secondary problems from radio-therapy. The breast is heavily vascular and prone to a series of events begin-ning with a haematoma or seroma, progressing through infection and delayed wound healing, and ending with fibrosis and scarring. When radiotherapy is given to a damaged breast and a damaged dermal lymphatic network, the potential for swelling of the whole or part of the breast is increased.[26]

The patient's perspective

Health professionals should recognise that a patient's distress in relation to what may seem to be a minor medical problem needs to be acknowledged. Although it is not life-threatening, breast lymphoedema can be a source of many concerns for the patient. These add to the challenge of coping with the diagnosis of breast cancer and its treatment. Concerns include:

- heaviness, discomfort, pain

- body image problems

- sexual difficulties

- social isolation
- depression
- delay in resuming previous social activities
- fear of recurrence
- difficulties of adjustment.

These issues are discussed elsewhere (*see* p.89).

Management

Management begins by identifying those most at risk (*see* p.97). Educating the patient about why they are at risk, and how to reduce the risk, is clearly important. All patients with lymphoedema of the breast or arm should be investigated to exclude the presence of cancer, either primary or recurrence.

Because lymphoedema is chronic and progressive, patients need to know what lymphoedema is and the implications of living with a chronic condition. Only then can they make informed choices. A multiprofessional approach is preferable. The multiprofessional team may include the general practitioner, surgeon, breast care nurse, oncologist, physiotherapist, prosthetic adviser and psychologist. The physiotherapist can advise on exercises to increase shoulder function and so help prevent scarring from surgery and/or radio-therapy. The prosthetic adviser can provide access to suitable brassieres and other clothing. Manual lymphatic drainage (MLD) and simple lymphatic drain-age (SLD) are helpful (*see* pp 203 and 217). The massage increases lymphatic drainage, softens the breast and disrupts the fibrosis caused by surgery and radiotherapy.

Advice regarding the care of the skin and prevention of infection is important. Acute inflammation of the breast can occur which is painful and distressing for the patient, who may well not be able to touch the area. Antibiotics should be prescribed (*see* p.130). If recurrent, long-term prophylaxis should be instituted.

Conclusion

Health professionals working with breast cancer patients need to be aware of the problems associated with breast lymphoedema. Recognition of the prob-lems and empathy are the first steps in assisting women with breast lymph-oedema. Surgeons and nurses should continue to scrutinise surgical techniques and procedures for wound care. Patients would also benefit if oncologists, breast care and other nurses incorporated the increasing research evidence on lymphoedema into clinical practice. Although there is still much to be discovered about how to manage lymphoedema of the breast, much can be done now through prevention, early diagnosis and supportive care.

References

1   Stanton AWB *et al.* (1996) Current puzzles presented by mastectomy oedema (breast cancer related lymphoedema). *Vascular Medicine.* **1**:213–25.
2   Maunsell E *et al.* (1992) Arm problems and psychological distress after surgery for breast cancer. *Canadian Journal of Surgery.* **36**:315–20.
3   Badger C and Regnard C (1989) Oedema in advanced disease: a flow diagram. *Palliative Medicine.* **3**:213–5.
4   Veitch J (1993) Skin problems in lymphoedema. *Wound Management.* **4**:42–5.
5   Woods M (1993) Patient's perceptions of breast cancer related lymphoedema. *European Journal of Cancer Care.* **2**:125–8.
6   Tobin M *et al.* (1993) The psychological morbidity of breast cancer-related arm swelling. *Cancer.* **72**:3248–52.
7   Kirshbaum M (1996) The development, implementation and evaluation of guidelines for the management of breast cancer related lymphoedema. *European Journal of Cancer Care.* **5**:246–51.
8   Mirolo B *et al.* (1995) Psychosocial benefits of postmastectomy lymphoedema therapy. *Cancer Nursing.* **18**:197–205.
9   Agur A (1991) *Grant's Atlas of Anatomy*, 9th edn. Williams and Wilkins, Baltimore.
10 McGregor AL (1986) *Lee McGregor's Synopsis of Surgical Anatomy*, 12th edn. GAG Decker and DJ du Pressis (eds). John Wright, Bristol.
11 Benson ET and Thorogood J (1986) The effect of surgical technique on the local recurrence rates following mastectomy. *European Journal of Surgical Oncology.* **12**:267–71.
12 Fisher B *et al.* (1985) Ten year results of a randomised clinical trial comparing radical mastectomy and total mastectomy with or without radiation. *New England Journal of Medicine.* **312**:674–81.
13 Siegel B *et al.* (1990) Level I and II axillary dissection in the treatment of early-stage breast cancer. *Archives of Surgery.* **125**:1144–7.
14 Warmuth M *et al.* (1998) Complications of axillary lymph node dissection for carcinoma of the breast. *Cancer.* **83**:1362–8.
15 Aiken D *et al.* (1984) Prevention of seromas following mastectomy and axillary dissection. *Surgery, Gynecology and Obstetrics.* **158**:327–33.
16 Tadych K and Donegan WL (1987) Postmastectomy seromas and wound drainage. *Surgery, Gynecology and Obstetrics.* **165**:483–7.
17 Morton DL *et al.* (1992) Technical details of intra-operative lymphatic mapping for early stage melanoma. *Archives of Surgery.* **36**:392–9.
18 Albertini JJ *et al.* (1996) Lymphatic mapping and sentinel node biopsy in the patient with breast cancer. *Journal of the American Medical Association.* **276**: 1818–22.

19   McIntosh SA and Purushotham AD (1998) Lymphatic mapping and sentinel node biopsy in breast cancer. *British Journal of Surgery*. **85**:1347–56.

20   Cox CE *et al.* (1998) Guidelines for sentinel node biopsy and lymphatic mapping of patients with breast cancer. *Annals of Surgery*. **227**:645–53.

21   McIntosh SA *et al.* (1999) Therapeutic implications of the sentinel lymph node in breast cancer. *Lancet*. **354**:570.

22   Ikner CL *et al.* (1998) Comparison of the homogeneity of breast dose distributions with and without the medial wedge. *Medical Dosimetry*. **23**:89–94.

23   Goodman M *et al.* (1997) Integumentary and mucous membrane alterations. In: SL Groenwald, MH Frogge, M Goodman, CH Yarbro (eds) *Cancer Nursing: Principles and Practice*, 4th edn. Jones and Barlett, Boston.

24   Bloomer W and Hellman S (1975) Normal tissue responses to radiation therapy. *New England Journal of Medicine*. **293**:80–3.

25   Porock D *et al.* (1998) Predicting the severity of radiation skin reactions in women with breast cancer. *Oncology Nursing Forum*. **25**:1019–29.

26   Kissin MW *et al.* (1986) Risk of lymphoedema following the treatment of breast cancer. *British Journal of Surgery*. **73**:580–4.

21 Male genital lymphoedema

Neil Haldar and David Cranston

The causes of male genital lymphoedema are the same as for lymphoedema in other parts of the body (Box 21.A).[1] Male genital lymphoedema may be an acute (reversible) phenomenon such as that following trauma, surgery, paraphimosis or scrotal cellulitis. More often it is a chronic (irreversible) state characterised by brawny oedema and rough thickened penoscrotal skin. The debilitating functional and cosmetic effects have significant psychological and social consequences for the patient (Figure 21.1).

Primary or idiopathic lymphoedema of the male genitalia is rare and generally also affects the lower or upper limbs, but may occur in isolation. It may be present at birth but more commonly manifests in the teens or early twenties. As the affected individual grows, the compromised lymphatics become increasingly unable to drain interstitial fluid and swelling eventually becomes evident.[2] Severe trauma to the groin can cause lymphoedema as a result of a major local loss of tissue including lymph nodes and lymphatics. This is seen particularly after degloving injuries of the scrotum.

In parts of Africa, India and South America, the commonest causes of male genital lymphoedema are infective in origin. Filariasis often affects the genital

---

Box 21.A Classification of groin lymphoedema[1]

Primary or idiopathic

Congenital (e.g. Milroy's disease).

Lymphoedema praecox (developing at puberty).

Lymphoedema tarda (developing after the age of 35 years).

Secondary or obstructive

Inflammatory:
   filariasis
   syphilitic chancroid, tuberculosis, leprosy.

Surgical:
   lymph node dissection of inguinal region
   scars in the groin.

Post-radiation destruction of lymphatics.

Blockage of lymphatics by cancer.

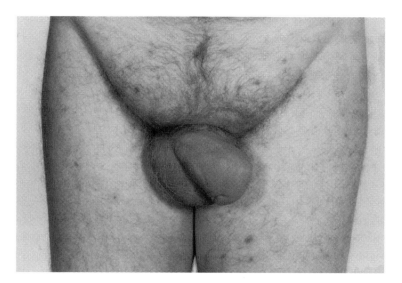

Figure 21.1   Male genital lymphoedema.

lymphatics leading to elephantiasis of the penis and scrotum. Bacterial infections, such as tuberculosis and syphilis, can also present with generalised lymphoedema of the genitals together with other typical clinical features.[3]

Lymphoedema of the genitalia is uncommon in countries where filiariasis is not endemic. In the Western world most cases of lymphoedema of the penis and scrotum are associated with cancer or trauma. Both testicular seminomas and testicular lymphomas may present with lymphoedema. Although any malignant process which spreads to lymph nodes of the groin can cause lymphoedema, it is more common after surgical resection or radiotherapy directed against nodal secondaries. Squamous cell cancer of the penis, testicular tumours and melanoma are often treated by block dissection or radiation. Lymphoedema after groin node dissection is as high as 25%.[4] The combination of radiotherapy and surgical block dissection carries a higher risk of lymphoedema than either treatment alone. Recurrent tumour may be responsible for lymphoedema developing some years after radiotherapy for the primary disease.

Groin lymphoedema should be differentiated from oedema produced by venous insufficiency secondary to medical causes, for example cardiac failure, end-stage renal failure, venous thrombosis and hypoproteinaemia. In recumbent patients, the genital region is particularly susceptible because of the effect of gravity.

Pathophysiology

Lymphography of the genital region has shown that most patients with genital lymphoedema have dilated obstructed lymphatic vessels in the genitalia and an insufficiency of regional lymph nodes and vessels.[5] Blockage of genital lymphatics is either a primary phenomenom as in Milroy's disease or secondary to infection, surgery or malignancy.

Obstruction of the lymphatics results in proximal dilation and valvular incompetence. Lymph backflow then occurs from the deep lymphatics into the dermal plexus, and this results in clinical lymphoedema. The high protein content of the lymphoedema leads to chronic inflammation and fibrosis with subsequent loss of elasticity. Superadded infection leads to further scarring and the oedematous, thick penile and scrotal skin is irreversibly altered. Fascial barriers and dependency exacerbate the situation.

The posterior and posterolateral aspects of the scrotum are often spared. The reason for this is unclear but may be due to collateral flow through perirectal lymphatics. In addition, the separation of the penile and scrotal lymphatic systems explains why penile and scrotal lymphoedema are not necessarily concomitant.

Clinical features

The abnormal retention of interstitial fluid and lymph in the skin and subcutaneous tissues of the penis and scrotum produces swelling, pain and possibly dysuria. Sexual dysfunction is common, often with painful erections. Genital oedema is generally a slowly progressive condition and can become enormous. The skin becomes coarse, thick and warty; lymphatic bullae and troublesome lymphorrhoea may occur. The penis can become buried in an elongated preputial sac which makes micturition difficult and predisposes to the development of preputial calculi, ulceration and even malignant transformation as a result of chronic irritation.

Investigation

Genital lymphoedema should be differentiated from oedema produced by venous insufficiency. Patients with chronic genital lymphoedema generally have a firm scrotum which does not indent easily with finger pressure. Further, the swelling is localised (i.e. does not involve the legs or the buttocks) unless it is associated with leg lymphoedema after cancer surgery and/or radiotherapy. In contrast, with venous oedema, the swelling is typically soft and pitting, and is present also in the legs and possibly the buttocks.

Detailed personal and family histories may identify the primary cause. Measurement of plasma albumin, urea, creatinine and electrolyte concentrations, and liver function tests should be obtained in all patients and will help exclude any underlying medical condition such as renal or hepatic failure, or hypoproteinaemia.

Physical examination will confirm a swollen scrotum and/or penis with thick oedematous skin and reveal any underlying abnormalities. Fungal infection in the groins and perineum are common and may cause erythema, itching and leakage of lymph. The groins should be palpated for pathologically enlarged lymph nodes and a rectal examination carried out. Blood, urine and aspirated lymph can be sent for microbiological investigation to identify any primary or secondary infection. CT or MRI may be indicated to confirm or exclude intrapelvic cancer, para-aortic lymphadenopathy or retroperitoneal fibrosis.

Lymphangiogram

Although many urologists are content to diagnose mild lymphoedema from the history and physical findings, a contrast or isotope lymphangiogram will distinguish between an obstructive cause and venous oedema. The lymphangiogram will usually reveal filling of the superficial and deep lymphatics with the appearance of ectatic (i.e. convoluted) lymphatic channels in both inguinal areas. Filling is often seen to be absent above the inguinal ligaments on both sides. Lymphangiography is essential before surgical options are pursued and is of some value in evaluating prognosis. Penile or scrotal skin biopsy, if performed, would confirm dilation of the subdermal and dermal lymphatics with diffuse fibrosis and hyperkeratosis of the epidermis.

If the underlying cause of the lymphoedema is thought to be malignant in origin, evaluation may include CT of the abdomen and pelvis and possibly a lymph node biopsy, chest radiograph, liver ultrasound, cystoscopy and urine cytology. Excretory urograms and cystoscopy will rule out any urinary abnormalities or urinary extravasation.

Management

Regardless of cause, chronic lymphoedema of the male genitalia can be extremely debilitating and difficult to manage. The objectives of treatment are to reduce swelling with the aim of restoring shape and function, and also to prevent acute inflammatory episodes (AIE). In cases of secondary lymphoedema of the groin, the underlying cause should be dealt with if possible. For example, in filiariasis, tuberculosis or syphilis, the appropriate antimicrobial agent should be commenced (see p.265).

Non-surgical treatment

Conservative non-surgical therapy may be beneficial for milder degrees of genital lymphoedema or in elderly individuals in whom the risk of surgery is prohibitive. Good skin hygiene, including a daily bath and the application of a moisturiser is of fundamental importance. Although compression is not a practical proposition, daily lymphatic massage and a scrotal support may help to limit the progression and discomfort of the lymphoedema. Advice on suitable clothing should be offered, such as cotton underpants changed daily and cycling shorts, which provide gentle pressure and support to the upper thighs and scrotum.

Antibiotics should be prescribed for cellulitis (see p.130). Control of recurrent AIE can be achieved through meticulous skin care (see p.118), a reduction in swelling and, when necessary, prophylactic antibiotics (see p.137). The use of diuretics for pure lymphoedema is physiologically unsound but may be helpful in oedema of mixed origin.

Benzopyrones have also been advocated for the treatment of genital lymph-oedema. These are drugs which stimulate circulatory macrophages to break down proteins to their constituent amino acids (see p.245).

Surgery

With the development of plastic surgical techniques and knowledge of normal and pathological lymphatic circulation, several surgical methods for the treatment of male genital lymphoedema have evolved. These may be divided into two broad categories. The first approach, termed physiological, is designed to rectify or improve abnormal lymphatic drainage.[6] The second is excisional and involves the removal of the brawny indurated areas (lymph-angiectomy) followed by the covering of the scrotal contents and penis with adjacent normal skin or split skin grafts.[7-9]

Physiological procedure (non-excisional surgery)

Physiological (non-excisional) procedures are only of occasional use in the management of genital lymphoedema. They generally involve the removal of the obstruction, correction of the circulatory defect, and the establishment of new lymphatic channels (lymphangioplasty). In general, these bridging and shunting procedures are complicated to perform and the results are often disappointing.

Excisional surgery

Excisional surgery with proper attention to technical details often yields a highly satisfactory functional and cosmetic outcome. There are two types of excisional surgery:

- complete (radical) excision with skin grafting
- excision of lymphoedematous tissue and reconstruction with penile skin without the use of skin grafts.

Opinions differ about which is the more effective.

Complete excision of the skin and the subdermal lymphoedema becomes mandatory in the presence of gross secondary cutaneous changes, such as ulceration, chronic lymph leakage, dermal lymph varices and vesiculation. However, even in the absence of these overt changes, relatively occult dermal involvement is often misjudged and can lead to recurrence of lymphoedema if penile skin flap reconstruction is used instead of radical excision. It is important to completely excise the lymphoedematous sub-cutaneous tissue from the penile flap to prevent a recurrence of lymph-oedema. Recurrence and contracture are less common following radical excision and skin grafting.

Although the appearance of the reconstructed penis after skin grafting is different in colour and texture, the eventual cosmetic and functional result is more acceptable. In an uncircumcised male, the inner lining of the prepuce is relatively uninvolved with lymphoedema and can be unfurled to cover the distal penis with split skin grafting, although a doughnut ring deformity may occur if more than a narrow rim of prepuce is used. The grafted area often remains dry because of the lack of secretory dermal glands. Patients are instructed to use emollients regularly. Postoperatively, most men are able to have erections sufficient for sexual intercourse. Indeed, after hospital discharge, erections are encouraged as they act as a natural tissue expander.

Scrotal reconstruction generally does not require split skin grafting, since the posterolateral scrotum and perineal areas generally remain free of lymph-oedema. The mobility and elasticity of the perineal skin allow it to be drawn forward as a pedicle skin flap and closed over the testicles and spermatic cords, even after extensive excision of scrotal lymphoedema. This posterior skin flap provides a superior cosmetic appearance because it utilises typical scrotal skin. However, some surgeons advocate the use of skin grafts, generally from the thigh, for scrotal reconstruction on the grounds that there is the possibility of recurrent lymphoedema if local genital tissue is used.

Summary

Male genital lymphoedema has many possible causes and results in significant debilitating functional, cosmetic and psychosocial sequelae. Management should initially be directed at the underlying cause (if correctable) and every effort should be made to prevent secondary complications. If surgical management is appropriate, whatever technique is chosen, one should strive for:

- a functional penis and scrotum that are cosmetically acceptable to the patient

- a minimal chance of recurrent lymphoedema of the penis and scrotum

- a penis with sensation for sexual activity.

References

1   Bulkley GJ (1962) Scrotal and penile lymphedema. *Journal of Urology.* **87**:422.
2   Fiens NR (1980) A new surgical technique for lymphoedema of the penis and scrotum. *Journal of Paediatric Surgery.* **15**:787–9.
3   Sylla C *et al.* (1998) Penile and scrotal elephantiasis in Senegal. *African Journal of Urology.* **4**:36–41.
4   Karakousis CP *et al.* (1983) Lymphedema after groin dissection. *American Journal of Surgery.* **145**:205–8.
5   May AR and Kinmonth JB (1976) Lymphographic studes of primary genital lymphoedema. *British Journal of Surgery.* **63**:655–70.
6   Huang GK *et al.* (1985) Microlymphaticovenous anastomosis for treating scrotal elephantiasis. *Microsurgery.* **6**:36–9.
7   Das S *et al.* (1983) Surgery of male genital lymphedema. *Journal of Urology.* **129**:1240.
8   Martinez RE *et al.* (1988) Primary lymphedema of the scrotum: surgical treatment and reconstruction. *Annals of Plastic Surgery.* **21**:354–7.
9   Ollapallil JJ and Watters DAK (1995) Surgical management of elephantiasis of male genitalia. *British Journal of Urology.* **76**:213–5.

22 Oedema in advanced cancer

Vaughan Keeley

Introduction

Most lymphoedema management is palliative rather than curative. In advanced cancer, any form of oedema can be problematic and, because of the patient's general condition and poor prognosis, the aims of treatment generally need to be more limited. The key principles of palliative care are of course all relevant:

- focus on quality of life including good symptom relief

- a whole-person approach taking into account the person's past life-experience and current situation

- care which encompasses both the person with life-threatening disease and those who matter to the person

- respect for patient autonomy and choice

- emphasis on open and sensitive communication with patients, relatives, other informal carers and professional colleagues.[1]

For most patients, oedema is only one of several problems. Patients may therefore benefit from referral to a specialist palliative care service:

> 'The active total care of patients with progressive, far-advanced disease and limited prognosis, and their families, by a multiprofessional team who have undergone recognised specialist palliative care training. It provides physical, psychological, social and spiritual support, and will involve practitioners with a broad mix of skills, including medical and nursing care, social work, pastoral/spiritual care, physiotherapy, occupational therapy, pharmacy and related specialties'.[1]

Many specialist palliative care services in the UK provide specific lymphoedema treatment as part of their remit.[2]

Causes

Oedema is a common symptom of advanced cancer.[3] It may affect only limbs, particularly the legs, or be more widespread, for example including the trunk as well as the legs. Several concurrent factors may contribute to the formation of oedema (Box 22.A). In advanced pelvic malignant disease, for example, lymph node infiltration and inferior vena caval compression may together cause leg swelling, possibly compounded by hypoproteinaemia, anaemia and immobility. Hypoproteinaemia and anaemia may also cause swelling of the legs as a result of a 'high output failure' of lymph drainage without any abnormality of the structure of the lymphatic system (*see* p.14).

Box 22.A Causes of oedema in advanced cancer

Local

Lymphatic obstruction/damage (secondary lymphoedema):
- surgery/radiotherapy
- metastatic tumour in lymph nodes or skin lymphatics
- infection.

Venous obstruction:
- deep vein thrombosis (DVT)
- superior vena caval obstruction
- inferior vena caval obstruction
- extrinsic compression by tumour
- thrombophlebitis migrans.

Lymphovenous oedema:
- immobility and dependency
- localised weakness due to neurological deficit.

General

Cardiac failure (which may be secondary to or exacerbated by anaemia).

Hypoproteinaemia:
- catabolic state
- hepatic disease
- nutritional deficiency
- nephrotic syndrome
- protein-losing enteropathy.

Late stage chronic renal failure.

Drugs:
- salt and water retention, e.g. NSAIDs and corticosteroids
- vasodilation, e.g. nifedipine.

Malignant ascites.

Specific conditions

Breast cancer

A particularly severe and intractable form of lymphoedema may occur in women with recurrent breast cancer. The deep lymphatic drainage of the arm may have already been compromised by surgery and radiotherapy to the axilla in the treatment of the primary disease. The situation is then made worse by axillary node recurrence, and the development of metastatic disease in the skin of the chest wall and upper arm results in extensive infiltration of the dermal and subcutaneous lymphatics and further lymphatic destruction (Figure 22.1). The tissues of the swollen arm tend to become tense and hard and the skin may be discoloured and inflamed. Lymph blisters (acquired lymphangiomas) are common and skin breakdown may result in lymphorrhoea and ulceration.

Deep venous obstruction of the arm alone, for example axillary vein thrombosis or narrowing due to extrinsic compression by tumour, may lead to arm oedema or exacerbate existing lymphoedema. Distended collateral veins (particularly around the shoulder) and cyanosis or mottling of the skin suggest venous obstruction. In some patients with extrinsic venous compression, the impairment of venous drainage may vary with arm position. With disease recurrence in the axilla, the brachial plexus may become infiltrated with tumour and lead to progressive altered sensation, pain and weakness of

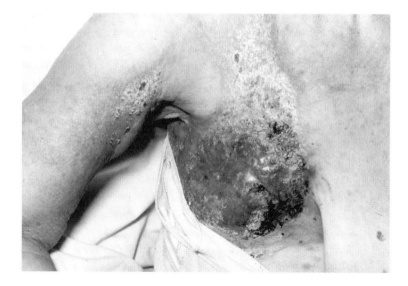

Figure 22.1 Metastatic breast cancer of chest wall and upper arm.

the arm. The weakness leads to immobility which will exacerbate any pre-existing oedema.

Pelvic malignant disease

Patients with advanced pelvic malignant disease, for example cancers of uterine cervix, ovary, prostate, bladder and rectum, may have leg and truncal oedema stemming from several factors (Figure 22.2).[4] As with breast cancer, lymphoedema may be the result of treatment. After radical hysterectomy (which includes excision of the pelvic lymph nodes) and postoperative radiotherapy for cancer of the cervix, about 40% of women develop lymphoedema.[5] In the presence of recurrent disease the following may be contributory:

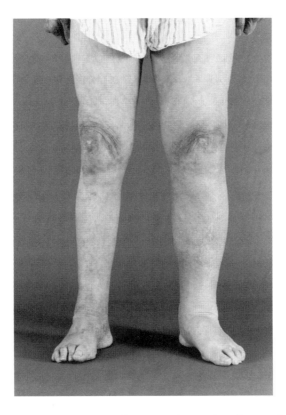

Figure 22.2   Lymphoedema secondary to advanced pelvic malignant disease arising from prostate cancer.

- lymphatic obstruction from malignant lymph nodes in pelvic and para-aortic regions

- extrinsic venous compression from enlarged lymph nodes/tumour masses

- inferior vena caval obstruction

- DVT

- hypo-albuminaemia

- drug-induced fluid retention, e.g. NSAID or corticosteroid

- ascites (see below).

Venous outflow obstruction leads to dilation of skin venules and the limb may appear cyanosed. Haemorrhage into the skin may occur and there may be dilated collateral vessels visible on the abdominal wall and flanks. Increasing leg oedema leads to immobility. This in turn increases venous hypertension and thence the capillary filtration rate. This further increases the oedema. The patient is at greater risk of developing DVT, causing even more swelling.

Malignant ascites

Ascites is most common in ovarian, colorectal, gastric, pancreatic and uterine cancers. Leg oedema may be a feature of malignant ascites.[6] The pathogenesis is complex and may be the result of:

- reduced outflow of fluid from the peritoneal cavity
   obstruction of diaphragmatic and peritoneal lymphatics by metastases
   radiotherapy-induced lymphatic damage (which may cause chylous ascites)

- increased production of peritoneal fluid
   release of cytokines by the tumour causing increased permeability of capillaries and leakage of albumin
   'leaky' tumour blood vessels
   liver metastases causing increased hepatic vein pressure due to compression, resulting in an increased production of renin and salt and water retention.

Hypo-albuminaemia

Hypo-albuminaemia is common in advanced cancer. It occurs particularly as a result of the altered metabolism seen in cachexia-anorexia syndrome, which includes decreased hepatic protein synthesis.[7]

Box 22.B Features of superior vena caval obstruction

Common presenting symptoms:
- dyspnoea   50%
- neck and facial swelling   40%
- trunk and arm swelling   40%
- a sensation of choking
- a feeling of fullness in the head
- headache.

Other symptoms include:
- chest pain
- cough
- dysphagia
- cognitive dysfunction
- hallucinations
- convulsions.

Common physical signs:
- thoracic vein distension   65%
- neck vein distension   55%
- facial oedema   55%
- tachypnoea   40%
- plethora of face   15%
- cyanosis   15%
- arm oedema   10%
- vocal cord paresis   3%
- Horner's syndrome.   3%

In severe cases:
- laryngeal stridor
- coma
- death.

Superior vena caval obstruction

Superior vena caval (mediastinal) obstruction is caused most commonly by extrinsic compression by metastases in the upper mediastinal lymph nodes (Box 22.B). It occurs in about 15% of patients with lung cancer, particularly small cell lung cancer. Indeed, lung cancer is responsible for 80% of cases. It also occurs in other malignant diseases such as lymphoma, breast cancer and testicular seminoma.[8,9] Secondary venous thrombosis may account for the acute onset in some patients.

Inferior vena caval obstruction

Inferior vena caval obstruction is usually due to extrinsic compression by hepatomegaly or retroperitoneal lymphadenopathy. It may also be caused by cancer of the kidney or postradiation fibrosis. Clinical features include oedema of the legs, abdomen and genitalia. If the obstruction is above the level of the hepatic veins, ascites may also occur. Dilated collateral veins are often visible on the abdominal wall.

General clinical features

The clinical features of lymphoedema and other forms of oedema in advanced cancer are mainly the same as those seen in other situations (*see* p.44). However, the following are particularly important:

- pain
- infection
- ulceration
- lymphorrhoea
- impaired function/mobility
- psychosocial impact.

Pain

Patients with lymphoedema and active cancer are more likely to experience pain (67%) and tightness (43%) in the affected limb than those with inactive disease.[10] Patients with active cancer are at risk of developing neuropathic pain as a result of nerve compression or destruction by tumour. This pain is often severe and tingling, burning and/or stabbing in character (*see* p.68). It is associated with altered sensation in the area of the pain, and light touch may be more painful than firm deep pressure (touch-evoked allodynia). There may be an associated motor deficit.

In severe arm oedema in advanced disease, the weight of the limb may cause significant pain and stiffness of the shoulder. Similarly with severe leg oedema, the effect on gait may result in hip and back pain. In the presence of secondary skin cancers and fungating lesions, pain may be exacerbated by inflammation and infection. Acute DVT or superficial thrombophlebitis may also increase pain.

Infection, ulceration and lymphorrhoea

The existing predisposition to infection in lymphoedema (*see* p.130) is increased in advanced disease by:

- increased portals of infection
    fragile, thin, dry stretched skin (particularly in elderly debilitated patients and those on corticosteroids)
    lymphorrhoea (leakage of lymph through the skin)
    secondary skin tumours
    fungating tumours/ulceration

- reduced resistance to infection
    from treatment, e.g. chemotherapy and radiotherapy
    a feature of progressive cancer.

Patients may present with increased swelling and pain, with redness and warmth of the affected area and influenza-like symptoms (*see* p.130).

Although ulceration is a more prominent feature of venous disease,[11] it can occur in lymphoedema particularly in advanced cancer (Figure 22.3). In this situation, the following may contribute to ulcer formation:

- fragility of the skin

- formation of lymph blisters (acquired lymphangiomas)

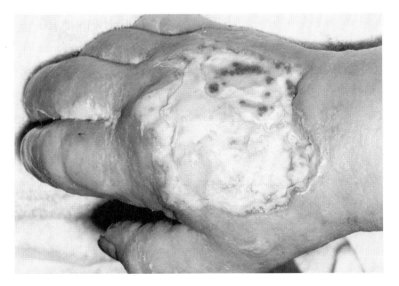

Figure 22.3 Ulceration in lymphoedematous hand following infection in advanced breast cancer.

- severe infection with blistering and desquamation

- fungating tumours

- concurrent venous disease

- skin damage as a result of poorly fitting compression garments or poorly applied support bandaging.

Lymphorrhoea may be associated with ulceration/fungating tumours or with rupture of lymph blisters (*see* p.45). The leakage can be profuse and a source of distress for patients, with soaking of clothing despite support bandaging. In some patients with ulceration or fungating tumours colonisation by anaerobic bacteria can lead to an unpleasant malodorous discharge and increased pain.

Impaired function and mobility

Most patients with advanced malignancy experience generalised weakness.[12] The additional burden of a heavy limb or limbs further impairs mobility. Severe limb oedema causes a reduction in the range of joint movement which will be exacerbated by weakness caused by neural injury by recurrent tumour, for example brachial plexus infiltration in breast cancer. Gross swelling of the hand causes weakness of grip and the hand can become virtually useless (Figure 22.4). An extremely swollen paralysed arm is a severe painful disability.

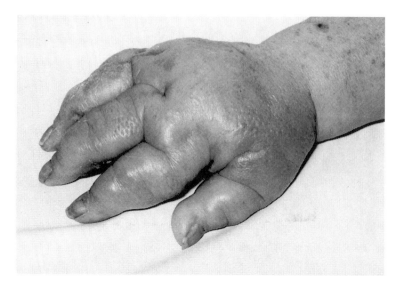

Figure 22.4 Grossly oedematous hand in advanced breast cancer.

Similarly, gross oedema of the legs and lower trunk (possibly including the genitalia) can cause severe difficulty in walking even without neural deficit. This may result in the patient spending much of the day, and sometimes the night, sitting in a chair. This then leads to further exacerbation of the swelling (see p.55).

Psychosocial impact

Lymphoedema secondary to treatment for breast cancer is commonly associated with significant psychological morbidity (see p.89).[13] For patients coping with oedema and advancing disease, the psychosocial aspects may be even greater. The symptoms and disabilities associated with the swelling are often worse and, in addition, patients and their families have to cope with psychological distress associated with terminal illness and the anticipation of death.

Evaluation

The evaluation of patients with oedema in advanced cancer should take into account the various causal factors (Box 22.A). History taking should aim to elicit the associated symptoms and psychosocial aspects of both the oedema and the underlying illness, including any recent acute inflammatory episodes (AIE).

The examination will look for the clinical signs (see p.344), for example skin condition, evidence of infection and limitation of function. Signs of DVT are not reliable but evidence of increased venous pressure (e.g. dilated collateral veins) should be sought. Patients with advanced cancer may develop DVT even when wearing compression garments and occasionally when apparently adequately anticoagulated after previous thrombotic episodes.

Provided the patient's general condition warrants it, investigations may help to define the cause(s) of the oedema and to detect any potentially reversible factors, such as anaemia. Investigations include:

- full blood count
- plasma electrolytes, urea and creatinine concentrations
- plasma albumin concentration
- ultrasound, CT or MRI to evaluate disease status and lymphadenopathy
- colour Doppler ultrasound and possibly venogram to evaluate venous function.

Management

When uncontrollable tumour is the main cause, the oedema is unlikely to respond well to treatment. Management should be focused on easing the symptoms rather than reducing the oedema. Emphasis is placed on:

- enhancing the quality of life
- respecting the patient's choices and priorities
- providing psychological support to the patient and family.

The burden of treatment must not exceed the benefit.[14] In some situations, such as mild ankle oedema in a patient with reduced mobility, early management may prevent the problem from becoming worse.[4]

Physical therapy

The range of physical therapies described in previous chapters may be used but will generally have to be adapted to the patient's particular needs in the light of their general condition and wishes. It is therefore important that the patient, and carers if possible, are involved in a discussion of the realistic outcomes of management and in the decisions about treatment. Management may include:[4]

- skin care
- support and positioning of the swollen limb(s)
- passive and active exercises to maintain range of movement, mobility and function
- massage in the form of simple lymph drainage (SLD)
- manual lymphatic drainage (MLD)
- support bandages or low compression garments
- pneumatic compression therapy (PCT)
- appliances to aid mobility and function.

Skin care

Skin care remains important in advanced disease, with the aim of preventing debilitating infections. This includes washing and carefully drying the affected limb(s), preferably every day. The use of moisturising creams, such as aqueous cream, and the avoidance of trauma are essential. If the skin is very thin, dry and fragile as a result of the oedema, disease process and/or corticosteroids, the use of elastic compression garments may make matters worse because of the shearing forces when putting the garment on and taking it off. In these situations, light support bandaging is more appropriate. Skin breakdown may occur because of tumour fungation.

With very fragile skin, any dressings should be non-adherent but, even so, will generally need to be soaked off with sterile saline to avoid further damage to the skin. Haemostatic dressings may be needed to control the bleeding (e.g. calcium alginate) or topical adrenaline (epinephrine) solution 1 in 1000 (1mg in 1ml) when dressings are changed.

Fungating lesions

Fungating lesions may be malodorous because of superadded anaerobic bacterial infection. Metronidazole is often helpful in this situation. This can either be applied topically as metronidazole 0.8% gel o.d.[15] or given orally b.d.. The usual oral regimen is metronidazole 400mg b.d. for 2 weeks but, sometimes, it needs to be continued indefinitely.

The choice of route depends on the clinical situation. Topical metronidazole is more expensive but, if applied adequately, generally relieves the odour in 2–3 days and is relatively free from adverse effects. Unfortunately, with large irregular fungating tumours, it may not be easy to apply the gel to the deeper crevices where the bacteria grow. Further, the gel is less effective if there is profuse discharge, presumably because it is flushed away or diluted by the discharge. Some patients develop anorexia and/or nausea with oral metronidazole and, if alcohol is consumed as well, occasionally develop an adverse reaction like that seen with disulfiram in the treatment of alcoholism (flushing of the face and neck, headaches, epigastric discomfort, nausea and vomiting, hypotension). Generally, however, a complete bar on alcohol is not necessary in patients taking metronidazole.[16] If patients experience nausea, a dose reduction to metronidazole 200mg b.d. may relieve it without loss of odour control.

Support and positioning

In very ill patients, the appropriate positioning and support of swollen limbs while lying in bed, for example using pillows, may aid comfort. In patients with arm oedema the use of a sling to support the arm is not generally recommended because it may cause pooling of fluid at the elbow and stiffness of the elbow and shoulder joint.[17] However, in ambulant breast cancer patients with gross arm oedema and weakness from brachial plexus damage, a sling which takes the weight away from the shoulder and neck and distributes it across the back (e.g. Polysling) often provides comfort. It may also improve mobility by improving balance. The sling should be removed when the patient is resting.

At rest, some patients benefit from placing the limb in specially made foam supports/splints so that the limb (including the hand) is fully supported in the horizontal position (Figure 22.5).[18] Similarly, patients with leg oedema may find elevation of the limbs comfortable while sitting. The back needs to be well-supported to prevent backache, ideally by using a reclining chair with the legs supported along their entire length.

Exercise

Exercise needs to be carefully tailored to the patient's abilities and general condition. However, even passive movements of a swollen limb (including hand and fingers or feet and toes) in a severely ill, bedbound patient can reduce stiffness and discomfort. In more active patients, exercise may maintain rather than improve function. A complex exercise regimen is rarely appropriate.

SLD and MLD

Specialised forms of massage are used in the management of lymphoedema (*see* pp 203 and 217). The presence of active cancer is often considered to be a contra-indication because stimulation of lymph flow around the site of a tumour might lead to metastasis.[19] There is no evidence to support this view

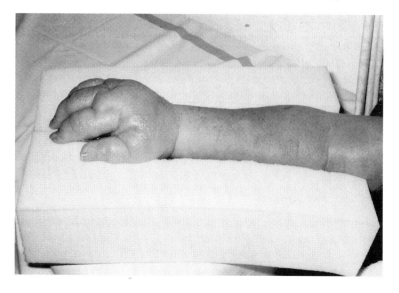

Figure 22.5 Foam support for severely oedematous arm in advanced breast cancer.

but, equally, none to contradict it. However, in the presence of advanced metastatic disease, the potential benefits of SLD and MLD, particularly for truncal oedema, outweigh any risk of inducing further metastatic spread. As always, treatment must be adapted to individual circumstances; MLD is time-consuming and could exhaust a debilitated patient. Massage is impractical and uncomfortable where there is cancerous cutaneous spread.

Support bandages and compression garments

As already stated, the aim in advanced cancer is often simply to provide comfort and to minimise further increases in volume rather than trying to reduce the oedema. Thus support from light bandages (possibly applied by an instructed relative) or from low compression garments may be appropriate. Bandages can sometimes be left on for more than 1 day but the skin condition needs to be checked regularly, particulary if there is impaired skin sensation.[4] Shaped Tubigrip is a useful alternative; it is easy to apply and causes less trauma than compression garments. A second layer can be used to give greater support if required. It is important to ensure that the Shaped Tubigrip does not form ridges or roll down the limb and act as a tourniquet because this can exacerbate the swelling and increase discomfort. Shaped Tubigrip is generally uncomfortable if the foot or hand is very swollen; it should *not* be used if the digits are swollen. The possibility of skin damage with firm bandaging must be borne in mind.

Bandaging helps to control lymphorrhoea. A sterile pad/gauze dressing is used to absorb the lymph. Sometimes the bandaging needs to be changed several times per day because of lymph soaking through. Bandaging alone may halt lymphorrhoea in 24–48 hours.[4] Other support devices, such as a Reid sleeve, can also be used to control lymphorrhoea.[20]

In some situations compression bandaging can increase the amount of fluid leakage. For example, in patients with fungating breast tumours in the axilla or chest wall, the application of pressure to the adjacent swollen arm may improve lymph drainage from the arm and increase the load on the neighbouring superficial lymphatics around the shoulder and chest wall. With damaged lymphatics exposed to the surface in fungating tumours, increased flow through these will result in increased leakage. In these circumstances, it may still be appropriate to apply compression to the arm to relieve symptoms, but the patient should be warned that the discharge from lesions in the chest wall or axilla may increase. Therefore, any dressings may need to be changed more than once a day, at least in the short-term.

Contra-indications

There are situations where compression of the swollen limbs is inappropriate or would cause more problems, for example cardiac failure and acute DVT.

There is, therefore, a need to decide on the underlying cause(s) of the oedema if possible. Even if the cause is pure lymphoedema, compression in advanced disease may cause difficulties elsewhere. For example, in advanced pelvic malignant disease with bilateral leg swelling, genital and truncal oedema, compression of the legs may lead to increased truncal and genital swelling. This may be reduced if massage is employed as well to improve lymph flow from the genitalia and lower trunk. The use of low compression garments such as support tights or maternity garments may be useful in this situation because they also provide some support to the genital area. Below knee bandaging may prevent lymphorrhoea and skin ulceration. Patients should be evaluated regularly and treatment adjusted according to patients' preference and physical condition.

Pneumatic compression therapy

Pneumatic compression therapy (PCT) is used less than in the past.[21] However, there is still a role for it in advanced disease (see p.236). It may soften a hard oedema and ease discomfort. It is particularly helpful in venous oedema but should be avoided in cardiac failure. There is a risk of increasing truncal or genital oedema if PCT is used alone. Care should also be taken if there is a neural deficit and the patient is unable to feel discomfort. The use of PCT without the use of support bandaging or a compression garment between applications is rarely helpful. A multichamber sequential intermittent pneumatic compression pump is preferable (see p.237). Near the end of life, a compression pump used on low pressure (20–30mmHg) can help by massaging the legs, preventing lymphorrhoea and reducing the need for bandaging.

Appliances to aid mobility and function

In order to enable patients to continue to function as normally as possible with severely swollen limbs, various appliances may be helpful. These include aids for walking and dressing for those with swollen legs, and special cutlery, tin openers, scissors etc. for those with grossly swollen and weak hands and arms. The advice of an occupational therapist should be sought.

Drug therapy

The use of drugs in managing oedema in advanced cancer will depend upon the underlying cause of the oedema. Agents which may be considered include:

- corticosteroids
- diuretics

- analgesics
- benzopyrones.

Corticosteroids

Systemic corticosteroids may have a role in the management of lymphoedema caused by cancer and associated symptoms such as nerve compression pain. The proposed mechanism of action is the reduction of inflammation and peritumour oedema. This in turn may relieve pressure on neighbouring structures such as lymphatics, veins and nerves.

Dexamethasone is a good choice and should be given initially for 1 week, for example dexamethasone 8–16mg daily.[16] If the trial is successful, the dose can then be gradually reduced until the lowest level which relieves the symptoms is reached. This may take some weeks, during which time adverse effects may manifest, for example fluid retention, Cushingoid facies, gastrointestinal disturbance, weight gain, proximal myopathy, diabetes mellitus and psychosis. Should any of these occur, the balance of benefit versus burden will need to be reviewed with the patient and a decision made whether to continue or gradually withdraw the drug. If the initial trial of a corticosteroid is not definitely helpful, the drug should be discontinued after 7–10 days.

Diuretics

Diuretics do not generally have a part to play in the management of pure lymphoedema (see p.244). However, they may have a role in the management of oedema of advanced cancer if partly caused by fluid retention, for example drug-induced or in cardiac failure. Furosemide (frusemide) is a good choice. The dose is adjusted according to effect and it may be helpful to monitor the plasma electrolytes, urea and creatinine to avoid further symptoms as a result of deteriorating renal function or hyponatraemia. In situations where there is increased activity of the renin-angiotensin system as in many cases of ascites, spironolactone is preferable.[16] The dose is titrated against effect and, again, it may be useful to monitor plasma biochemistry.

Analgesics and other drugs for pain relief

Patients with pain associated with oedema in advanced cancer may benefit from various analgesics, the choice depending on the underlying cause of the pain (see p.68).

Benzopyrones

Some have suggested that benzopyrones have a role in the management of lymphoedema in advanced disease.[22] However, because the benefit is seen only after 3–6 months, there is little place for benzopyrones in advanced disease (*see* p.245).

Psychosocial support

Psychosocial support for patients and carers is important in advanced cancer whether or not oedema is a problem. Any problems associated with oedema, for example altered body image, reduced function/mobility and loss of independence, will add to the patient's distress. Support from a multi-professional specialist palliative care team may be helpful and referral as a priority should be considered.

Treatment of specific conditions

The treatment of any potentially reversible factors should be considered in the light of the patient's general condition.

Anaemia

Anaemia of chronic disease may be treated by blood transfusion or erythro-poietin, whereas iron deficiency anaemia will respond to oral iron therapy.

Heart failure

Heart failure may respond to conventional treatment which includes diuretics, digoxin, and ACE-inhibitors.

Fluid-retaining drugs

Fluid-retaining drugs (e.g. NSAIDs and corticosteroids) which exacerbate the oedema should be withdrawn if possible, unless clearly needed for the relief of other symptoms.

Hypo-albuminaemia

The treatment of hypo-albuminaemia is generally unrewarding in advanced cancer. Increasing the protein intake in the diet does not help and infusions of human albumin provides only short-lived benefit, if any.

Malignant ascites

Reduction in ascites, if present, can improve associated leg oedema. Treatment options include:

- anticancer therapy, e.g. in ovarian cancer
- paracentesis
- diuretic therapy, e.g. with spironolactone with or without furosemide (frusemide)[23]
- peritoneovenous shunt.

Superior vena caval obstruction

Superior vena caval obstruction (SVCO) with severe symptoms is an oncological emergency. The usual treatment consists of high-dose corticosteroids (e.g. dexamethasone 16mg o.d./8mg b.d. PO) and urgent radiotherapy to the mediastinum. Corticosteroids reduce peritumour oedema and thereby relieve extrinsic compression. Chemotherapy may be used for patients with lymphoma and small cell lung cancer.

The insertion of a self-expanding metal stent into the superior vena cava via a venous puncture is a recently introduced form of treatment.[24] Thrombolysis may need to be performed prior to stent insertion, but the immediate and long-term results are good, with over 90% of patients dying without recurrence of SVCO.

Inferior vena caval obstruction

Inferior vena caval obstruction (IVCO) may be helped by a trial of corticosteroids (see above) and possibly by specific anticancer treatment. Metal stents have also been used but are less successful than with SVCO.[24] Symptomatic relief is slower and there is a greater risk of pulmonary embolism.

Deep vein thrombosis

The management of DVT with anticoagulants in patients with advanced cancer needs careful consideration.[25] The presence of existing bleeding from tumours such as fungating breast lesions is a contra-indication, and changes in other drugs may make maintaining stable anticoagulation with warfarin difficult. Even if patients are anticoagulated to a routine level with warfarin (INR = 2–3), they may still develop further thrombo-embolic events. Anticoagulation to an INR of 3–4 is sometimes recommended but this is not without risk, particularly in debilitated patients.[26]

Use of the newer, more expensive low molecular weight heparins (e.g. dalteparin) makes anticoagulation easier but there is still a need to consider the appropriateness of such treatment in the light of the patient's general condition and prognosis. Dalteparin is given in a dose of 200 units/kg by SC injection o.d. (maximum daily dose 18 000 units).[16] The dose can be reduced to 100 units/kg if the patient is at greater risk of haemorrhage.[26] Treatment can continue for some months and generally no laboratory monitoring is required.

Anticancer treatment

In some situations of oedema associated with advancing cancer, specific palliative anticancer treatment, may be appropriate:

- radiotherapy
- chemotherapy
- hormone treatment.

Radiotherapy to enlarged metastatic lymph nodes may help to reduce the size of the nodes and improve lymphatic and venous flow. However, radiotherapy itself causes damage to lymphatics and may therefore limit improvement in the long-term. Further, improvement may only be temporary because of subsequent recurrence.

Palliative chemotherapy for diseases such as breast cancer, ovarian cancer and lymphomas may shrink the tumour and thereby improve lymphatic and venous flow, but perhaps only temporarily.

Hormone therapy, for example for breast and prostate cancer, may also help improve oedema by reducing tumour size. These options should be considered by the appropriate oncological team if the patient's general condition is good enough and if they wish to explore them.

Conclusion

The palliative care of oedema in advanced cancer is often complex and referral to a specialist palliative care team is frequently appropriate. The aims are:

- to optimise the patient's quality of life
- to provide psychosocial support
- to ensure that the benefits of treatment are not outweighed by the burdens.

References

1   NHS Executive EL(96)85 (1996) A Policy Framework for Commissioning Cancer Services: Palliative Care Services.
2   British Lymphology Society Directory of Lymphoedema Treatment Services 1999/2000.
3   Badger C and Regnard C (1989) Oedema in advanced disease: a flow diagram. *Palliative Medicine.* **3**:213–5.
4   Mortimer PS *et al.* (1998) Lymphoedema. In: D Doyle, G Hanks, N Macdonald (eds) *Oxford Textbook of Palliative Medicine,* 2nd edn. Oxford, pp 657–65.
5   Werngren-Elgström M and Lidman D (1994) Lymphoedema of the lower extremities after surgery and radiotherapy for cancer of the cervix. *Scandinavian Journal of Plastic Reconstructive and Hand Surgery.* **28**:289–93.
6   De Simone GG (1999) Treatment of malignant ascites. *Progress in Palliative Care.* **7**:10–16.
7   Jaskowiak NT and Alexander HR (1998) The pathophysiology of cancer cachexia. In: D Doyle, G Hanks, N Macdonald (eds) *Oxford Textbook of Palliative Medicine,* 2nd edn. Oxford Medical Publications, Oxford, pp 534–48.
8   Tabbarah HJ *et al.* (1988) Intrathoracic complications. In: DA Casciato and BB Lowitz (eds) *Manual of Clinical Oncology,* 2nd edn. Little Brown, Boston, Massachusetts, pp 435–52.
9   Kee ST *et al.* (1998) Superior vena cava syndrome: treatment with catheter-directed thrombolysis and endovascular stent placement. *Radiology.* **206**:187–93.
10 Badger CMA *et al.* (1988) Pain in the chronically swollen limb. *Progress in Lymphology.* **11**:243–6.
11 Chant ADB (1992) Hypothesis: Why venous oedema causes ulcers and lymphoedema does not. *European Journal of Plastic Surgery.* **6**:427–9.
12 Neuenschwander H and Bruera E (1998) Asthenia. In: D Doyle, G Hanks, N Macdonald (eds). *Oxford Textbook of Palliative Medicine,* 2nd edn. Oxford Medical Publications, Oxford, pp 573–81.
13 Tobin MB *et al.* (1993) The psychological morbidity of breast-cancer related arm swelling. *Cancer* **72**:3248–52.
14 British Lymphology Society (1997) *Definitions of Need Document.* BLS Publication, Caterham, Surrey.
15 Newman V *et al.* (1989) The use of metronidazole gel to control the smell of malodorous lesions. *Palliative Medicine.* **3**:303–5.
16 Twycross R *et al.* (1998) *Palliative Care Formulary.* Radcliffe Medical Press, Oxford.
17 Badger C (1987) Lymphoedema: management of patients with advanced cancer. *Professional Nurse.* **2**:100–2.
18 O'Brien A and Hickey J (1995) Poster. British Lymphology Interest Group Annual Conference, Oxford.
19 Wittlinger H and Wittlinger G (1995) Absolute contraindications. In: *Textbook of Dr Vodder's Manual Lymph Drainage Vol. 1. Basic Course.* 5th edn. Haug International, Brussels, p. 74.
20 Szuba A *et al.* (1996) A novel therapy for lymphoedema complicated by lymphorrhoea. *Vascular Medicine.* **1**:247–50.

21   Gray R (1987) The management of limb oedema in patients with advanced cancer. *Physiotherapy.* **73**:504–6.

22   Casley-Smith JR and Casley-Smith JR (1997) *Venous Disease, Ulcers, Palliative and Geriatric Care and Acute Injuries in Modern Treatment for Lymphoedema,* 5th edn. The Lymphoedema Association of Australia, pp 280–1.

23   Twycross R (1997) *Symptom Management in Advanced Cancer,* 2nd edn. Radcliffe Medical Press, Oxford.

24   Renwick I (1999) Metallic stents in palliative care. *CME Bulletin Palliative Medicine.* **1**:41–4.

25   Johnson MJ and Sherry K (1997) How do palliative physicians manage venous thromboembolism? *Palliative Medicine.* **11**:462–8.

26   British National Formulary (1999) *British National Formulary.* British Medical Association, Royal Pharmaceutical Society of Great Britain, March.

23 Lymphoedema in cancer: an Indian perspective

MR Rajagopal

When the resources of the people and of the hospitals are limited as in India, management has to be modified. Dealing with lymphoedema in cancer is challenging because of many factors (Box 23.A). On the positive side, an extended family is still the norm. Very often relatives are willing to learn basic nursing skills and to give the needed time.

Box 23.A   Challenges in the management of cancer-related lymphoedema in India

Medical practice is generally geared to curative treatment; palliation of incurable problems like lymphoedema is neglected.

Specialised care for lymphoedema is rarely available.

Patients are less likely to seek help early; medical help is often sought only at an advanced stage of the disease.

Even when patients seek help, continuing care is difficult because of:
• poor roads
• poor facilities for communication
• financial problems.

Hypoproteinaemia is common, although the relevance of this in lymphoedema is unclear.

Lack of knowledge prevents doctors from using basic management techniques.

Even where facilities for special care exist, referrals are uncommon.

It is necessary to devise a low-cost management strategy; the aim must be to reach as many people as possible.

There are not enough professional carers.

Devising a low-cost strategy

The following low-cost strategy is suggested:

• increased awareness
• a realistic management plan.

A two-pronged educational awareness programme on palliative care aimed at the public and health professionals is necessary. Education about lymphoedema should be part of such a programme. When planning management, the following questions should be borne in mind:

- is the patient's life-span limited? (If not, more active efforts at reduction of lymphoedema are indicated)

- can the patient perform self-massage?

- what is the family situation?

- are there complications that have to be addressed first, e.g. infection and pain which are preventing effective manual drainage?

- is there an associated correctable problem which is exacerbating the lymphoedema, e.g. cardiac failure, renal failure, or drug-induced fluid retention?

In relation to the family, it is necessary to find out who is available to help the patient and whether they are willing and able to spend adequate time with the patient on a regular basis. Sensitivity is needed here; it is easy to place a heavy burden on a carer who is already hard-pressed for time and to add the burden of guilt when they fail to do all that is requested of them.

Because of limited financial resources, we do not use compression machines, garments or bandages at the Pain and Palliative Care Clinic in Calicut. Further, both bandages and compression garments are difficult to wear in a hot climate. The emphasis is therefore on prevention of complications and on treatment modalities which can be easily learnt.

Explanation and education

The first step is education of the patient and the relative about prophylaxis against complications. They are advised to:

- keep the skin moisturised with a bland cream or ointment

- avoid all trauma to the limb, including heat (e.g. sunburn), injections and venepuncture

- prevent prolonged periods of limb dependency, keeping the limb elevated as much as possible

- perform exercises which do not involve heavy muscular effort but which permit a wide range of movement.

It is essential to give adequate explanations to the patient. Unless expectations are realistic, the patient and the relatives will find it difficult to accept limited long-term improvement. This will result in poor adherence to treatment.

One of the first steps is to identify the relatives who appear to be most willing to and capable of learning simple lymphatic drainage (SLD). The education of the patients and carers in Calicut is generally performed by a trained non-professional volunteer. This is necessary because of a lack of trained nurses.

After checking that pain relief is adequate, the volunteer measures the limb circumference and commences treatment.[1] The volunteer then proceeds to perform SLD. The relative watches this on the first day and learns how the massage is performed. The whole procedure is planned to last about 1 hour. Measurement is repeated at the end of the procedure.

On the second day, the volunteer and the relative do the massage together. Over the next few days, the relative gradually takes over the massage completely. Our experience shows that SLD performed by a relative is successful whenever one is available who is motivated and can find the time. This strategy works only if the patient can first be made pain-free. If pain prevents massage, a vicious circle follows in which increasing oedema increases pain. On the other hand, light massage eases discomfort in some patients.

Case history 1

A 17-year-old girl who had a chondrosarcoma over the hip underwent radiotherapy. She developed severe oedema of the lower limb and was in intense pain. Sitting with the lower limb dependent and kept straight was the only position she could rest in. A horizontal position was not tolerated even for a minute, in spite of analgesics including oral morphine. Unless the dependent position could be abandoned, we were at an impasse.

An epidural cannula was inserted in the lumbar region and 0.25% bupivacaine was administered initially as a bolus, followed by a continuous infusion with a syringe pump. This made her feel slightly better; but still did not enable her to lie horizontally. The next day, the concentration of the epidural infusion of bupivacaine was increased to 0.5%. This worked and, for the first time in 2 weeks, she could lie on a bed. SLD was started. In 3 days, the limb became much smaller, the requirement of the epidural bupivacaine reduced and she could move about comfortably in a wheelchair. She became so much better that the epidural cannula was removed after 1 week and she thanked the doctors for 'working a miracle' on her leg.

When a limb with lymphoedema has been neglected and untreated for a long time, infection can become a serious complication. However, there is still scope for improvement in most cases, as shown by the following case history.

Case history 2

A 45-year-old woman had undergone a radical cystectomy for cancer of the bladder. Postoperatively she developed bilateral lymphoedema of the legs. When first seen at the Pain and Palliative Care Clinic, she had blisters on both legs below the knees with a foul-smelling purulent discharge. She was given morphine for her pain and was started on antibiotics. SLD was possible only above the knees. This was started, and the thighs became smaller and softer, and the legs started to heal. With continued skin care and SLD, the relatives managed to keep her lymphoedema under control for the rest of her life.

Drug therapy

Corticosteroids are prescribed when the lymphoedema is thought to be secondary to obstruction by tumour. Diuretics are avoided because they do not help true lymphoedema. In addition, they can cause hypovolaemia and electrolyte disturbances which may be missed because of limited facilities for follow-up.

Monitoring

The patient needs to be monitored at least once a month. In addition to checking the state of the limb, the massage technique is reviewed for any lapse or error. Although manual lymphatic drainage (MLD) necessitates a skilled practitioner,[2] we have found that motivated relatives can achieve a significant reduction in limb size with SLD.

Summary

In summary, where resources and manpower are limited, the following can still offer valuable palliation to patients with lymphoedema in cancer:

- evaluation to assess the extent of the problem and to exclude associated correctable exacerbating factors
- explanation and counselling to enable the patient and relatives to understand and accept the situation

- pain relief and the control of infection if present
- instituting preventive measures against complications
- identifying relatives who can undertake the task of SLD for about 1 hour a day
- measurement of the circumference of the limb to monitor progress
- review at least once a month.

References

1 Sitzia J (1995) Volume measurement in lymphoedema treatment: examination of formulae. *European Journal of Cancer Care.* **4**:11–16.
2 Mitchell HS (1995) Breast cancer and arm lymphoedema – what can be done? *Journal of Cancer Care.* **4**:61–7.

Index

abdominal massage in SLD
  arm oedema 229–30
  leg oedema 233
acne 311–12
acute inflammatory episode(s) (AIE), see
    inflammation
addresses, useful xiii
adherence to self-care regimens 110
adipositas spongiosa, see lipoedema
adjuvant analgesics 77, 85
adolescents, management 113, 304
advice, see education
aesthetics, compression garments 187–9
aetiology, see causes; classification;
    pathophysiology
age of onset 23, 293–4
albendazole 265–6
allergy 124
anaemia in advanced cancer 354
analgesics 75, 76–85
  in advanced cancer 353
  mastectomy patient 69
anastomosis, lymphovenous 288
aneuploidy 28–9
angio-osteohypertrophy syndrome 28
angiosarcoma, post-mastectomy
    (Stewart–Treves syndrome) 50
ankle, compression garment fit at 191
anthelmintics 265–7
antibiotics, AIE 136, 137–8, 310
anticoagulants
  intravenous, in DVT management in
    advanced cancer 356
  oral
    coumarins as 247
    in DVT management in advanced
      cancer 355–6
antifungals 126, 134
anti-oxidants
  oxerutins as 253
  proanthocyanadins as 263
aplasia 23, 24, 25
  radiological appearance 302
arm (upper limb)
  compression garments, see sleeves

exercises 153–6
  at home 160–2
  positioning 148–9
  see also limbs and specific parts
arm oedema
  breast cancer 33, 68–71
    pain 68–71
    psychosocial issues 194
    SLD 220
    supporting arm 348–9
  exercises in, see arm
  functional effects 93
  MLD in post-traumatic oedema 211–12
  pain
    in advanced cancer 344
    in breast cancer (and its treatment)
      68–71
  SLD 223–30
    breast cancer 220
  see also limbs
armchair legs 55–6
arterial supply
  exercise and 140
  insufficiency, MLLB 174
arthritis, inflammatory 39
ascites 17
  malignant 342
    management 355
assessment, see evaluation
axillary lymph nodes 321–3
  anatomy 321–5
  dissection, complications 324–5
  massage 225–6, 231
  sampling/biopsy 35, 325

back massage
  lower 233
  upper 228–9
bacterial infections 37
  acute inflammatory reactions with 133–4
  of fungating lesions 349
  male genital lymphoedema 331
bandages
  compression, see compression bandages
  historical use 166

multilayer, *see* multilayer lymphoedema
    bandaging
    supportive, in advanced cancer 351–2
bath oil 122–3
bed rest, AIE 136–7
benzopyrones 245–64, 267
    DCT and 261–3
    in lymphoedema 255–61
        in advanced cancer 354
        clinical trials 257–61
        of head and neck 317
        of male genitalia 335
    in venous insufficiency 252–5
biopsy, axillary node 35, 325
blood, exercise effects on circulation
    40–3
blood supply, *see entries under* arterial;
    circulation; venous
body image 90–1, 194
body presentation 91–3
brachial plexopathy 73
    post-mastectomy 69–71
breast 321–30
    cancer (and its treatment) 33–5, 321–30,
        340–1
        acute inflammatory reaction 133
        advanced/metastatic disease, *see*
            metastases
        arm oedema, *see* arm oedema
        DCT 109
        description of breast lymphoedema
            321
        diagnosis of lymphoedema in 53
        management of breast lymphoedema
            328
        psychosocial aspects 327–8, 347
        radiotherapy 326–7
        surgical treatment, *see* mastectomy;
            surgery
    lymphatic drainage 321–3
breathing, deep, *see* relaxation
British Lymphology Society
    address xiii
    chronic oedema management groups 97,
        98
British Standard specification for
    Graduated Compression Hosiery
    (1985) 190
Brugia spp. 38
by-pass procedures
    enteromesenteric bridge 288–9
    omental, *see* omental by-pass

calcium dobesilate 264
calcium etamsylate 264–5
calf muscle (venous leg) pump 141
    exercises, in stockings 193
'call-up' technique, *see* inciting technique
cancer (malignant disease) 32–6
    advanced/metastatic, *see* metastases
    brachial plexopathy and 69–71, 73
    breast, *see* breast
    cervical, *see* cervical cancer
    as complication 50–1
        immunodeficiency and 132
    in India 359–63
    PCT in patients with, cautions 239–40
    pelvic 341–2
    recurrent
        brachial plexopathy with 74
        head and neck oedema with 316, 317
        local, palliative therapy 104–7
    skin, *see* skin
    squamous cell 51
    sympathetically-maintained pain 71
    TENS in patients with 273–80
    treatment
        advancing disease 356
        pain management 75
        radiotherapy, *see* radiotherapy
capillary filtration capacity 12
capillary pressure/capillary hydrostatic
    pressure 12, 14
    increased 15–17
capillary surface area, increased 18
cardiology, *see* heart
carers, family as, *see* family
(+)-catechin 248
causes (of oedema) 22–43, 51–2
    in advanced cancer 338–9
    of male genital lymphoedema 331–2
    surgery as 285
    see also pathophysiology
caval vein obstruction, *see* vena caval
    obstruction
cellulitis 37
    classical 131
    lymphoedema and, differences 132
cervical cancer 35
    hysterectomy and radiotherapy 341
cervical lymph nodes (neck nodes)
    anatomy 307–9
    metastases 307, 307–10
    management 310
Charles' operation 287

cheilitis granulomatosa 311
chemotherapy, palliative 356
    in head and neck cancer recurrence 317
chest massage
    lower 229–30
    upper 226–8
children 112–13, 293–305
    associated features 294, 295–6
    early-onset/congenital forms, see
        congenital lymphoedema
    examination 301
    history-taking 293–6
    investigations 301–3
    late-onset primary lymphoedema
        299–300
    management 112–13, 303–5
    psychosocial dimensions 6, 113, 304
chromone, structure 247
chromosomal aneuploidy 28–9
chronic condition, psychological impact
        89–90
chronic oedema management groups 97, 98
chylous reflux 47
    clinical manifestations 24, 47
    surgical management 290–1
circular knit compression garments 187
circular movements
    in MLD 206–8
    in SLD 221–2
circulation, exercise effects 140–7
classification 22–43, 293
    of chronic oedema into management
        groups 97, 98
    grading 44, 45
clinical features (symptoms and signs) 3,
        44–67
    in advanced cancer
        of lymphoedema 344–7
        of superior vena caval obstruction 343
    of breast lymphoedema 321
    of chylous reflux 24
    of lipoedema vs lymphoedema 58
    of male genital lymphoedema 333
clothing 91–2, 111–12
    see also footwear
codeine 78–9
cold creams 123
colloid osmotic pressure (interstitial) 12, 14
    fall/decrease 14–15, 17
colloid osmotic pressure difference 13
colour Doppler ultrasound 64
compliance, interstitial 15

complications 48–51
    cutaneous, see skin
compression (external) 106–7, 165
    effects on lymph flow 14
    pneumatic, see pneumatic compression
        therapy
compression bandages
    in advanced cancer 351
    elastic 168, 170, 171
    multilayered, see multilayer lymphoedema
        bandaging
compression garments (elastic garments) 7,
        92–3, 106, 111, 166, 186–98
    actions 192
    in advanced cancer 352
    application 196
    children 303–4
    contra-indications 194
    cost and availability 197–8
    evaluation for use 193
    evidence of efficacy 193
    indications 194
    lower-class 112
    patient instruction/information 196–7
    pneumatic, see pneumatic compression
        therapy
    psychosocial issues 194–5
    rationale for use 191
    starting with 195–6
computed tomography 62–3
    male genital lymphoedema 334
concentric muscle work 145
congenital heart disease 296
congenital lymphoedema (lymphoedema
        congenita) 24, 25, 26, 27–32,
        296–9
    age of onset 23, 293–4
    associated features 294, 295–6
    inheritance 294
    see also genetics
conjunctival oedema 313
contact dermatitis 39, 124, 126–7
    treatment 127
contractions, muscle 145
contrast lymphography, see lymphography
cording 34–5
corticosteroids 245
    as adjuvant analgesics 85
    in advanced cancer 353
        in India 362
    adverse effects 127
    in dermatitis 127

cost
  compression garments 197
  lymphoedema management in cancer in
      India 359–60
  MLLB 185–6
coumarin 245
  clinical trials 258, 259, 260–1
      in filaritic lymphoedema 266
  DCT and 262
  hepatotoxicity 249
  oxerutin and, see oxerutin
coumarols 245
  sources 246
COX inhibitors
  COX-2 inhibitors
      preferential 79
      specific 78, 79
  non-specific 79
creams 123–4
cromoglicate 245
cutaneous problems, see skin
cyclo-oxygenase inhibitors, see COX
      inhibitors
cytotoxic drug therapy in head and neck
      cancer recurrence 317

dalteparin 356
debulking surgery 285–7
decongestive lymphoedema therapy (DLT)
      7, 103–11
  benzopyrones and 261–3
  factors influencing outcome 101
  historical aspects 102
  intensive phase, see management
  maintenance phase, see management
deep vein thrombosis, see thrombosis
dermatitis 135
  contact, see contact dermatitis
dermatology, see skin
dermatolymphangio-adenitis, episodic 135
dermis 118
dexamethasone 245
  in advanced cancer 353
diagnosis 58
  differential, see differential diagnosis
'die-back' phenomenon 24, 26
diethylcarbamazine (DEC) 266–7
differential diagnosis 51–8
  male genital (groin) lymphoedema 332,
      333
diosmetin 247
diosmin 247, 252

disability, physical 48, 93–4
distal obliteration of lymphatics 24–5
distichiasis 31, 295, 299–300
diuretics 244
  in advanced cancer 353
      in India, avoidance 362
  head and neck oedema 317
  male genital lymphoedema 335
dobesilate 264
doctor–patient relationships 4–7, 95
domiciliary exercise programmes 160–4
Doppler ultrasound, colour 64
Down's syndrome 29
drainage, see lymph, drainage; lymph nodes,
      drainage; lymphatic drainage
dressings, advanced cancer 349
drug therapy 244–70
  in advanced cancer 352–4
      contra-indicated drugs 354
  in India 362
  head and neck oedema 317
  male genital lymphoedema 335

eccentric muscle work 145
education (incl. advice/information) in self-
      care 110
  cancer patients (and relatives) in India
      360–1
  compression garments 196–7
  exercise 150–1
  head and neck oedema 316
  male genital lymphoedema 335
  MLLB 175
  skin care 121, 122
  SLD 219–20
elastic compression bandages 168, 170,
      171
elastic compression garments, see
      compression garments
elastic properties of bandages 171
elbow exercises 155
  at home 161
elephantiasis
  endemic/non-filarial 39
  filarial, see filariasis
elephantiasis nostras 311
emollients, see moisturisers
employment, see occupation
endocrine (hormone) therapy in advanced
      cancer 356
enteromesenteric bridge by-pass 288–9
erysipelas 37

erythema ab igne 48
erythrocyanosis frigida 56
etamsylate 264–5
evaluation/assessment (incl. examination)
    97–102
  children 301
  for compression garment use 193
  exercise/movements and 147
  male genital lymphoedema 334
  ongoing 110
  of pain 71–4
  of skin 120–1
exercise 107, 140–64
  in advanced cancer 350
  calf muscle pump, in stockings 193
  circulation and effects of 140–7
  evaluation regarding 147
  passive 150
  programmes 149–51, 153–64
    home 160–4
exotoxins, streptococcal pyogenic 133
eyelashes, in-growing (distichiasis) 31, 295,
    299–300
eyelid oedema 312–13

factitious lymphoedema 40
family/relatives (as carers)
  Indian cancer patients 360, 361–2, 362
  SLD by 219, 361–2, 362
family history with children 294–5
females
  genetic forms of lymphoedema in 296
  gynaecological cancer 35
fibrosis
  PCT cautions relating to 240
  radiation-related 327
  retroperitoneal 40
fibrous histiocytoma, malignant 51
filariasis, lymphatic 38, 135
  anthelmintics 265–7
  male genital lymphoedema 331–2
fingers (patient's)
  bandaging 179
  exercises 155
    at home 161
fingers (therapist's), movements in MLD
    206, 207–8
flaps
  causing head and neck oedema 310–11
  in treatment of lymphoedema
    head and neck oedema 318–19
    male genital lymphoedema 336

flat bed knit compression garments 187
flavan (and derivatives) 245
flavonoids 245, 252
  in grape seed extracts 263–4
  structures 247, 248
fluid (interstitial)
  excess accumulation, *see* oedema;
    swelling
  exchange, Starling principle 12–13
  nature/composition 11
  pressure, *see* hydrostatic pressure
  volume, homeostasis 14–19
fluid-retaining drugs in advanced cancer,
    withdrawal 354
fluorescence lymphangiography 64
foam padding 177
Foldi, E 102, 103
folliculitis 128
foot bandaging 182–3
footwear/shoes 92, 111
  children 113
free radical scavengers, oxerutins as 253
frusemide, *see* furosemide
functional impairment in advanced cancer
    346–7
  management 352
fungal infections 126
  AIE and 134
fungating tumours 349
furosemide (frusemide) 244
  in advanced cancer 353

gender and genetic forms of lymphoedema
    296
  see also females; males
genetics (of congenital lymphoedema)
    27–32, 294–5, 296–300
  management considering 304–5
  modes of inheritance 294
genitalia
  cancer (females) 35, 341
  oedema (groin lymphoedema in males)
    331–7
    causes/classification 331–2
    clinical features 333
    investigation 333–4
    management 291, 334–6
    pathophysiology 333
    with PCT 240
girdle, shoulder, exercises 154–5, 156
glucocorticoids, *see* corticosteroids
gonadal dysgenesis 298–9

grading
  of lymphoedema 44, 45
  of skin condition 120
grafts, skin, *see* skin flaps and grafts
grape *seed* extract 263–4
groin lymph nodes
  dissection 36, 332
  massage
    in MLD 210–11
    in SLD 229, 232
groin lymphoedema, *see* genitalia
gynaecological cancer 35, 341

haematoma, breast cancer surgery 325
hand
  bandaging 179, 180
  compression garment 188
  exercises 155
    at home 161
  oedema in advanced cancer 346
head and neck oedema 306–20
  anatomy relevant to 307–10
  management, *see* management
  pathophysiology 306–7
health professional–patient relationships
    4–7, 95
heart
  congenital disease 296
  failure 17
    in advanced cancer 354
helminths 38
heparin, low molecular weight, in advanced
    cancer 356
hepatic disease 17
hepatotoxicity, coumarin 249
hereditary disorders 27–32
heredity, *see* genetics
hesperetin 248
hesperidin 248, 252
high-frequency ultrasound 64
high-output failure 52
high-protein oedema 19
histiocytoma, malignant fibrous 51
history of therapy 102, 166
  pneumatic compression 237
history-taking 100
  children 293–6
  medical, multilayer bandaging
    and 175
Homans' operation 286
  modified 287
home exercise programmes 160–4

homeostasis of interstitial fluid volume
    14–19
hormone therapy in advanced cancer 356
hydrangin 246
hydraulic conductance 12
hydrodynamic pressure and venous return
    142
hydrostatic pressure
  capillary, *see* capillary pressure
  interstitial fluid (= interstitial fluid
    pressure) 12
  rise 14
  venous return and 142
hydrostatic pressure difference 13
7-hydroxycoumarin 246
hydroxyethylrutosides, *see* oxerutin
hygiene in head and neck oedema 317
hyperkeratosis 44, 45, 119
  management 125
hyperplasia 23–4, 25, 26
  radiological appearance 302
hypertrophy, limb 52
hypo-albuminaemia 342, 354
hypoplasia 23, 24, 25
  radiological appearance 302
hypoproteinaemia in advanced cancer 339
hysterectomy, radical 341

idiopathic lymphoedema, *see* primary
    lymphoedema
imaging 59–64
  children 301
    appearance 302–3
  lipoedema 57
  see also specific modalities
immobility, chronic leg oedema 55–6
immune response, local alterations
    49, 132
inciting ('call-up') technique 205–6
  specific movements of 206–8
India, lymphoedema in cancer 359–63
infants
  management 303
  newborn, investigations 302
infections 37–8
  acute inflammatory reaction caused by
    133–4
  in advanced cancer in lymphoedema,
    predisposition 345
  children 301
  fungal, *see* fungal infections
  of fungating lesions 349

groin lymphoedema with 331–2
recurrent, head and neck oedema
    secondary to 311
inflammation 38–40
  acute inflammatory episode(s) (AIE;
    secondary acute inflammation) 49,
    130–9
    atypical 131
    causes 133
    clinical characteristics 130–2
    definition 130
    diagnosis 136
    history of 100
    management 136–8, 174, 310, 317,
    335
    predisposing factors 134–5
    prevalence 132–3
    recurrent 131, 137–8
  oedema of 18–19
    head and neck oedema with recurrent
    inflammation 311
information, see education
inheritance, see genetics
injury, traumatic 40
  arm oedema following, MLD 211–12
  head and neck oedema following 310–11
inspection, skin 120
intercostal neuralgia 70
International Society of Lymphology
  address xiii
  definitions of primary vs secondary
    lymphoedema 22
  grading classification 44, 45
interstitial compartment
  compliance 15
  fluid, see fluid
  nature 11
investigation of lymphoedema 58–65
  children 301–3
  head and neck oedema 316
  male genital lymphoedema 333–4
isometric contraction 145
isotonic contraction 145
isotope scans, see lymphoscintigraphy
ivermectin 266–7

job, see occupation

kaempferol 247
Kaposi's sarcoma
  as cause 36
  as complication 51

keratolytics 125
Klinefelter's syndrome 29
Klippel–Trenaunay–Weber
  syndrome 28

Laplace's law 170
LASER therapy, low-level 282–3
layers of bandages, number 171
leg(s) (lower limb)
  bandaging 181–5
  compression garments, see stockings
  exercises 156–9
    at home 162–4
  massive obesity of lower leg
    56–7
  MLD 209–11
  positioning 148
    resting in elevation 142, 147–8, 148
  venous pump, see calf muscle pump
  see also limbs and specific parts
leg oedema
  in advanced cancer 347
    supporting leg 350
  chronic, with immobility 55–6
  exercises in, see legs
  functional effects 93–4
  SLD 231–8
Letessier–Meig syndrome 30, 299
lifestyle, education regarding 150–1
limbs
  hypertrophy 52
  positioning 148–9
    in advanced cancer 349–50
    in MLLB 178
    resting in elevation 142, 147–8, 148
  surgical reduction 285–7
  volume and circumference
    bandaging reducing 173
    benzopyrones reducing 257–61
    LASER therapy reducing 283
    measurement 114
    sub-bandage pressure with MLLB and
    172
    TENS reducing 273–80
  see also arm; leg
lipodermatosclerosis 54
lipodystrophy, see lipoedema
lipoedema (lipodystrophy; massive obesity of
    lower legs; painful fat syndrome)
    56–7
  management 168
liposarcoma 51

liver
    coumarin toxicity 249
    disease, colloid osmotic pressure fall 17
local support groups 9
Long-term Medical Conditions Alliance 8
lotions 124
lower limb, see leg
lymph
    drainage (= physiological flow) 13–14
        defective 19
        increased 15
    drainage procedures (surgical) 287–90
    leakage through skin, see lymphorrhoea
lymph node(s)
    axillary, see axillary lymph nodes
    cervical, see cervical lymph nodes
    drainage in MLD 208
    groin, see groin lymph nodes
lymph node dissection (in cancer)
    cervical nodes 310, 314
    groin nodes 36, 332
lymphadenitis 37
lymphangiography
    child 302
    direct 59
    fluorescence 64
    isotope, see lymphoscintigraphy
    male genital lymphoedema 334
lymphangiomas 45–7, 119
lymphangiosarcoma 50–1, 121
lymphangioscintigraphy, see
        lymphoscintigraphy
lymphangitis 37
lymphatic drainage (= lymphatic
        system/return)
    breast 321–3
    exercise effects 143–4
    obliteration, see obliteration
    obstruction/damage in advanced cancer
        339
lymphatic drainage (methods), see manual
        lymphatic drainage; simple
        lymphatic drainage
lymphoedema ab igne 47–8
lymphoedema–distichiasis 31, 295,
        299–300
lymphoedema praecox 26
    defined 23, 293, 294
Lymphoedema Support Network 6, 8–9
    address xiii
    role 8–9
    typical cases from files 1–2

lymphoedema tarda 26
    defined 23, 293
lymphography, indirect/contrast
    lipoedema 57
    primary lymphoedema 23, 24
lymphorrhoea (lymph leakage through skin
        e.g. from lymphangiomas) 49,
        127–8
    in advanced cancer 346
    treatment 128, 135
lymphoscintigraphy (isotope scans) 60–2
    in lipoedema 57
    qualitative 61
    quantitative 61
lymphostasis verrucosis 55–6
lymphovenous anastomosis 288
lymphovenous oedema in advanced cancer
        339

magnetic resonance imaging (MRI) 63
    male genital lymphoedema 334
males
    genetic forms of lymphoedema in 296
    genital oedema, see genitalia
malignancy, see cancer
management/treatment of lymphoedema
        97–117, 140–284
    access to treatment 6–7
    in advanced/metastatic disease, see
        metastases
    AIE 136–8, 174, 310, 317, 335
    breast lymphoedema 328
    children 112–13, 303–5
    combined methods 203
    containment in 165–202
    evaluation in, see evaluation
    future prospects 114–15
    head and neck lymphoedema 315–19
        primary lymphoedema 310
        secondary lymphoedema (various
            causes) 311, 312, 313
    historical aspects, see history
    inadequate provision 3–4
    intensive phase (complex DLT; complex
        physical therapy) 104–7, 108–10
        bandaging, see multilayer
            lymphoedema bandaging
    maintenance phase 104–7, 110
        compression garments in, see
            compression garments
    monitoring treatment 101
        in advanced cancer 362

outcome, see outcome
patient-centred approach 99–102, 113
prevention of lymphoedema 102–3
self-care, see self-care
skin, see skin, care
strategies 97–117
see also specific methods
manual lymphatic drainage (MLD)
    (lymphatic drainage massage)
    105–6, 108, 203–16
in advanced cancer 350–1
contra-indications 218
examples 209–13
failure 204
in head and neck oedema 317–18
place of 204
results 213
simple form, see simple lymphatic
    drainage
techniques 204–8
massage, lymphatic drainage, see manual
    lymphatic drainage; simple
    lymphatic drainage
mastectomy (sequelae) 324–5
AIE 133
compression sleeves 193
LASER therapy 283
lymphangioma (Stewart–Treves syndrome)
    50
MLD with lymphoedema 212–13
pain 68–71
seroma 34, 325
Meig's syndrome 30, 299
melanoma 51
Melkersson–Rosenthal syndrome 311
Memorial Sloan Kettering levels of neck
    lymphatics 309
men, see males
metastases (and advanced disease in general)
    98, 338–63
brachial plexopathy with 73, 74
breast cancer 53, 340–1
    routes of lymphatic spread 323
causes of oedema 338–9
cervical lymph node, see cervical lymph
    nodes
clinical features of lymphoedema 344–7
dissemination risk
    with MLD 318
    with PCT 239–40
palliative care/management 348–56
    physical therapies 174, 348–52

pelvic cancers 341–2
    psychosocial impact 347, 354
methadone 83
metronidazole 349
microsurgery, head and neck lymphoedema
    318
Milroy's disease 27, 31, 296–7
mobility in advanced cancer
    appliances aiding 352
    impaired 346–7
moisturisers (incl. emollients) 121–5
    in hyperkeratosis 125
    sensitivity to 125
morbidity, see quality of life
morphine 76, 77, 79–82
    adverse effects 82–3, 84
    opioid dose equivalents to 81
    starting 80
movements (patient's)
    circulation and effects of 144–7
        lymphatic return and 144
        venous return and 141, 142
    evaluation 147
    see also mobility
movements (therapeutic)
    in MLD 206–8
    in SLD 221–2
        in self-massage 223–35
multilayer lymphoedema bandaging (MLLB)
    106, 109–10, 165, 166–86
    application protocol 175–85
    contra-indications and cautions 174–5
    cost/availability 285–6
    evidence of efficacy 172–3
    indications 174
    personal impact 185–6
    physical principles 170
    principal effects 165, 168
    rationale/reasons for use 167, 168–9
muscle activity
    and circulation 144–7
        agonists 145, 146
        antagonists 145, 146
        fixators 145, 146
        synergists 145, 146
    definitions of 145–7
    lymphatic return and 144
    venous return and 141, 142
myxoedema, pretibial 39–40

nails, dystrophic yellow, see yellow nail
    syndrome

nasal lymphoedema 312
neck
    exercises 154
    lymph nodes, see cervical lymph nodes
    massage (SLD) 223–5
    oedema, see head and neck oedema
needs, patients' 89
neonatal investigations 302
neoplasms, see tumours
nerve blocks 85–6
nerve damage, see neuropathic pain
neuropathic pain (incl. nerve injury pain)
    causes 72
    management 85
    post-mastectomy 69–71
newborn, investigations 302
non-adherence to self-care regimens 110
nonsteroidal anti-inflammatory drugs
        78, 79
Nonne–Milroy type hereditary lymphoedema
        (Milroy's disease) 27, 31, 296–7
Noonan's syndrome 30, 297–8
nose, lymphoedema 312
NSAIDs 78, 79
nurses, specialist 102

obesity 151
    of lower legs, massive, see lipoedema
obliteration of lymphatic system 22
    distal 24–5
    proximal 25, 26
occupation (employment; job; vocation;
        work)
    advice regarding 150–1
    effects on 94
oedema
    genital, with PCT 240
    leg, chronic, immobile patients 55–6
    pathogenesis, see cause; pathophysiology
oil
    bath 122–3
    emulsions of water in 123
    in SLD, contra-indicated 221
oil-in-water emulsions 123
ointments 124
Olszewski's classification 26
omental by-pass 289–90
    head and neck oedema 318–19
opioids 76, 77, 78–85
    adverse effects 82–3, 84
    doses 79–82
    strong 79–85

tolerance 83
    weak 78–9
outcome of lymphoedema and its treatment
    DCT 101
    measures 114
    see also quality of life
overweight, see obesity
oxerutin (hydroxyethylrutosides) incl.
        troxerutin/tri-oxerutin 245
    in lymphoedema 256
        clinical trials 258, 259
    pharmacological properties 253–4
    structure 248
    in venous insufficiency 252–5
oxerutin + coumarins (incl. troxerutin/
        tri-oxerutin) 248–9, 249
    clinical trials 258, 260
    dose 251
Oxford pressure monitor 172

padding in MLLB 176–7
    applying
        arm 179
        leg 182
pain 48, 68–88
    in advanced cancer and lymphoedema
        344, 353
    characteristics 68–71
    control/management 74–85
        drug, see analgesics
        non-drug 75
    evaluation 71–4
    incidence 68
painful fat syndrome, see lipoedema
palliative therapy
    advanced/metastatic cancer, see
        metastases
    locally recurrent cancer 104–7
palpation, skin 120
panty tights 189
papillomatosis 45, 46, 119
passive exercise 150
pathophysiology 11–21, 167
    head and neck oedema 306–7
    male genital lymphoedema 333
    see also cause
patient-centred care 99–102, 113
pelvic malignant disease, advanced 341–2
penicillin, AIE 136, 137–8
penis, reconstruction 336
peritoneal cavity fluid accumulation, see
        ascites

pharmacotherapy, *see* drug therapy
physical disability 48, 93–4
physical therapy
  advanced cancer 174, 348–52
  AIE 138
  combinations of 203
  complex, *see* management, intensive
    phase
physiology of interstitial fluid formation
  11–21
platelet function and NSAIDs 78, 79
pneumatic compression therapy (PCT)
  236–43
  in advanced cancer 352
  contra-indications/cautions 239–40, 241
  definitions 236
  guidelines for use 240–2
  history 237
  indications 239
  pump types 237–9
podoconiosis 39
positioning (patient)
  limbs, *see* limbs
  in SLD 221
post-thrombotic syndrome 55
posture and exercise 150
pressures
  colloid osmotic, *see* colloid osmotic
    pressure
  hydrostatic, *see* hydrostatic pressure
  in MLLB 168, 169–72, 177
  Starling principle of fluid exchange and
    12–13
  see also compression
pretibial myxoedema 39–40
prevention of lymphoedema 102–3
primary (idiopathic) lymphoedema 23–32,
  293
  children 296–300
  clinical classification 32
  definition 22
  head and neck 310
  lower limb, MLD 209
  male genitalia 331
proanthocyanadins 263–4
prophylactic management 102–3
prostate cancer 36, 341
protein levels, *see* high-protein oedema;
  hypoproteinaemia
Proteus syndrome 53
proximal obliteration of lymphatics 25, 26
psychological treatment, pain 75

psychosocial dimensions 48, 89–96
  in advanced cancer 347, 354
  breast/breast cancer-related lymphoedema
    327–8, 347
  children/adolescents 6, 113, 304
  compression garments 194–5
  MLLB 185–6
  quantifying psychological morbidity 114
'pumpkin head' oedema 314, 316, 319
pumps
  lymphatics, intrinsic and extrinsic 143–4
  pneumatic compression, types 237–9
  venous leg, *see* calf muscle pump
pyrones, structure and derivatives
  α-pyrones 245
  γ-pyrone 246
  see also benzopyrones

quality of life (impact on incl. morbidity)
  2–4, 90
  measures 90
  see also outcome
quercetin 245
  structure 247
    of derivatives 248

radio-isotope scans, *see* lymphoscintigraphy
radiology, *see* imaging
radiotherapy 46
  in advanced cancer 356
  brachial plexopathy with 73–4
  in breast cancer 326–7
  in cervical cancer 341
  head and neck (incl. nodes) 310, 313–15
re-absorption technique, *see* resorption
  technique
reduction operations 285–7
reflection coefficient 13
rehabilitation 97
relatives, *see* family/relatives
relaxation/deep breathing
  exercise followed by 156, 159
    at home 162
  in SLD
    post-treatment 228, 230, 233
    pre-treatment 223
reproductive tract, *see* genitalia
resorption (re-absorption) technique 204–5
  specific movements of 206–8
rest
  AIE 136–7
  limbs elevated at 142, 147–8, 148

retroperitoneal fibrosis 40
rhinophyma 312
ringworm, foot (tinea pedis) 134
rosacea 311–12
rutin 245, 252
    hydroxethylation, see oxerutin
    structure 248

sarcomas
    as complication 50–1
    Kaposi's, see Kaposi's sarcoma
scarring, lymphoedema secondary to
        310–11
scintigraphy, see lymphoscintigraphy
scrotal reconstruction 336–7
secondary lymphoedema 32–40, 293
    children 300–1
    definition 22
    lower limb, MLD 210–11
    male genitalia 331–2
segmental compression garments 237, 238
self-care/management 4
    adherence 110
    education in, see education
self-massage 221, 223–5
sensitisation of skin 124–5
sequential compression garments 237, 238
seroma, breast cancer surgery 34
sex, see females; gender; males
sex-linked (X-linked) conditions 299
sexual relationships 95
Shaped Tubigrip 351
shoes, see footwear
short-stretch bandages, see multilayer
        lymphoedema bandaging
shoulder exercises 154–5, 156
    at home 160
simple lymphatic drainage (SLD) 108,
        217–38
    in advanced cancer 350–1
    contra-indications 218
    factors influencing success 217
    indications 217–18
    method 221–2
    relatives performing 219, 361–2,
        362
    self-massage 221, 223–5
    training of staff 218–19
skimmetin 246
skin 118–29
    cancer of/affecting (as complication) 51
        examination for 121

care 105, 108, 118–29
    in advanced cancer 348–9
    aims 121–5
    children 113
    patient information/advice 121, 122
complications affecting 44–8, 119,
        125–8
    management 125–8
evaluation 120–1
functions 118–19
lymph leakage through, see lymphorrhoea
movement between and underlying
        tissues and, and lymphatic return
        144
radiation effects 327
sensitisation 124–5
skin flaps and grafts
    head and neck oedema 319
    male genital lymphoedema 336
sleeves, elastic 187, 188
    compression classes 191
    fit at wrist 191
    post-mastectomy 193
slings 349–50
Sloan Kettering levels of neck lymphatics
        309
soap substitutes 123
social dimensions 94–5
sodium cromoglicate 245
specialist nurses 102
squamous cell cancer 51
Starling principle of fluid exchange
        12–13
steroids, see corticosteroids
Stewart–Treves syndrome 50
stockinette, application
    arm 178–9
    foam padding after 177
    leg 181
stockings, elastic 187, 189
    calf muscle pump exercises in 193
    compression profile and classes
        190, 191
    cost/availability 197
    fit at ankle 191
streptococcal pyogenic exotoxins 133
stretches 156
sub-bandage pressure 170–2, 177
support (limb)
    in advanced cancer 349–50
    with bandages 351–2
    effects 165

support (patient)
  organisations 7–9
    addresses xiii
    role 7–9
  social 94–5
surgery (as cause of lymphoedema) 285,
    313–15, 316
  in breast cancer
    complications 324–5
    radical surgery, *see* mastectomy
  lymph node, *see* lymph node dissection
surgery (in lymphoedema treatment)
    285–91
  children, contra-indicated 303
  head and neck lymphoedema 318–19
    eyelid lymphoedema 313
    nasal lymphoedema 312
  male genital lymphoedema 291,
    335–7
swelling
  differential diagnosis 51–8
  mechanism 11–21
  see also oedema
sympathetically-maintained pain
  cancer patient 71
  management 86
symptoms, *see* clinical features

teaching, *see* education
teenagers/adolescents, management 113,
    304
tenosynovitis 40
TENS, *see* transcutaneous electrical nerve
    stimulation
tension, bandage 170–1
therapist–patient relationships 4–7, 95
therapy, *see* management
thigh stocking 189
Thompson's operation 287
thrombosis, deep vein 49–50
  in advanced cancer 347
    management 355–6
  syndrome (post-thrombotic)
    following 55
thumb movements in MLD 207–8
tinea pedis 134
toe bandage 181
training, staff, SLD 218–19
transcutaneous electrical nerve stimulation
    (TENS) 271–82
  advantages/disadvantages 281
  contra-indications/complications 282

equipment 271–2
  in head and neck oedema 318
  practical experiences 272–80
traumatic injury, *see* injury
treatment, *see* management
tri-oxerutin, *see* oxerutin
trisomy-21 29
troxerutin, *see* oxerutin
Tubigrip, Shaped 351
tumours
  malignant, *see* cancer
  swelling/enlargement caused
    by 52
Turner's syndrome 28–9, 298

ulceration in advanced cancer 345–6
ultrasound 63–4
  colour Doppler 64
umbeliferone 246
unguentum lymphaticum 265
upper limb, *see* arm
uterine cervix, cancer, *see* cervical
    cancer

valvular incompetence, congenital 25
vanishing creams 123–4
vasculature, *see* entries under arterial;
    circulation; venous
vena caval obstruction (in cancer)
  inferior 344
    management 355
  superior 343
    management 355
venous leg pump, *see* calf muscle pump
venous system (venous return)
  blood pooling, garments reducing 193
  chronic disease/insufficiency
    54–5, 167
    benzopyrones in 252–5
    male genital (groin) lymphoedema
      differentiated from 332, 333
  exercise and 140–2
  lymphatic system surgically anastomosed
    to 288
  obstruction in advanced cancer 339
    breast cancer 340–1
    pelvic cancers 342
    vena caval obstruction, *see* vena caval
      obstruction
  thrombosis, *see* thrombosis
vis a tergo 143
vocation, *see* occupation

volume
    interstitial fluid, homeostasis
        14–19
    limb, see limbs
vulval cancer 35

walking 151
warfarin 248
    in deep vein thrombosis 355
    oxerutin and, see oxerutin
weight, excessive, see obesity
width of bandages 171–2
Winiwarter, Felix von 102
women, see females

work (job), see occupation
work (muscle) 145
wrist
    compression garment fit at 191
    exercises 155, 156
        at home 161
Wucheria bancrofti 38

X-linked conditions 299
XO karyotype 28–9, 298
XXY karyotype 29

yellow nail syndrome 30, 300
    eyelid oedema 313